T0180551

Advances in Intelligent Systems and Computing

Volume 526

Series editor

Janusz Kacprzyk, Polish Academy of Sciences, Warsaw, Poland
e-mail: kacprzyk@ibspan.waw.pl

About this Series

The series "Advances in Intelligent Systems and Computing" contains publications on theory, applications, and design methods of Intelligent Systems and Intelligent Computing. Virtually all disciplines such as engineering, natural sciences, computer and information science, ICT, economics, business, e-commerce, environment, healthcare, life science are covered. The list of topics spans all the areas of modern intelligent systems and computing.

The publications within "Advances in Intelligent Systems and Computing" are primarily textbooks and proceedings of important conferences, symposia and congresses. They cover significant recent developments in the field, both of a foundational and applicable character. An important characteristic feature of the series is the short publication time and world-wide distribution. This permits a rapid and broad dissemination of research results.

More information about this series at http://www.springer.com/series/11156

Marek Gzik · Ewaryst Tkacz
Zbigniew Paszenda · Ewa Piętka
Editors

Innovations in Biomedical Engineering

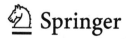 Springer

Editors
Marek Gzik
Faculty of Biomedical Engineering
Silesian University of Technology
Gliwice
Poland

Zbigniew Paszenda
Faculty of Biomedical Engineering
Silesian University of Technology
Gliwice
Poland

Ewaryst Tkacz
Faculty of Biomedical Engineering
Silesian University of Technology
Zabrze
Poland

Ewa Piętka
Faculty of Biomedical Engineering
Silesian University of Technology
Gliwice
Poland

ISSN 2194-5357   ISSN 2194-5365   (electronic)
Advances in Intelligent Systems and Computing
ISBN 978-3-319-47153-2   ISBN 978-3-319-47154-9   (eBook)
DOI 10.1007/978-3-319-47154-9

Library of Congress Control Number: 2016952908

Printed on acid-free paper

This Springer imprint is published by Springer Nature
The registered company is Springer International Publishing AG
The registered company address is: Gewerbestrasse 11, 6330 Cham, Switzerland

Preface

During the last two decades, it is not hard to observe unusual direct progress of civilization in many fields concerning conditionality coming up from technical theories or more generally technical sciences. We experience extraordinary dynamics of the development of technological processes including different fields of daily life which concerns particularly ways of communicating. We are aspiring for disseminating of the view that the success in the concrete action is a consequence of the wisdom won over, collected and appropriately processed. They are talking straight about the coming into existence of the information society.

In such a context the meeting of the specialists dealing with the widely understood innovations in biomedical engineering would give a new dimension associated with promoting something like the new quality. Because having the innovative approach as a pointer in today's world of changing attitudes and socioeconomic conditions can be perceived as one of the most important advantages. It results from the universal globalization letting one to observe surrounding world. Thanks to the development of new biotechnologies rising from the rapid progress in biomedical sciences, by comprehending the contemporary needs of surrounding world it may be said almost without any risk that life without biomedical sciences would stopped existing.

At present, as it seems, implementing the universal standardization of the transfer and the processing of information is the most important issue which in a significant way influences for expanding the circle of biomedical applications. It is a kind of challenge to put the proper weight into particular branches covered by biomedical engineering and therefore we decided to edit the book as a four-part elaboration covering biomaterials, biomechanics, biomedical informatics and last but not least biomedical signals processing. One should aspire to its permanent integration rather than the disintegration to progress in the context of the technological development. Hence, the constant observation and the appropriate problem analysis of biomedical sciences as well as checking the technologies development and their applications is picking up great importance.

The monograph returned to hands of readers being a result of meeting specialists dealing with the above-mentioned issues should contribute in a significant way to the success in implementing consequences of human imagination into the social life. We believe being aware of a human weakness and an imperfection that the monograph presenting a joint effort of the increasing crowd of professionals and enthusiasts will influence the technology development further regarding generally understood biomedicine with constantly expanding spectrum of its applications.

The last part of this preface will be devoted to express our great thanks and appreciation to all the contributors of this book, which were listed in the special section as "Contributor's List" and to persons who gave us unusual help in final editing process. Special thanks to Dr. Barbara Mika and Dr. Paweł Kostka for incredible engagement and help in creating the final version of this book.

October 2016

Ewaryst Tkacz
Marek Gzik
Zbigniew Paszenda
Ewa Pietka

Contents

Modelling and Simulations in Biomechanics

Signal Analysis

List of Contributors

Wojciech Adamczyk
Biomedical Engineering Lab, Institute of Thermal Technology,
Silesian University of Technology, Gliwice, Poland

Magdalena Antonowicz
Faculty of Biomedical Engineering, Department of Biomaterials and Medical Devices
Engineering, Silesian University of Technology, Zabrze, Poland

Alicja Balin
Biomechatronics Department, Silesian University of Technology, Zabrze, Poland

Marcin Basiaga
Faculty of Biomedical Engineering, Department of Biomaterials and Medical Devices
Engineering, Silesian University of Technology, Zabrze, Poland

Bohdan Bączkowski
Department of Prosthetic Dentistry, Medical University of Warsaw, Warsaw, Poland

Andrzej Bieniek
Department of Biomechatronics, Silesian University of Technology, Zabrze, Poland

Maria J. Bieńkowska
Faculty of Automatic Control, Electronics and Computer Science, Silesian University
of Technology, Gliwice, Poland

Andrzej Blazejewski
Technical University of Koszalin, Koszalin, Poland

Damian Borys
Institute of Automatic Control, Silesian University of Technology, Gliwice, Poland

Jan Borys
Faculty of Medicine, Medical University of Białystok, Białystok, Poland

Zbigniew Budzianowski
Faculty of Biomedical Engineering, Department of Biosensors and Biomedical Signals
Processing, Silesian University of Technology, Gliwice, Poland

Piotr Buliński
Biomedical Engineering Lab, Institute of Thermal Technology,
Silesian University of Technology, Gliwice, Poland

Michał Burkacki
Department of Biomechatronics, Faculty of Biomedical Engineering,
Silesian University of Technology, Zabrze, Poland

Igor Buzalewicz
Bio-Optics Group, Faculty of Fundamental Problems of Technology,
Department of Biomedical Engineering, Wrocław University of Science
and Technology, Wrocław, Poland

Marta Danch-Wierzchowska
Institute of Automatic Control, Silesian University of Technology, Gliwice, Poland

Jan Ryszard Dąbrowski
Department of Materials and Biomedical Engineering,
Bialystok University of Technology, Bialystok, Poland

Zofia Drzazga
Department of Medical Physics, Institute of Physics, University of Silesia, Katowice,
Poland; Silesian Center for Education and Interdisciplinary Research, Chorzów, Poland

Anna Filipowska
Faculty of Automatic Control, Electronics and Computer Science, Silesian University
of Technology, Gliwice, Poland

Wojciech Filipowski
Faculty of Automatic Control, Electronics and Computer Science, Silesian University
of Technology, Gliwice, Poland

Aldona Giec-Lorenz
Laboratory of Magnetic Resonance Imaging,
Helimed Diagnostic Imaging Sp. z o.o., Katowice, Poland

Ewelina Głąb
Faculty of Biomedical Engineering, Department of Biomaterials and Medical Devices
Engineering, Silesian University of Technology, Zabrze, Poland

Sebastian Glowinski
Technical University of Koszalin, Koszalin, Poland

Adam Golda
Department of Cardiology, Gliwice Medical Centre, Gliwice, Poland

Kamil Gorczewski
Department of PET Diagnostics, Maria Skłodowska-Curie Memorial Cancer Center
and Institute of Oncology, Gliwice, Poland

Piotr Grabiec
Polish-Japanese Academy of Information Technology,
Warsaw, Poland

Katarzyna Gruszczyńska
Department of Radiology and Nuclear Medicine, School of Medicine in Katowice,
Medical University of Silesia, Katowice, Poland

Magdalena Grygiel-Pradelok
Department of Biomaterials and Medical Devices Engineering,
Faculty of Biomedical Engineering, Silesian University of Technology, Zabrze, Poland

Marek Gzik
Department of Biomechatronics, Faculty of Biomedical Engineering,
Silesian University of Technology, Zabrze, Poland

Bożena Gzik-Zroska
Department of Biomaterials and Medical Devices Engineering, Faculty of Biomedical
Engineering, Silesian University of Technology, Zabrze, Poland

Norbert Henzel
Institute of Medical Technology and Equipment ITAM, Zabrze, Poland

Jacek Hermanson
Janusz Daab Provincial Hospital of Orthopaedics
and Traumatology in Piekary Śląskie, Piekary, Śląskie, Poland

Agnieszka Hyla
Faculty of Biomedical Engineering, Department of Biomaterials and Medical Devices
Engineering, Silesian University of Technology, Zabrze, Poland

Ewa Jasek-Gajda
Department of Histology, Jagiellonian University Medical College, Cracow, Poland

Katarzyna Jochymczyk-Woźniak
Department of Biomechatronics, Faculty of Biomedical Engineering,
Silesian University of Technology, Zabrze, Poland

Kamil Joszko
Department of Biomechatronics, Faculty of Biomedical Engineering,
Silesian University of Technology, Zabrze, Poland

Aleksandra Juraszczyk
Faculty of Biomedical Engineering, Silesian University of Technology, Zabrze, Poland

Jacek Jurkojć
Department of Biomechatronics, Silesian University of Technology, Zabrze, Poland

Marcin Kaczmarek
Department of Biomaterials and Medical Devices Engineering, Faculty of Biomedical
Engineering, Silesian University of Technology, Zabrze, Poland

Anita Kajzer
Faculty of Biomedical Engineering, Department of Biomaterials and Medical Devices
Engineering, Silesian University of Technology, Zabrze, Poland

Wojciech Kajzer
Department of Biomaterials and Medical Devices Engineering, Faculty of Biomedical
Engineering, Silesian University of Technology, Zabrze, Poland

Ilona Karpiel
Department of Medical Physics, Institute of Physics, University of Silesia, Katowice, Poland; Silesian Center for Education and Interdisciplinary Research, Chorzów, Poland

Jacek Kawa
Faculty of Biomedical Engineering, Silesian University of Technology, Zabrze, Poland

Edyta Kawlewska
Department of Biomechatronics, Faculty of Biomedical Engineering, Silesian University of Technology, Zabrze, Poland

Marcin Klekotka
Department of Materials and Biomedical Engineering, Bialystok University of Technology, Bialystok, Poland

Bogdan Koczy
Janusz Daab Provincial Hospital of Orthopaedics and Traumatology in Piekary Śląskie, Piekary, Śląskie, Poland

Ilona Kopyta
Department of Paediatrics and Developmental Age Neurology, Chair of Paediatrics, Medical University of Silesia, Katowice, Poland

M. Kot
AGH University of Science and Technology, Cracow, Poland

Marta Krzesińska
Department of Biosensors and Biomedical Signals Processing, Faculty of Biomedical Engineering, Silesian University of Technology, Zabrze, Poland

Tomasz Krzyzynski
Technical University of Koszalin, Koszalin, Poland

Przemyslaw Kurtyka
Department of Biomaterials and Medical Devices Engineering, Faculty of Biomedical Engineering, Silesian University of Technology, Zabrze, Poland

Jurgen M. Lackner
Joanneum Research Forschungsges MbH, Institute of Surface Technologies and Photonics, Functional Surfaces, Niklasdorf, Austria

Dawid Larysz
Department of Radiotherapy, Maria Sklodowska-Curie Memorial Cancer Center and Institute of Oncology, Gliwice, Poland

Aneta Liber-Kneć
Crakow University of Technology, Crakow, Poland

Anna M. Lipowicz
Institute of Anthropology, Wrocław University of Environmental and Life Sciences, Wrocław, Poland

Sylwia Łagan
Crakow University of Technology, Crakow, Poland

Karina Maciejewska
Department of Medical Physics, Institute of Physics, University of Silesia, Katowice, Poland

Justyna Majewska
Department of Biosensors and Biomedical Signals Processing, Faculty of Biomedical Engineering, Silesian University of Technology, Zabrze, Poland

Bogusław Major
Institute of Metallurgy and Materials Science, Polish Academy of Sciences, Crakow, Poland

L. Major
Institute of Metallurgy and Materials Science, Polish Academy of Sciences, Krakow, Poland

Roman Major
Institute of Metallurgy and Materials Science, Polish Academy of Sciences, Crakow, Poland

Jan Marciniak
Department of Biomaterials and Medical Devices Engineering, Faculty of Biomedical Engineering, Silesian University of Technology, Zabrze, Poland

Tomasz Marciniak
Faculty of Telecommunications, Computer Sciences and Electrical Engineering, University of Science and Technology, Bydgoszcz, Poland

Patrycja Mazgaj
Department of Medical Physics, Institute of Physics, University of Silesia, Katowice, Poland; Silesian Center for Education and Interdisciplinary Research, Chorzów, Poland

Bartłomiej Melka
Institute of Thermal Technology, Biomedical Engineering Lab, Silesian University of Technology, Gliwice, Poland

Robert Michnik
Department of Biomechatronics, Faculty of Biomedical Engineering, Silesian University of Technology, Zabrze, Poland

Michał Mielnik
Janusz Daab Provincial Hospital of Orthopaedics and Traumatology in Piekary Śląskie, Piekary, Śląskie, Poland

Żaneta Anna Mierzejewska
Mechanical Faculty, Białystok University of Technology, Białystok, Poland

Andrzej W. Mitas
Department of Informatics and Medical Equipment, Faculty of Biomedical
Engineering, Silesian University of Technology, Gliwice, Poland

Alicja Mondrzejewska
Institute of Medical Technology and Equipment ITAM,
Zabrze, Poland

Andrzej Myśliwiec
Department of Kinesitherapy and Special Methods of Physiotherapy,
Academy of Physical Education in Katowice, Katowice, Poland

Adrian Nowak
Polish-Japanese Academy of Information Technology,
Warsaw, Poland

Andrzej J. Nowak
Institute of Thermal Technology, Biomedical Engineering Lab,
Silesian University of Technology, Gliwice, Poland

Katarzyna Nowakowska
Department of Biomechatronics, Faculty of Biomedical Engineering,
Silesian University of Technology, Zabrze, Poland

Wojciech Oleksy
Faculty of Biomedical Engineering, Department of Biosensors and Biomedical Signals
Processing, Silesian University of Technology, Gliwice, Poland

Ziemowit Ostrowski
Biomedical Engineering Lab, Institute of Thermal Technology,
Silesian University of Technology, Gliwice, Poland

Zbigniew Paszenda
Faculty of Biomedical Engineering, Department of Biomaterials and Medical Devices
Engineering, Silesian University of Technology, Zabrze, Poland

Marcin Paszkuta
Institute of Informatics, Silesian University of Technology, Gliwice, Poland

Zbigniew Pilecki
Chorzów Pediatrics and Oncology Center, Chorzów, Poland

Halina Podbielska
Bio-Optics Group, Faculty of Fundamental Problems of Technology,
Department of Biomedical Engineering, Wrocław University of Science
and Technology, Wrocław, Poland

Grzegorz Prajsnar
Janusz Daab Provincial Hospital of Orthopaedics
and Traumatology in Piekary Śląskie, Piekary, Śląskie, Poland

Bartłomiej Pyciński
Faculty of Biomedical Engineering, Silesian University of Technology, Zabrze, Poland

W. Rakowski
AGH University of Science and Technology, Cracow, Poland

Łukasz Rodak
Janusz Daab Provincial Hospital of Orthopaedics and Traumatology
in Piekary Śląskie, Piekary, Śląskie, Poland

Marek Rojczyk
Institute of Thermal Technology, Biomedical Engineering Lab,
Silesian University of Technology, Gliwice, Poland

Piotr Rozentryt
Silesian Center for Heart Disease, Zabrze, Poland

Bartłomiej J. Sawaryn
Department of Biosensors and Biomedical Signals Processing, Faculty of Biomedical
Engineering, Silesian University of Technology, Zabrze, Poland

Jacek Semenowicz
Janusz Daab Provincial Hospital of Orthopaedics and Traumatology in Piekary Śląskie,
Piekary, Śląskie, Poland

Jarosław Sidun
Mechanical Faculty, Białystok University of Technology, Białystok, Poland

Damian Sołtan
Department of Biomechatronics, Faculty of Biomedical Engineering,
Silesian University of Technology, Zabrze, Poland

Ewa Stachowiak
Biomechatronics Department, Silesian University of Technology, Zabrze, Poland

Paula Stępień
Faculty of Automatic Control, Electronics and Computer Science,
Silesian University of Technology, Gliwice, Poland

Sławomir Suchoń
Department of Biomechatronics, Faculty of Biomedical Engineering,
Silesian University of Technology, Zabrze, Poland

Agnieszka Szczęsna
Institute of Informatics, Silesian University of Technology, Gliwice, Poland

Janusz Szewczenko
Faculty of Biomedical Engineering, Department of Biomaterials and Medical Devices
Engineering, Silesian University of Technology, Zabrze, Poland

Sandra Śmigiel
Faculty of Telecommunications, Computer Sciences and Electrical Engineering,
University of Science and Technology, Bydgoszcz, Poland

Agnieszka Świerkosz
AGH University of Science and Technology, Kraków, Poland

Andrzej Swierniak
Institute of Automatic Control, Silesian University of Technology, Gliwice, Poland

Mateusz Tajstra
Silesian Center for Heart Disease, Zabrze, Poland

Ewaryst Tkacz
Department of Biosensors and Biomedical Signals Processing,
Silesian University of Technology, Zabrze, Poland

Klaudia Trembecka-Wojciga
Institute of Metallurgy and Materials Science, Polish Academy of Sciences,
Crakow, Poland

Agnieszka Trojankowska
Department of Medical Physics, Institute of Physics, University of Silesia,
Katowice, Poland

Paweł Ulrych
Laboratory of Magnetic Resonance Imaging,
Helimed Diagnostic Imaging Sp. z o.o., Katowice, Poland

Witold Walke
Faculty of Biomedical Engineering, Department of Biomaterials and Medical Devices
Engineering, Silesian University of Technology, Zabrze, Poland

Agata M. Wijata
Department of Informatics and Medical Equipment, Faculty of Biomedical
Engineering, Silesian University of Technology, Gliwice, Poland

Piotr Wilczek
Bioengineering Laboratory, Heart Prosthesis Institute, Zabrze, Poland

Piotr Wodarski
Department of Biomechatronics, Silesian University of Technology, Zabrze, Poland

Marzena Wojciechowska
Polish-Japanese Academy of Information Technology,
Warsaw, Poland

Elżbieta Wojtyńska
Department of Prosthetic Dentistry, Medical University of Warsaw, Warsaw, Poland

Wojciech Wolański
Department of Biomechatronics, Faculty of Biomedical Engineering,
Silesian University of Technology, Zabrze, Poland

Tomasz Wróbel
Faculty of Mechanical Engineering, Department of Foundry,
Silesian University of Technology, Gliwice, Poland

Anna Ziębowicz
Faculty of Biomedical Engineering, Department of Biomaterials and Medical Devices
Engineering, Silesian University of Technology, Zabrze, Poland

Bogusław Ziębowicz
Department of Biomedical Materials Engineering, Silesian University of Technology,
Gliwice, Poland

Engineering of Biomaterials

Electrochemical Properties of TiO_2 Oxide Layer Deposited on Ti6Al7Nb Alloy

Marcin Basiaga$^{(\boxtimes)}$, Janusz Szewczenko, Witold Walke, Zbigniew Paszenda, Magdalena Antonowicz, and Agnieszka Hyla

Faculty of Biomedical Engineering, Department of Biomaterials and Medical Devices Engineering, Silesian University of Technology, Roosevelta 40, Zabrze, Poland
Marcin.Basiaga@polsl.pl

Abstract. One way to increase the biocompatibility of the surface of titanium alloys is to produce a surface layer with better physicochemical properties of the whole set than the base. The most popular methods of surface modification used in medical products include: chemical methods (eg. sol-gel method, atomic layer deposition (ALD)) and electrochemical (eg. anodic oxidation, fluorescent processing). Therefore, authors of this paper carried out a comparative analysis of TiO_2 layers produced both using chemical (ALD) and electrochemical (anodic oxidation) methods. The study was performed based on evaluation of electrochemical properties of produced TiO2 layer on the Ti6Al7Nb substrate alloy. As a part of electrochemical properties testing, potentiodynamic, potentiostatic and impedance studies were performed. All the tests were carried out in simulated physiological Ringer's solution in $T = 37 \pm 1^{\circ}C$ temperature. Based on the results it was found that the most favorable set of electrochemical properties characterises TiO_2 layer deposited by ALD method.

Keywords: TiO_2 · ALD method · Anodic oxidation · Electrochemical properties · Surface morfology

1 Introduction

Biomedical engineering is an interdisciplinary field of study, which touches numerous different aspects of medical science, such as different ways to modify surfaces of biomaterials intended for implants. There is an endless search for new better solutions, the goal of which is to correct implant's features by improving e.g. electrochemical properties of surfaces in contact with biological fluids environment. Implant's surfaces may be modified using many different methods. Each of available technologies has it's advantages and disadvantages. The latter usually disqualify them from the general use on most kinds of surfaces. Therefore, despite wide range of surface treatments, new technologies are still in development. Scientists' aim is to improve solutions used so far or discover innovative ones. Optimal treatments are being sought, those with highest covering accuracy in case of various surfaces, also with complicated geometry.

© Springer International Publishing AG 2017
M. Gzik et al. (eds.), *Innovations in Biomedical Engineering*, Advances in Intelligent Systems and Computing 526, DOI 10.1007/978-3-319-47154-9_1

Another approach is developing recurrent methods with the prospect of use in mass production. Amongst other methods on the research stage, the prognosis of wide use has been made for two technologies: anodic oxidation and thin layers deposition Atomic Layer Deposition (ALD) [1–7]. These methods have a number of advantages including low temperature process, the immutability of geometric features and process repeatability. Authors' earlier work has shown that layers prepared both by anodic oxidation and the ALD method are characterised by favorable performance properties of the substrate-layer system compared to the substrate itself. However, a basic condition for success is selecting the right surface layer. Thin film coatings based on metal oxides for many years are very popular, i.e. Al_2O_3, TiO_2, ZnO or SiO_2 [8–12]. One of most frequently used materials for such kinds of substrates is titanium oxide (TiO_2). The literature does not clearly indicate which of the above methods of application is more favorable. Therefore, the authors decided to conduct a comparative analysis of two methods of applying the layer of TiO_2 to determine the method which gives a layer characterized by the most beneficial set of electrochemical properties.

2   Materials and Methods

Samples used in the study were obtained from a Ti6Al7Nb rod with a diameter of d = 14 mm. Samples were subjected to preliminary surface modification that consist of vibratory processing conducted using suitable ceramic blocks required to obtain a constant surface roughness ($Ra \leq 0,3\mu m$) and then a layer of TiO_2 was deposited in two ways: by anodic oxidation and ALD. Anodic oxidation was carried out in an electrolyte based on phosphoric and sulfuric acids (TitanColor from POLIGRAT GmbH) at a potential of 97V. ALD process was carried out with the participation of two precursors: $TiCl_4$ and H_20, at 2500 cycles and T = 200°C. Parameters of both deposition processes were selected based on authors' earlier studies [13–16], which showed a similar thickness of TiO_2 layer (approximately 200 nm). At the final stage, samples were subjected to steam sterilization in an autoclave at a temperature T = 134°C at a pressure of p = 2,1 bar for t = 12 min.

In order to evaluate electrochemical properties of Ti6Al7Nb alloy with modified surface authors proposed potentiodynamic, potentiostatic nd impedance studies. In addition to surface preparation described above, an assessment of their topography was conducted.

Pitting corrosion resistance study was performed by recording of potentiodynamic polarization curves according to ASTM F2129 standard [17,18]. Measuring set consisted of a potentiostat VoltaLab PGP201, reference electrode (saturated calomel electrode NEK KP-113), the auxiliary electrode (platinum electrode type PtP-201), the anode (the test sample) and a PC with VoltaMaster 4 software. Before approaching Surface tests of every prepared sample, they were all purified in 96 % ethyl alcohol using an ultrasonic bath SONICA 1200M for approx. t = 6 min. Corrosion tests started from indicating the opening potential E_{OCP} at electroless conditions. Anodic polarization curves were recorded from the starting potential $E_{start} = E_{OCP} - 100\,mV$. Potential value changed in the direction of the anode at a rate of $0.167\,\mathrm{mV/s}$. When anodic current density reached $1\,mA/cm^2$, polarisation direction was changed.

Crevice corrosion resistance study was performed using a potentiostatic method, by recording the change in current density at a potential of $+800\,\mathrm{mV}$ during 15 min. The study used the same measurement system as in the case of potentiodynamic test [19].

In order to obtain additional information on analysed samples' electrochemical properties of the surface, research using electrochemical impedance spectroscopy was also carried out. The measurements that were performed using an AutoLab PGSTAT 302N measuring system equipped with a FRA2 module (Frequency Response Analyser). Measuring system that was used enables research in the frequency range $10^4 \div 10^{-3}\,Hz$. The voltage amplitude of the sinusoidal excitation signal was 10 mV. During the study the impedance spectrum was determined and obtained data were matched to the equivalent circuit. On this basis, the numerical values of the resistance R and the capacitor C of the analyzed system were established. Impedance spectra of the test system was shown as a Nyquist diagram for different values of frequency and as a Bode diagram. Collected EIS spectra were interpreted by the least-squares fitting to the electrical equivalent circuit. All the electrochemical tests were performed in the physiologic Ringer's solution at a temperature of $\mathrm{T} = 37^{\pm}1°C$ and pH $= 6, 8 \pm 0, 2$.

Additionally, a surface morphology study of thus prepared samples was performed using an atomic force microscope with a non-contact mode. The scanned area was $10 \times 10\ \mu m$, resolution of 256×256 was used. Samples were also subjected to observation using scanning electron microscope - ZEISS SUPRA 35 with type SE (Secondary Electrons) detector for secondary electrons in the magnification range of $1000 \div 100000x$.

3   Results

Pitting corrosion study results of all subjected samples were presented in Fig. 1. Based on the results it was found that the corrosion potential in the initial state (after vibration treatment) received the mean value of $E_{corr} = -186mV$. Anodic polarization curves designated that way, indicated the existance of a passive range of up to the potential value E $= +4000$ mV. In this case, there was no sudden increase of the anodic current density to indicate that the process of pitting corrosion has been initiated. Additionally, polarization resistance value equal to $R_p = 134k\Omega cm^2$ was determined using the Stern method.

Then the analysis of the results obtained while testing samples with TiO_2 layer, deposited both using ALD and anodic oxidation, was conducted.

Based on the survey, it was found that regardless of the application method depositing TiO_2 layer on the samples' surface was advantageous to increase the corrosion potential E_{corr} and polarization resistance R_p with respect to the samples in the initial state. The values of individual parameters characterizing

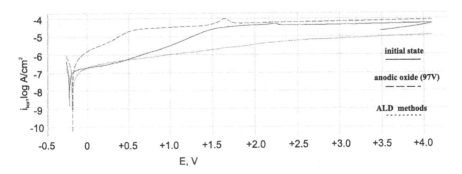

Fig. 1. Exemplary polarization curves for the Ti6Al7Nb with modified surface

the corrosion resistance were respectively: $E_{corr} = -173mV$, $R_p = 643k\Omega\,cm^2$ (anodic oxidation), $E_{corr} = -174mV$, $R_p = 1020k\Omega\,cm^2$ (ALD).

Based on the study of resistance to crevice corrosion it was found that regardless of the method used to prepare the surface, Ti6Al7Nb alloy is resistant to this type of corrosion - Fig. 2. The results confirmed the formation of a compact oxide barrier layer on the surface, separating the substrate from the corrosive environment in which the tests were performed.

To identify the nature of the oxide layer formed on the surface of chosen biomaterial in the next step the measurements were performed using electrochemical impedance spectroscopy. Examples of the impedance spectra recorded or the Ti6Al7Nb alloy with modified surface are shown in Fig. 3.

Electric values obtained based on the spectra are summarized in Table 1. It was found, that regardless of the method used to modify the alloy's surface, impedance module of tested systems decreases with increasing frequency, and phase angle also changes with the change of frequency.

Table 1. EIS results

Surface modification	E_{OCP}	R_s	R_{pore}	C_{PORE}	R_{ct}	CPE_{dl}	
Methods	mV	Ωcm^2	$k\Omega cm^2$	F	$M\Omega cm^2$	Y_0, $\Omega^{-1}cm^{-2s-n}$	n
Initial state	-197	20	-	-	5.45	0.2158	0.93
Anodic oxidation	-291	20	-	-	25.00	0.1846	0.97
ALD	-159	17	16	2.95	43.10	0.1778	0.90

The best fit of the modeled spectra to the impedance spectra determined during the study in Ringer's solution in case of samples in initial state and after anodic oxidation is provided by a simple equivalent circuit of a single time constant consisting of three electric components - Fig. 4a. In the circuit element R_s models electrolyte's (Ringer's solution) resistance - characterises resistance of transfering an electric charge at the TiO_2 - Ringer's solution interface, CPE_{dl} - electric properties of a double layer at the interface. The analysis of experimentally determined impedance spectra of corrosive systems of Ti6Al7Nb with a layer of TiO_2 deposited by ALD, uses equivalent electric circuit which is shown in

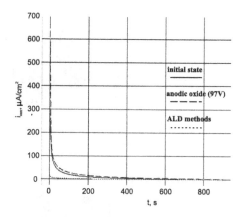

Fig. 2. Exemplary polarization curves showing the relations between the current density and time for Ti6Al7Nb alloy with modified surface

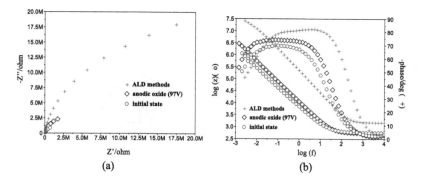

Fig. 3. Impedance spectra of Ti6Al7Nb alloy sample with modified surface: (a) Nyquist diagram, (b) Bode diagram

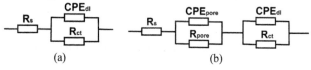

Fig. 4. Equivalent electric circuit for Ti6Al7Nb – TiO2 layer – Ringer's solution system

Fig. 4b. Impedance spectra were in this case interpreted by comparison to equivalent electric circuit pointing out presence of a double layer (two time constants shown in the chart), where R_s - Ringer's solution resistance, R_{pore} - resistance of electrolyte in porous phase, C_{pore} - capacity of double layer (porous and surface), R_{ct} and CPE_{dl} - electric charge transfer resistance and capacity of oxide layer. The use of two constant phase elements in an electric circuit influenced positively the quality of experimentally determined curves fit.

On the basis of observation using a scanning electron microscope and the atomic force microscope, it was found that the process of applying the layers by

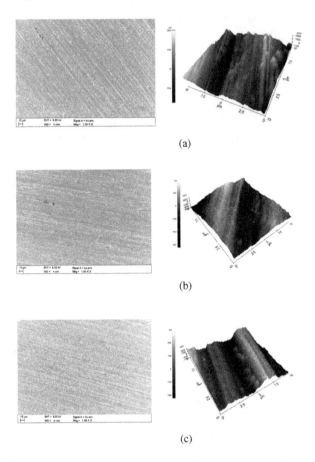

(a)

(b)

(c)

Fig. 5. Modified surface topography of Ti6Al7Nb alloy, SEM, AFM: (a) initial state, (b) anodic oxidation, (c) ALD

anodic oxidation and ALD does not affect on a large degree the quality of the surface topography - Fig. 5.

4   Conclusion

Rating electrochemical properties of metallic biomaterials used for implants to bone is the primary criterion for their suitability for this type of medical devices. Electrochemical properties of the product are reflected in the preparation of its surface. A suitable method for preparing the surface of the implant, which is in direct contact with the bone tissue, is essential for the proper conduction of the treatment process. Safety of the implant is also influenced by the chemical composition of the surface layer. During contact with body fluids a thin oxide layer mostly created out of main alloy element: Ti, Al, Nb, builds itself up on the surface of Ti6Al7Nb. In order to prevent the formation of the oxide layer with the participation of Al, the authors have proposed applying to the surface of titanium alloy Ti6Al7Nb a TiO_2 layer using methods of anodic oxidation and ALD. This type of surface treatment allowed the formulation of a thin layer of TiO_2 under controlled conditions, thereby removing Al and Nb. Based on the obtained results a beneficial effect of the applied layer of TiO_2 on improving the electrochemical properties regardless to the method of application. Potentiodynamic studies have shown that for every case, there was no sudden increase of the anodic treatment in terms of the potential to +4000 mV, meaning initiation of the process of pitting corrosion. This was confirmed in EIS studies, which did not detect a Warburg impedance proving a diffusion phenomena initiation. On the other hand potentiostatic studies have shown that regardless of the method of application of the test sample is resistant to crevice corrosion. The study of surface topography (AFM) revealed that the type of the method of surface treatment (anodic oxidation, ALD) does not change the roughness of the metal substrate which is quite favorable.

To summarize, the preferred set of electrochemical properties characterizes a layer of TiO_2 deposited by ALD. Both in potentiodynamic and impedance studies the layer has obtained the highest value of polarization resistance and charge transfer resistance which proves its high density and electrochemical stability. Therefore, in the case of implants for bone tissue contact, ALD method for applying TiO_2 oxide on the surface of the Ti6Al7Nb alloy it is justified and fully useful for improving the corrosion resistance.

References

1. Li, P.H., Chu, P.K.: Thin film deposition technologies and processing of biomaterials. In: Thin Film Coatings for Biomaterials and Biomedical Applications, pp. 3–28 (2016)
2. Basiaga, M., Walke, W., Paszenda, Z., Kajzer, A.: The effect of EO and steam sterilization on mechanical and electrochemical properties of titanium grade 4. Materiali Tehnologije **50**(1), 153–158 (2016)
3. Marin, E., Lanzutti, A., Lekka, M., Guzman, L., Ensinger, W., Fedrizzi, L.: Chemical and mechanical characterization of TiO_2/Al_2O_3 atomic layer depositions on AISI 316 L stainless steel. Surf. Coat. Technol. **211**, 84–88 (2012)
4. Shan, C.X., Hou, X., Choy, K.L.: Layers on implantable titanium alloys. Optica Applicata **43**(1), 173–180 (2008)
5. Szewczenko, J., Jaglarz, J., Kurzyk, J., Paszenda, Z.: Optical methods applied in thickness and topography testing of passive layers on implantable titanium alloys. Optica Applicata **43**(1), 173–180 (2013)
6. Babilas, D., et al.: On the electropolishing and anodic oxidation of Ti-15Mo alloy. Electrochimica Acta **205**, 256–265 (2016)
7. Lia, X., Chena, T., Hua, J., Lib, S., Zouc, Q., Lia, Y., Jianga, N., Lia, H., Lia, J.: Modified surface morphology of a novel Ti-24Nb-4Zr-7.9Sn titanium alloy via anodic oxidation for enhanced interfacial biocompatibility and osseointegration. Colloids Surf. B Biointerfaces **144**, 265–275 (2016)
8. Wang, W.K., et al.: Nanotribological properties of ALD-processed bilayer TiO_2/ZnO films. Microelectron. Reliab. **54**(12), 2754–2759 (2014)

9. Borgese, L., Bontempi, E., Gelfi, M., Depero, L.E., Goudeau, P., Geandier, G., Thiaudière, D.: Microstructure and elastic properties of atomic layer deposited TiO2 anatase thin films. Acta Materialia **59**(7), 2891–2900 (2011)

10. Aarik, L., Arroval, T., Rammula, R., Mändar, H., Sammelselg, V., Aarik, J.: Atomic layer deposition of TiO_2 from $TiCl_4$ and O_3. Thin Solid Films **542**, 100–107 (2013)

11. Saleem, M.R., Silfsten, P., Honkanen, S., Turunen, J.: Thermal properties of TiO_2 films grown by atomic layer deposition. Thin Solid Films **520**, 5442–5446 (2012)

12. Zhong, Q., Yan, J., Qian, X., Zhang, T., Zhang, Z., Lia, A.: Atomic layer deposition enhanced grafting of phosphorylcholine on stainless steel for intravascular stents. Colloids Surf. B Biointerfaces **121**, 238–247 (2014)

13. Basiaga, M., Jendruś, R., Walke, W., Paszenda, Z., Kaczmarek, M., Popczyk, M.: Influence of surface modification on properties of stainless steel used for implants. Arch. Metall. Mater. **60**(4), 2965–2969 (2015)

14. Basiaga, M., Staszuk, M., Walke, W., Opilski, Z.: Mechanical properties of ALD TiO_2 layers on stainless steel substrate. Materialwissenschaft Werkstofftechnik **47**(5), 1–9 (2016)

15. Kiel, M., Szewczenko, J., Nowińska, K.: Technological capabilities of surface layers formation on implants made of Ti-6Al-4V alloy. Acta Bioeng. Biomech. **17**(1), 31–37 (2015)

16. Marciniak, J., Szewczenko, J., Kajzer, W.: Surface modification of implants for bone surgery. Arch. Metall. Mater. **60**(3), 2123–2129 (2015)

17. ASTM F2129: Standard Test Method for Conducting Cyclic Potentiodynamic Polarization Measurements to Determine the Corrosion Susceptibility of Small Implant Devices (2015)

18. Kajzer, A., Kajzer, W., Dzielicki, J., Matejczyk, D.: The study of physicochemical properties of stabilizing plates removed from the body after treatment of pectus excavatum. Acta Bioeng. Biomech. **2**, 35–44 (2015)

19. ASTM F746–04: Standard Test Method for Pitting or Crevice Corrosion of Metallic Surgical Implant Materials (2009)

Laboratory Evaluation of the Fit of Anti-rotational Elements at the Hybrid Implant Abutments Used in Prosthetic Dentistry

Bohdan Bączkowski[1]([✉]), Anna Ziębowicz[2], Bogusław Ziębowicz[3],
and Elżbieta Wojtyńska[1]

[1] Department of Prosthetic Dentistry,
Medical University of Warsaw, Nowogrodzka 59, 02-006 Warsaw, Poland
bohdanb@wp.pl
[2] Department of Biomaterials and Medical Devices Engineering,
Silesian University of Technology, Roosevelta 40, 41-800 Zabrze, Poland
anna.ziebowicz@polsl.pl
[3] Department of Biomedical Materials Engineering,
Silesian University of Technology, Konarskiego 18a, 44-100 Gliwice, Poland
boguslaw.ziebowicz@polsl.pl

Abstract. Hybrid implant abutments join the features of standard metal-ceramic implant abutments and custom made pure ceramic ones. They are made of zirconium oxide in CAD/CAM technology and are combined with a base made of titanium, supplied by the manufacturer of the implants. The aim of the study was to evaluate the marginal seal at the border of the implant and hybrid abutment, as well as the degree of fit of these elements. Both marginal seal and the degree of matching between the Replace Select 4.3 (Nobel Biocare, Sweden) implant and the hybrid abutment fall within the limits described in the literature.

Keywords: Implant · Hybrid implant abutment

1   Introduction

The discovery of osseointegration in bones allowed for the use of predictable and long-term treatment with dental implants for patients with missing teeth. The development of CAD/CAM technology at the end of the 20th century made it possible to obtain customised implant abutments made of zirconium oxide. The use of the ceramic abutments creates a possibility to obtain geometry that is similar to the shape of the prepared tooth and allows for customised shaping of the emergence profile. The disadvantage of these fillers is, however, the difficulty of establishing proper thickness of the abutments' walls due to characteristic features of the material they are made of. The long-term success of the prosthetic rehabilitation by using dental implants is determined by a number of factors,

© Springer International Publishing AG 2017
M. Gzik et al. (eds.), *Innovations in Biomedical Engineering*, Advances in Intelligent
Systems and Computing 526, DOI 10.1007/978-3-319-47154-9_2

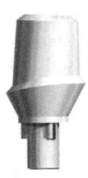

Fig. 1. Standard hybrid abutment

including tightness and stability of the connection between the implant and the prosthetic abutment [1,2].

Standard hybrid abutments are commonly made by joining titanium base with a ceramic ring, most frequently made of zirconium dioxide (Fig. 1). The process of combining these two is completed by using chemo- and light-curing composite cements such as Panavia F (Kuraray, Japan), Multilink Implant (Ivoclar Vivadent, Liechtenstein) or Vita Duo Cement (VITA, Germany) [3,4].

Hybrid implant abutments join the features of standard metal-ceramic implant abutments and custom made pure ceramic ones. They are made of zirconium oxide in CAD/CAM technology and are combined with a base made of titanium, supplied by the manufacturer of the implants (Fig. 2). The advantage of this method is the possibility of full customisation of the abutments' shape.

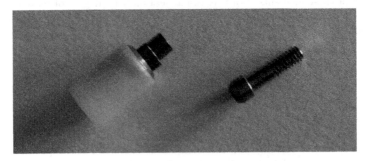

Fig. 2. Custom made hybrid abutment

2   Methodology

The aim of the study was to evaluate the marginal seal at the border of the implant and hybrid abutment, as well as the degree of fit of these elements. To determine the degree of fit, the scanning with the electron microscope (SEM) Zeiss Supra 35 with the SE type detector was used in the study. Due to the lack of conductivity of the tested samples, their surfaces were subjected to a process of spraying with a layer of gold. The study involved the system consisting of an implant and a hybrid abutment. It included an analysis of the connection surface of the Replace implant platform with a hybrid abutment made of Robo-cam material. The analysis was conducted at a random point of connection and then the measuring point was changed, and the pitch angle of the measurement amounted to 120°. The analysis of the dimensions of the implant socket and the stabilising element of the abutment was based on the measurements of the inner diameter of the socket of the implant (tube), the outer diameter of the stabilising element (tube), and the linear dimensions - width (D) and height (H) of the anti-rotational elements (Figs. 3 and 4).

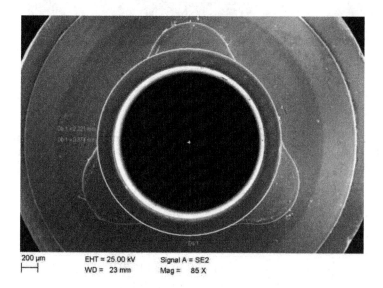

Fig. 3. Measurement of diameter of the socket of the anti-rotational element (tube) in the hybrid abutment

3   Results

Based on the survey, differences in the width of the gap (d) between the implant platform and the abutment were found. For a hybrid abutment the average width of the connection amounted to 16.37 [μm], (min.10.12 [μm], max 21.68 [μm]) (Δ = 11.56 [μm]) (Table 1). The internal diameter of the inlet socket of the implant and the outer diameter of the stabilising element (tube) of the abutments (Table 2) were also subjected to comparison. Additionally, the linear dimensions of anti-rotational elements and sockets in the implants were compared. In the conducted test, the differences in the diameters of stabilising element (tube)

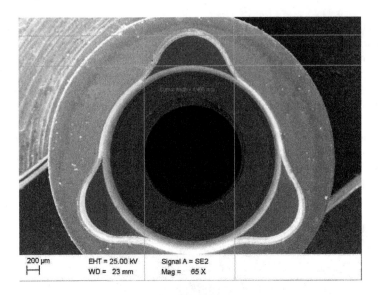

Fig. 4. Measurement of linear dimensions of the anti-rotational element (ear) in the implant Replace Select 4.3 (Nobel Biocare, Sweden)

Table 1. The width of the gap between the implant platform and abutment in micrometres. A, B, C – consecutive positions of the measurements, pitch angle of the measurement at 120°

Implant - hybrid abutment			
No.	A	B	C
1.	21.68	14.37	18.90
2.	12.47	14.43	18.90
3.	11.96	10.12	17.71
4.	18.21	12.31	13.27
5.	15.24	20.31	11.68
6.	18.14	17.44	19.10
7.	15.67	14.88	17.72
8.	15.12	12.11	17.99
9.	10.45	15.54	16.39
10.	10.45	15.01	13.79
Average	**15.52**	**15.02**	**16.37**

between the tested abutment and the groove of the implant were shown. These values amounted respectively for the hybrid abutment to min. 2.215 [mm], max. 2.315 [mm] ($\Delta = 2.241$ [mm]), while the diameter of the groove implant Replace Select 4.3 (Nobel Biocare, Sweden amounted to min. 2.676 [mm], max. 2.688 [mm] ($\Delta = 2.680$ [mm]).

Table 2. The fit degree comparison obtained by measuring the diameter of the external and internal anti–rotational elements

No.	External diameter hybrid abutment, mm	Internal diameter implant, mm
1.	2.221	2.681
2.	2.229	2.676
3.	2.227	2.678
4.	2.215	2.688
Average	**2.241**	**2.680**

Table 3. Comparison of fit degree of external and internal anti–rotation elements

No.	Linear measurements: hybrid abutments		Linear measurements: implant	
	D_h	H_h	D_i	H_i
1.	1.165	353.5	1.430	478.8
2.	1.105	324.4	1.427	447.4
3.	1.090	320.2	1.468	478.6
4.	1.127	350.7	1.432	466.1
5.	1.109	330.0	1.429	457.3
Average	**1.123**	**335.7**	**1.437**	**465.6**

The height (H) of the element and the length at its base (D) were also measured. For the hybrid abutment, the length of the rotation element measured at the base D_h amounted to min. 1.090, max. $1.185 (\Delta = 1,123)$, and the height H_h of the element measured from its base to the tangent running to its edge amounted to min. 320.2 [mm], max. 353.5 [mm] $(\Delta = 335.7)$.

The measurement of the length of the internal anti-rotational D_i elements of the implant Replace Select 4.3 (Nobel Biocare, Sweden) amounted to min. 1.427 [mm], $max. 1.468$ [mm] $(\Delta = 1.437)$, while its height H_i amounted to min. 447.4 [mm], $max. 478.8$ [mm] $(\Delta = 335.7)$ (Table 3).

4   Conclusions

Implant abutments used in dental prosthodontics play an important role in achieving positive results during long-term implant prosthetics treatment. Prevention of the prosthetic failures, such as the loosening of the superstructure, fractures or several biological complications may depend on proper adjustment of the connecting elements, geometry, the size of the abutment and the crown, as well as the distribution of forces exerted to the construction [5–7]. The marginal seal tests conducted in the present study showed differences between the values achieved at different points of measurement for the hybrid abutment. According to different authors, the satisfactory gap ranges from 23 to 150 [μm] [8,9].

Therefore, the results obtained in this study can be considered as very good. The degree of the implant fit with the abutments' connection should allow for longitudinal rotation by 3°, which can prevent brittle fracture, but at the same time it can lead to greater risk of deformation during chewing. Subsequently, this can lead to periodic expansion of the marginal gap and transferring more pressure to the *abutments'* screw [10,11]. The authors consider the distance between 0 and 300 [μm] as a good result, therefore the average distance for a hybrid abutment obtained in this study should be regarded as satisfactory. Both marginal seal and the degree of matching between the Replace Select 4.3 (Nobel Biocare, Sweden) implant and the hybrid abutment fall within the limits described in the literature.

References

1. Al-Turki, L.E., Chai, J., Lautenschlager, E.P.: Changes in prosthetic screw stability because of misfit of implant-supported prostheses. Int. J. Prosthodont. **15**, 38–42 (2002)
2. Ziębowicz, A., Bączkowski, B.: Numerical analysis of the implant – abutment system. In: Piętka, E., Kawa, J. (eds.) ITIB 2012. LNCS, vol. 7339, pp. 341–350. Springer, Heidelberg (2012). doi:10.1007/978-3-642-31196-3_34
3. Vita Enamic Implant-supported Crowns Working Instructions, Vita GmbH, Germany
4. Martínez-Rus, F., Ferreiroa, A., Özcan, M.: Marginal discrepancy of monolithic and veneered all-ceramic crowns on titanium and zirconia implant abutments before and after adhesive cementation: a scanning electron microscopy analysis. Int. J. Oral Maxillofac. Impl. **3**, 480–487 (2013)
5. Scarano, A., Assenza, B., Piattelli, M.: A 16-year study of the microgap between 272 human titanium implants and their abutments. J. Oral Implantol. **31**, 269–75 (2005)
6. Tesmer, M., Wallet, S., Koutouzis, T., Lundgren, T.: Bacterial colonization of the dental implant fixture-abutment interface: an in vitro study. J. Periodontol. **80**, 1991–1997 (2009)
7. Baldassari, M., Hjerppe, J., Romeo, D.: Marginal accuracy of three implant-ceramic abutment configuration. Int. J. Oral Maxillofac. Impl. **27**, 537–543 (2012)
8. Sumi, T., Braian, M., Shimada, A.: Characteristics of implant-CAD/CAM abutment connections of two different internal connection systems. J. Oral Rehab. **39**(5), 391–398 (2012)
9. Jemt, T.: Three-dimensional distortion of gold alloy castingsand welded titanium frameworks. Measurements of the precision of fit between completed implant prostheses and the master casts in routine edentulous situations. J. Oral Rehabil. **22**, 557–564 (1995)
10. Prisco, R., Santagnta, M., Vigolo, P.: Effect of aging and porcelain sintering on rotational freedom of internal hex one-piece zirconia abutments. Int. J. Oral Maxillofac. Impl. **1**, 1003–1008 (2013)
11. Coelho, A.L., Suzuki, M., Dibart, S.: Cross-sectional analysis of implant-abutment interface. J. Oral Rehab. **34**(7), 508–516 (2007)

Corrosion Resistance of Surface Treated NiTi Alloy Tested in Artificial Plasma

Marcin Kaczmarek$^{(\boxtimes)}$ and Przemyslaw Kurtyka

Department of Biomaterials and Medical Devices Engineering,
Faculty of Biomedical Engineering,
Silesian University of Technology, Zabrze, Poland
marcin.kaczmarek@polsl.pl

Abstract. Application of equiatomic NiTi alloys in cardiovascular system has been expanding over last decades. By modification of chemical and phase composition the limit of biocompatibility has been reached. Further development is connected with surface modification. Among many methods of surface treatment of NiTi alloys, passivation has been often chosen as the first choice method. Resistance to pitting and crevice corrosion of the surface modified NiTi alloy in artificial plasma was investigated by means of electrochemical methods (potentidynamic polarization and chronoamperometric method respectively). The obtained results indicate that the proposed surface treatment ensures good corrosion resistance in artificial plasma and can be applied in shaping final functional properties of NiTi alloys used in cardiovascular system.

Keywords: NiTi shape memory alloy · Surface treatment · Pitting and crevice corrosion · Artificial plasma

1 Introduction

Nearly equiatomic nickel-titanium alloys have been attracting both scientific and engineering interest for biomedical applications due to their unique mechanical properties and performance (shape memory and superelasticity), and biocompatibility. The shape memory effect is based on a phase transformation induced by the temperature or applied stresses. When a shape memory alloy is in its cold state (below As), the material can be easily deformed into a variety of new shapes and will remain in this shape until it is heated above the transition temperature (Af). After heating, the material recovers its original shape. Superelasticity refers to the ability of the alloy to undergo large elastic deformations, during mechanical loading-unloading cycles performed at constant temperatures.

Nowadays, due to the mentioned unique properties, NiTi shape memory alloys are widely used in numerous biomedical applications, focused mostly on minimally invasive procedures (e.g. orthodontics - orthodontic archives, endodontic files; orthopaedics - staples for foot surgery, bone plates, intramedullary nails; urology and gastroenterology). The use of NiTi alloys in

© Springer International Publishing AG 2017
M. Gzik et al. (eds.), *Innovations in Biomedical Engineering*, Advances in Intelligent Systems and Computing 526, DOI 10.1007/978-3-319-47154-9_3

biomedical application results from the unique functional properties and performance considering: elastic deployment, thermal deployment, kink resistance, biocompatibility, constant unloading stresses, biomechanical compatibility, dynamic interference, hysteresis, MR compatibility, fatigue resistance and uniform plastic deformation [1]. However, the most common is the application of these alloys in a cardiovascular field (e.g. vena cava filters, atrial septal occlusion device, ablation devices) with the special attention focused on stents. Stenting has become the standard procedure in treatment of cardiovascular diseases. Intravascular stents are extensively used in conjunction with conventional angioplasty to improve the final outcome of percutaneous revascularization procedures.

In spite of the mentioned interesting properties and application in biomedical field, special attention should be put concerning the implantation of alloys containing Ni. Although nickel is considered as the nutrition, trace element which plays important role in metabolic processes, it is well known that Ni is also considered as allergic, toxic, and carcinogenic element [2–6]. Therefore, describing the biocompatibility of NiTi alloys, nickel release should be taken into account. Since biocompatibility is strongly correlated with corrosion resistance, it is extremely important for alloys to exhibit excellent electrochemical, protective properties. Issues of corrosion resistance of metal biomaterials and its influence on functional properties have been widely described in the literature [7–16].

Good corrosion resistance and associated good biocompatibility can be ascribed to a passive oxide layer formed spontaneously on the alloy surface. The passive layer consist mostly of TiO_2. Depending on its structure, phase composition, stability and thickness the layer may act as a barrier against Ni release. Native oxide layers consisting mostly of TiO_2 seem to be the most appropriate in cardiovascular applications, especially taking into account deformability of surface layers corresponding to phenomenon of superelasticity. Thus issues of surface treatment of NiTi alloys play extremely important role in their biocompatibility. Different methods and protocols have been used for surface treatments - mechanical and electrochemical treatments, chemical etching, heat treatments, physical and chemical plasma methods, ion implantation, laser and electron-beam irradiation. Many studies of corrosion resistance of NiTi alloys in simulated body fluids have been reported [17–24]. However, due to diverse test regimes, and what is the most important different surface treatments applied, the obtained results are incomparable and questionable.

2   Materials and Methods

The aim of the study was evaluation of pitting and crevice corrosion resistance of the surface treated NiTi alloy. Due to possible cardiovascular applications, corrosion studies were carried out in artificial plasma - Table 1 - according to the requirements enclosed in the ISO 10993-15 and ASTM F746 standards. The chemical composition of the alloy (Ni - 55,5 %, Ti - balance) met the requirements of the ASTM 2063 standard. The tests were carried out on flat samples ($10 \times 10 \times 1\,mm$).

In order to evaluate the influence of diverse methods of surface modification on the corrosion resistance of the alloy, the following subsequent surface treatments were applied:

- grinding - abrasive paper (#600 grit).
- electropolishing,
- H_2O chemical passivation,
- H_2SO_4 electrochemical passivation.

Since passivation is often considered as the first choice surface treatment assuring formation of the dense, stable TiO_2 oxide layer, different methods of passivation were adopted in the study. Both chemical and electrochemical methods were adopted. The applied methods of surface treatment and their parameters were presented in Table 2.

Table 1. Chemical composition of the artificial plasma

Concentration of components, g/l						
NaCl	CaCl$_2$	KCl	NaHCO$_3$	NaH$_2$PO$_4$	MgSO$_4$	Na$_2$HPO$_4$
6.800	0.00	0.400	2.200	0.026	0.100	0.126

Table 2. Parameters of the applied surface modifications

Surface treatment	Applied baths	Time, min	Temp., °C	Potencial, V
Grinding	–	–	–	–
Electropolishing	HF-based	15	60	50
Chemical	H$_2$O	60	boiling	–
Electrochemical	H$_2$SO$_4$	3–20	10–30	25

The electrochemical tests of the investigated alloy were performed with the use of a potentiodynamic method by recording of anodic polarization curves. In the tests the scan rate was equal to 1 mV/sec. The PGP 201 (Radiometer) potentiostat with the software for electrochemical tests was applied. The saturated calomel electrode (SCE) was applied as the reference electrode and the auxiliary electrode was a platinum wire. All samples were immersed in the artificial plasma for 60 min before the scanning started at a potential of about 100 mV below the recorded open circuit potential (EOCP). The scanning direction was reversed when the anodic current density reached $1000\,\mu A/cm^2$. The tests were carried out at the temperature of $37 \pm 1°C$. On the basis of the recorded curves characteristic values describing the resistance to pitting corrosion i.e.: corrosion potential Ecorr (V), breakdown potential Eb (V) or transpassivation potential Etr (V), polarization resistance Rp ($\Omega*cm^2$) and corrosion current density (A/cm^2) were determined. To determine the value of polarization resistance

Rp the Stern method was applied. Corrosion current density was determined from the simplified formula: icorr = 0.026/Rp.

The ASTM F746 standard test method was applied to assess crevice corrosion resistance. According to the standard, stimulation of localized corrosion is marked by one of the following conditions: the polarization current density exceeds 500 $\mu A/cm^2$ instantly; the current density does not exceed 500 $\mu A/cm^2$ within 20 s, but is increasing in general; these two conditions are not met in the first 20 s, but are met in a period of 15 min. The crevice corrosion tests were carried out at the temperature of 37°C. The corrosion potential of the sample was continuously monitored for 1 h, starting immediately after immersion in the electrolyte. According to the ASTM standard, damage of the passive film is performed electrochemically by applying a potential of +800 mV versus SCE for durations up to 15 min on a creviced sample. If during 15 min localized corrosion is not stimulated the test is terminated and the material is considered resistant to localized corrosion, otherwise a voltage step back to a preselected potential is conducted. The test consists of alternating steps between stimulation at +800 mV and repassivation to a preselected potential up to a critical potential, for which repassivation does not take place, is attained (the increase of the preselected potential value between the steps is 50 mV).

3   Results

The electrochemical tests carried out in the artificial plasma showed diverse resistance of NiTi alloy to pitting corrosion, depending on the applied surface treatment. Results of the pitting corrosion tests for the ground, electropolished and passivated with the use of both chemical and electrochemical methods samples are presented in Table 3 and in Fig. 1. The results presented in the tables are mean values.

Table 3. Results of the pitting corrosion studies of the treated NiTi alloy

Surface treatment	Ecorr, mV	Etr, mV	Rp, k$\Omega \times$ cm^2	icorr, nA/cm^2
Grinding	−235	+ 346 (Eb)	66	394
Electropolishing	−81	+ 1357	37	688
H$_2$O passivation	+ 87	+ 1372	135	211
H$_2$SO$_4$ passivation	+ 121	+ 1395	143	172

Similarly to the results of pitting corrosion, the results of the crevice corrosion tests showed also diverse resistance of NiTi alloy to crevice corrosion depending on the applied surface treatment. The results of the crevice corrosion resistance for the ground, electropolished, and passivated samples are presented in Table 4 and in Fig. 2.

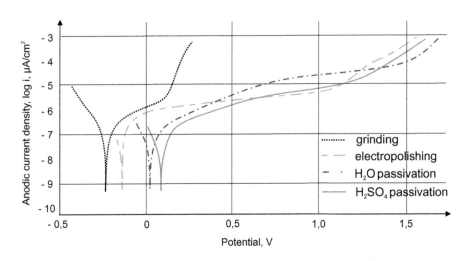

Fig. 1. Examples of anodic polarization curves for the treated NiTi alloy

Table 4. Results of the crevice corrosion studies of the NiTi alloy

Surface treatment	Ecorr, mV	Ecc, mV	Crevice corrosion resistance
Grinding	−235	+ 400	−
Electropolishing	−81	> + 800	+
H₂O passivation	+ 87	> + 800	+
H₂SO₄ passivation	+ 121	> + 800	+

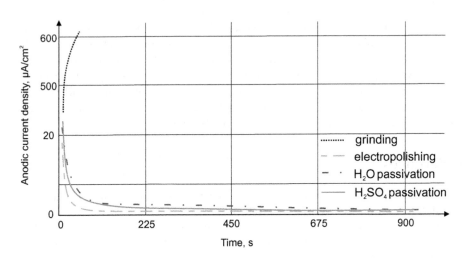

Fig. 2. Example results of chronoamperometric studies of the surface treated NiTi alloy

4 Discusion

Assessment of corrosion resistance is essential in determining biocompatibility of metal implant materials. By changes in chemical and phase composition the given level of biocompatibility has been reached. Further development of biocompatibility is related with surface modification. Different surface treatment methods have been applied in order to enhance corrosion resistance and biocompatibility in consequence. Due to application of shape memory alloys as cardiovascular implants, appropriate methods of surface treatment must be applied. Since the implants are miniaturized the only method ensuring required surface roughness and chemistry is electropolishing. And due to ease of oxidation of NiTi alloys the next first choice surface treatment is passivation. Passivation can be realized by means of both chemical and electrochemical methods.

In the presented work the following subsequent surface treatment methods were applied: grinding, electropolishing, H_2O chemical passivation and H_2SO_4 electrochemical passivation.

The potentiodynamic method is widely used in determining the susceptibility of alloys to both pitting and crevice corrosion. Thus both, the polarization method and the chromoamperometry method were applied respectively.

In general the obtained results of pitting corrosion showed that all the NiTi alloy samples were characterized by high resistance to this type of corrosion with the exception of the ground samples. For the electropolished and the passivated samples transpassivation values above $+1300\,\mathrm{mV}$ were recorded whereas for the ground samples the breakdown potential was observed ($+346\,\mathrm{mV}$). The applied passivation both chemical and electrochemical significantly increased polarization resistance of the tested NiTi alloy. The mechanism of improving corrosion resistance in reference to ground and even electropolished samples is related to the formation of thicker and denser oxide layers.

Similar behavior of the tested NiTi samples was observed in the crevice corrosion studies. Resistance to this type of corrosion is important because of the geometry of cardiovascular implants (for example stents). The obtained results have shown that grinding does not ensure resistance to this type of corrosion. The applied surface treatment, consisting of the electropolishing and the two types of passivation, significantly increased resistance to crevice corrosion. For all these samples no signs of corrosion were observed on their surfaces.

References

1. Duerig, T., Pelton, A., Stoeckel, D.: An overview of nitinol medical applications. Mater. Sci. Eng. **A273–275**, 149–160 (1999)
2. Symeonides, P.P., Paschologlou, C., Papageorgiou, S.: An allergic reaction after internal fixation of a fracture using a vitallium plate. J. Allergy Clin. Immunol. **51**, 251 (1973)
3. Elves, M.W., Wilson, J.N., Scales, H.S., Kemp, S.B.: Incidence of metal sensitivity in patients with total joint replacements. British Med. J. **4**, 376 (1975)

4. Veien, N.: In: Maibach, H., Menne, T. (eds.) Nickel and the Skin: Immunology and Toxicology, pp. 165–178. CRC, Boca Raton (1989)
5. Pulletikurthi, C., Munroe, N., Gill, P., Pandya, S., Persaud, D., Haider, W., Iyer, K., McGoron, A.: Cytotoxicity of Ni from surface-treated porous nitinol (PNT) on osteoblast cells. J. Mater. Eng. Perform. **20**, 824–829 (2011)
6. Rocher, P., et al.: Biocorrosion and cytocompatibility assessment of NiTi shape memory alloys. Scripta Materialia **50**, 255–260 (2004)
7. Basiaga, M., Jendrus, R., Walke, W., Paszenda, Z., Kaczmarek, M., Popczyk, M.: Influence of surface modification on properties of stainless steel used for implants. Arch. Metall. Mater. **60**(4), 2965–2969 (2015)
8. Basiaga, M., Staszuk, M., Walke, W., Opilski, Z.: Mechanical properties of ALD TiO2 layers on stainless steel substrate. Materialwissenschaft & Werkstofftechnik **47**(5), 1–9 (2016)
9. Kajzer, A., Kajzer, W., Dzielicki, J., Matejczyk, D.: The study of physicochemical properties of stabilizing plates removed from the body after treatment of pectus excavatum. Acta Bioeng. Biomech. **2**, 35–44 (2015)
10. Kajzer, A., Kajzer, W., Golombek, K., Knol, M., Dzielicki, J., Walke, W.: Corrosion resistance, EIS and wettability of the implants made of 316 LVM steel used in chest deformation treatment. Arch. Metall. Mater. **61**(2a), 767–770 (2016)
11. Szewczenko, J., Marciniak, J., Kajzer, W., Kajzer, A.: Evaluation of corrosive resistance of titanium alloys used for medical implants. Arch. Metall. Mater. **61**(2a), 695–770 (2016)
12. Basiaga, M., Walke, W., Paszenda, Z., Karasinski, P.: Research on electrochemical properties SiO2 layer intended for contact with blood deposited by sol-gel method. Eur. Cells Mater. **26**, 157 (2013)
13. Marciniak, J., Szewczenko, J., Kajzer, W.: Surface modification of implants for bone surgery. Arch. Metall. Mater. **60**(3), 2123–2129 (2015)
14. Szewczenko, J., Pochrzast, M., Walke, W.: Evaluation of electrochemical properties of modified Ti-6Al-4V ELI alloy. Przeglad Elektrotechniczny **87**(12b), 177–180 (2011)
15. Marciniak, J., Szewczenko, J., Walke, W., Basiaga, M., Kiel, M., Manka, I.: Biomechanical analysis of lumbar spine stabilization by means of transpedicular stabilizer. In: Pietka, E., Kawa, J. (eds.) Information Technologies in Biomedicine, pp. 529–536. Springer, Berlin (2008). Advances in Soft Computing, vol. 47, pp. 1615–3871
16. Kiel-Jamrozik, M., Szewczenko, J., Basiaga, M., Nowińska, K.: Technological capabilities of surface layers formation on implant made of Ti-6Al-4V ELI alloy. Acta Bioeng. Biomech. **17**(1), 31–37 (2015)
17. Vojtech, D., Fojt, J., Joska, L., Novak, P.: Surface treatment of NiTi shape memory alloy and its influence on corrosion behavior. Surf. Coat. Technol. **204**, 3895–3901 (2010)
18. Khalil-Allafi, J., Amin-Ahmadi, B., Zare, M.: Bio-compatibility and corrosion behavior of the shape memory NiTi alloy in the physiological environments simulated with body fluids for medical applications. Mater. Sci. Eng. C **30**, 1112–1117 (2010)
19. Chan, C.W., Man, H.C., Yue, T.M.: Susceptibility to stress corrosion cracking of NiTi laser weldment in Hanks' solution. Corros. Sci. **57**, 260–269 (2012)
20. Zhenga, C.Y., Niea, F.L., Zhenga, Y.F., Chengc, Y., Weid, S.C., Ruand, L., Valiev, R.Z.: Enhanced corrosion resistance and cellular behavior of ultrafine-grained biomedical NiTi alloy with a novel $SrO - SiO_2 - TiO_2$ sol-gel coating. Appl. Surf. Sci. **257**, 5913–5918 (2011)

21. Freiberg, K.E., Bremer-Streck, S., Kiehntopf, M., Rettenmayr, M., Undisz, A.: Effect of thermo-mechanical pre-treatment on short- and long-term Ni release from biomedical NiTi. Acta Biomaterialia **10**, 2290–2295 (2014)
22. Pound, B.G.: The electro-chemical behavior of nitinol in simulated physiological solutions. J. Biomed. Mater. Res. **85A**, 1103–1113 (2008)
23. Michiardi, A., Aparicio, C., Planell, J.A., Gil, F.J.: Electro-chemical behaviour of oxidized NiTi shape memory alloys for biomedical applications. Surf. Coat. Technol. **201**, 6484–6488 (2007)
24. Warner, C.P.: The effect of exposure to simulated body fluids on breakdown potentials. JMEPEG **18**, 754–759 (2009)

Corrosion Resistance of Stabilizers for Funnel Chest Treatment

Anita Kajzer[1]([⊠]), Ewelina Głąb[1], Wojciech Kajzer[1], Tomasz Wróbel[2],
and Magdalena Antonowicz[1]

[1] Faculty of Biomedical Engineering,
Department of Biomaterials and Medical Devices Engineering,
Silesian University of Technology, Roosevelta 40, Zabrze, Poland
`Anita.Kajzer@polsl.pl`
[2] Faculty of Mechanical Engineering, Department of Foundry,
Silesian University of Technology, Towarowa 7, 44-100 Gliwice, Poland

Abstract. The paper presents results of physicochemical properties of
the plates used for the treatment of pectus excavatum after implantation.
Within the research, chemical analysis, macroscopic evaluation of the
surface, electromechanical analysis, wettability and surface energy tests
were conducted. On the basis of obtained results, it can be stated that
the reduction of corrosion resistance is influenced by mechanical damage
of the surface and laser marking, as well as by producing stabilizers
made of various types of steel. This caused the decrease of corrosion
resistance of the plate with reduced content od Cr, Ni and Mo. It was
also stated that the analysed surfaces were hydrophilic with an average
surface wettability, on which overgrowth of the tissue was not observed,
which is an essential condition for short-term implants.

Keywords: Corrosion resistance · Wettability · Stainless steel ·
316LVM

1 Introduction

The development of implantology is connected with numerous accomplishments
of interdisciplinary fields of science and technique; with the increased knowledge
about the anatomy of the organs and physiological processes, as well as with
introducing innovative processes of treatment, diagnostics and therapy. Therefore, it is extremely important to place great demands on the used implants at
all of the stages of design, production and exploitation. Only complying all the
requirements and demands will guarantee correct stabilization and will ensure
health and safety of the patients. One of many very important subspecialties
of surgery, in which metal materials are priority, is thoracic surgery. It includes
surgical treatment of chest deformations. The deformation of anterior surface of
the chest causes many cardiovascular disorders. Left-sided heart displacement
is also connected with the disclosure of the right hilum and the change of the

© Springer International Publishing AG 2017
M. Gzik et al. (eds.), *Innovations in Biomedical Engineering*, Advances in Intelligent
Systems and Computing 526, DOI 10.1007/978-3-319-47154-9_4

heart shape which becomes similar to mitral heart. It is difficult to state how far cardiovascular disorders are dependent on the location of a heart and large blood vessels, and how far on the asthenic physique [1–4].

In order to minimize complications and postoperative pain in the treatment of chest deformations, minimally invasive Nuss technique is used [5]. In this method, a plate appropriately profiled to the anatomical curvature of the chest is introduced. Due to the fact that stabilization lasts up to 2 years, for this type of stabilizers steel CrNiMo [6] with good corrosion resistance in the tissue environment is used. Corrosion resistance is a result of precise selection of the amount of alloy elements. Above chrome concentration, within 13 %, we can observe a sudden change in electrochemical potential of steel from negative $(-0,6V)$ to positive $(0,2V)$. As a result, corrosion resistance increases in oxidizing areas and material itself gains ability of passivation similar to chrome. Nickel is responsible for stabilization of austenite phase. This results in the increase of stacking-fault energy and more persistent passive layer. In addition, due to presence of molybdenum, corrosion resistance is increased [7]. Mechanical damage of the surface which occurs during the process of implantation can cause interruption in the passive layer and at the same time, decrease of corrosion resistance, which as a consequence, leads to inflammations in the implant area [8,9]. Improvement of corrosion resistance can be obtained by applying surface layers [10] or using alternative steel biomaterials with higher biocompatibility, eg. titanium alloy [11–13]. Taking implantation technique into consideration, it is extremely important to conduct tests of physiochemical properties, both before and after implantation, in order to evaluate if the implant, which is present in the body from 12 to 24 months, fully ensures correct stabilization without reactions and inflammations. Therefore, in the research we conducted the analysis of the influence of mechanical surface damage on physiochemical properties on two plates used for the treatment of pectus excavatum, – PG1 and PG2, removed from the body after 28 months from the surgical procedure.

2   Materials and Methods

In order to conduct the tests, 2 plates used for the treatment of pectum excavatum were selected. The implants were placed in the body of a patient (male) for 28 months. During clinical observations periosteal reactions we observed. Such reaction of periosteum is most frequently caused by inflammation in the bone area. The plates were produced from austenitic stainless steel 316LVM with mechanical properties in the line with ISO 5832-1 recommendations [6]. As a surface treatment, electrochemical polishing, chemical passivation and steam sterilization were used. The plates were marked appropriately: PG1 – 320 mm long and PG2 – 360 mm long. Next, the plates were subsequently cut into samples with the use of Discotom – 6 mechanical cutter produced by Struers – Fig. 1.

The material for testing was divided into three groups of samples: containing mechanical damage in the form of numerous scratches – group 1, with undamaged surface – group 2 and with an engraving on the surface made for identification – group 3. From each group, 3 samples were selected for tests. Prior to

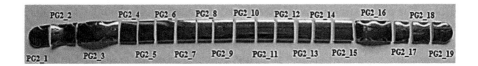

Fig. 1. The plate selected for the tests

the tests, the samples were cleansed in 96 % ethyl alcohol in ultrasonic baths BANDELIN Sonorex Digitec for 10 min.

2.1   Chemical Compostion Test

Researches of chemical composition of the implants were made using LECO GDS500A emission spectrometer. As a result of the glow discharge of studied areas of samples were obtained recording of complete emission spectrum from 165 nm to 460 nm using photosensitive Charge Coupled Device (CCD). Next, by using the method of comparison with reference standards appropriate for a group of stainless steel and NWA Quality Analyst software was determined from three measurements for each sample, the average concentration of the individual elements in the chemical composition of the implants. During the researches, the following work parameters of the spectrometer are used: voltage 1250V voltage, current intensity 45mA, pressure of argon 2 Tr and vacuum 0,1 Tr.

2.2   Wettability Test

In order to determine the surface wettability of the selected samples, the wetting angle and surface free energy were evaluated with the use of Owens-Wendt method. The wettability angle measurement were performed with two liquids: distilled water (θ w) (by Poch S.A.) and diiodomethane (by Merck). Measurements with a drop of liquid and diiodomethane spread over the sample surface were carried out at room temperature ($T = 23°C$) at the test stand incorporating SURFTENS UNIVERSAL goniometer by OEG and a PC with Surftens 4.5 software to assess the recorded drop image. 10 drops of distilled water and diiodomethane each, 1.0 μl volume, were placed on the surface of each of the samples. Duration of a single measurement was 60 seconds at the sampling frequency 1 Hz. The mean values of the wetting angle θ_{av} and the surface free energy γ_S were presented in tabular form.

2.3   Potentiodynamic Test

The tests were carried out as recommended by ISO 10993-15 standard. The test stand comprised of the VoltaLab PGP201 potentiostat, the reference electrode (saturated calomel electrode SCE), the auxiliary electrode (platinum wire), the anode (test sample) and a PC with VoltaMaster 4 software. The corrosion tests started with determination of the open circuit potential E_{OCP} during the first

120 min. The polarization curves were recorded starting with the initial potential value, $E_{init} = E_{OCP} - 100\,mV$. The potential changed along the anode direction at the rate of 3 mV/s. Once the anodic current density reached the value of $1mA/cm^2$, the polarization direction was reversed. On the basis of the curves the corrosion potential E_{corr}, the breakdown potential E_b, the repassivation potential E_{cp}, were determined along with the value of the polarization resistance R_p, calculated with the use of Stern method. Electrochemical test were carried out in the environment of 250 ml Ringer solution supplied by Baxter at the temperature $T = 37 \pm 1°C$ and pH $= 7 \pm 0.2$.

2.4 Macroscopic Observation

Evaluation of the surface using a stereomicroscope SteREO Discovery V8 from Zeiss with software AxioVision was carried out. Observations before and after the pitting corrosion resistance test were performed with total magnification: $9, 6x$ and $25x$.

3 Results and Discussion

3.1 Chemical Composition Test

Results of chemical composition test are presented in (Table 1).

On the basis of obtained results it can be stated, that due to the differences in percentage participation of individual alloy elements, the plates were produced from 2 different steel alloys. The diversified content of individual elements can influence on various properties of the implants. Steel with chrome concentration above 13 % proves better passivating properties, which is connected with the increase of corrosion resistance. Higher content of nickel fosters the increase of resistance to stress corrosion. Furthermore, molybdenum content of 2 %–4 % improves resistance to pitting corrosion. Comparing both plates in relation to all the described elements, less of their content was observed in steel used to produce plate PG1. For this steel higher concentration of carbon was observed in comparison to implant PG2.

3.2 Wettability Test

The results of wettability and surface energy calculations and examples of drops dripped in the surface of samples are presented in (Table 2). Higher average value

Table 1. The content of chemical elements

Elements	C%	Cr%	Ni%	Cu%	Mo%	S%	Si%	P%
Plate PG1	0.039	16.7	13.0	0.062	2.65	0.001	0.394	0.033
Plate PG2	0.029	17.1	13.4	0.057	2.72	0.00	0.373	0.029
ISO 5832-1	0.030 max	17.0-9.0	13.0-5.0	0.50 max	2.25-3.0	0.010 max	1.0 max	0.025 max

Table 2. Results of the wettability and surface energy

Plate number	Contact angle, θ_{avr}°		Surface energy $\gamma_s, mJ/m^2$
	Distilled water	Diiodomethane	
PG1	40.23 ± 3.73	42.40 ± 3.90	56.61 ± 2.10
PG2	36.10 ± 1.72	40.28 ± 2.80	59.49 ± 1.61

of contact angle was observed for PG1 plate. Obtained results for both plates were not significantly different from each other. On the basis of obtained values of wetting angles θ, hydrophylic character of the surface of the plate of average wettability was stated. The values of surface energy γ are comparable for both implants.

Obtained results of wetting angles are lower in comparison to the literature [9,14]. Therefore, it can be stated, that the contact of the stabilizer made of CrNiMo steel with body fluids influenced the increase of the surface wettability. The authors of the paper obtained the following results for steel CrNiMo: [14] value $\theta = 73.67^{\circ}$ for distilled water and value $\theta = 39.48^{\circ}$ for diiodomethane. On the other hand, the authors of the paper [9] state, that the average values of wetting angles change in the range of 76.44° to 81.95°. It can also be stated that there are insignificant differences in the values of surface energy for both plates with regards to the paper of the authors [15,16] in which for the analysed steel they were accordingly: $\gamma_s = 53.2 \ mJ/m^2$ and $\gamma_s = 44.1 \ mJ/m^2$.

3.3   Potentiodynamic Test

Results of potentiodynamic tests carried out to evaluate the pitting corrosion resistance are presented in (Table 3) and Fig. 2(a) and (b).

The values of selected parameter for both plates are different. The biggest differences were observed for breakdown potential E_{np}. Analysing appropriate

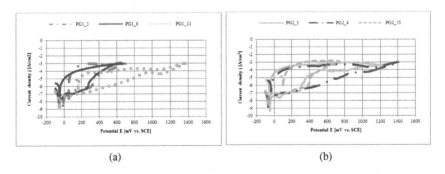

(a)   (b)

Fig. 2. Examples of polarization curves: (a) PG1_3 - mechanical damage, PG1_11 - undamaged, PG1$_8$ - engraving, (b) PG2_2 – mechanical damage, PG2_4 – undamaged, PG2_8 – engraving

groups of samples, it can be stated that the value of E_{np} is dependent on in the tested surface. The highest values were obtained for the samples from group 2 - with minor or complete lack of mechanical damage. Average values are: $E_{npav} = +1023$ mV for PG1 plate and $E_{npav} = +1318$ mV for PG2 plate. On this basis, it can be stated that passive layer in the areas of the least damage is the best protective barrier. The presence of mechanical damage in the form of scratches and burrs influences the decrease of the average value of breakdown potential, which for the samples from group 1 amounts to: $E_{npav} = +919$ mV for PG1 plate and $E_{bsr} = +1214$ mV for PG2 plate. However, the biggest influence on the decrease of corrosion resistance was noticed for laser marking. The layer was damaged, as a result of which the average value E_b in the group of 3 samples is the lowest in comparison to the rest of the samples and for the plate PG1 is +919 mV and for the plate PG2 +831 mV. It can be concluded that on the basis of the course of polarizations curves, the analysed material has the ability to repassivate in the body fluids environment. What is more, the highest average value of polarization resistance R_p was observed for the samples without any mechanical damage, which for plate PG1 came to $R_{pav} = 592 \, k\Omega cm^2$ and for plate PG2 - $R_{pav} = 1128 \, k\Omega cm^2$. The values reviewed differ, depending on the discussed plate. This is connected with the diversified content of alloy elements in both plates. In the previous paper of the authors [9] a negative influence of the surface damage on the corrosion resistance of the implants in comparison to the samples taken from implants in the initial state was also observed. The increase of corrosion resistance of steel CrNiMo was obtained by the authors of the paper [17] who covered the steel with SiO_2 layer. For the surface prepared in such way, the values of breakdown potential E_b ranged from +1543 mV +1518 mV for the samples subjected to ethylene oxide sterilization.

Table 3. The results of pitting corrosion tests

Surface condition	E_{corr}, mV	E_b, mV	E_{cp}, mV	$R_p, k\Omega cm^2$
PG1 plate				
Surface damage	-20 ± 16	$+919 \pm 318$	-19 ± 101	437 ± 38
Undamaged	-78 ± 46	$+1023 \pm 247$	$+60 \pm 89$	592 ± 224
Engraved	-83 ± 33	$+919 \pm 269$	$+57 \pm 94$	373 ± 116
PG2 plate				
Surface damage	-2 ± 40	$+1214 \pm 39$	$+129 \pm 302$	355 ± 123
Undamaged	-42 ± 24	$+1318 \pm 61$	-21 ± 37	989 ± 185
Engraved	-56 ± 14	$+831 \pm 234$	$+92 \pm 15$	323 ± 96

3.4   Macroscopic Observation

In the result of macroscopic evaluation, deep mechanical damage was observed for both PG1 plate (Fig. 3a) and PG2, in the end area of the implant, in the

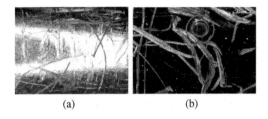

(a)   (b)

Fig. 3. Sample of surface: (a) before corrosion test – stereomicroscop mag. 9.6x and (b) after corrosion test with example of pitting – stereomicroscop mag. 25x

point of locking. Samples taken from the middle part of the plates had few or no damage. In case of both implants, no corrosion processes were observed. After pitting corrosion resistance tests, another macroscopic evaluation of the surface was carried out. Corrosion changes in the form of pitting were observed (Fig. 3(b)).

4 Conclusion

On the basis of macroscopic the biggest number of damage was observed in the end area of the implant, at the point of locking with bars. This is the area, where the plates were modelled in order to adjust the geometry to the anatomical shape of the chest. Numerous mechanical damage on the surface of the implants but, above all, laser marking technique had a huge impact on the decrease of the pitting corrosion resistance. As a result of the analysis of the obtained polarization curves, it can be concluded that for the samples with numerous mechanical surface damage hysteresis loops are wide. This proves slow repassivation. What is more, reduced breakdown potential can be observed for these samples. The decreased resistance in the places of frequent mechanical damage was probably caused by periosteal reactions in the tissues surrounding the implant, which was proved by clinical tests. In the most damaged areas, as well as in the areas of laser marking, changes in the form of corrosion pittings were observed. Furthermore, as a result of conducted tests of wettability and surface energy, the values of wetting angles of the plates PG1 and PG2 were similar. The higher the value of the wetting angle, the more hydrophobic the analyzed material. The values of wetting angles for plates PG1 and PG2 always reach the result below $90°$. On this basis, hydophylic but averagely wettable surface is observed. The wettability is determined by the level of absorption and aggregation of the material. During the observation of the implants no tissue adhesion was observed. This indicates beneficial for short-term implants low ability to adhesion and reaction of the surface to the osteoblasts activity [14, 18].

References

1. Szlachcińska, A., Kozak, J.: Wyniki leczenia szewskiej klatki piersiowej metoda Nussa. Kwartalnik Ortopedyczny, pp. 417–418 (2011). (in Polish)
2. Bohosiewicz, J., Kudela, G., Izwaryn, U.: Leczenie lejkowatej klatki piersiowej. Polski Przegląd Chirurgiczny, pp. 175–187 (2009). (in Polish)
3. Białas, A.J., Jabłoński, J.: Lejkowata klatka piersiowa u dzieci. Przegląd pediatryczny, pp. 112–115 (2010). (in Polish)
4. Korlacki, W., Grabowski, A., Dzielicki, J.: Metoda Nussa w leczeniu deformacji asymetrysznych i mieszanych klatki piersiowej. Kardiochirurgia Torakochirurgia Polska 8, 354–360 (2011). (in Polish)
5. Nuss, D., Kelly, R.E.: Indications and technique of nuss procedure for pectus excavatum. Thorac Surg. Clin. 20, 583–597 (2010)
6. ISO 5832-1.: Implants for surgery - Metallic materials, Part 1: Wrought stainless steel
7. Marciniak, J.: Biomateriały. Gliwice, Wydawnictwo Politechniki Śląskiej 15–17(158–159), 180–190 (2013). (in Polish)
8. Świeczko-Żurek, B., Serbiński, W., Szumlański, A.: Analysis of the failure of fixator used in bone surgery. Adv. Mater. Sci. 8(2), 84–88 (2008)
9. Kajzer, A., Kajzer, W., Dzielicki, J., Matejczyk, D.: The study of physico-chemical properties of stabilizing plates removed from the body after treatment of pectus excavatum. Acta Bioeng. Biomech. 2, 35–44 (2015). doi:10.5277/ABB-00140-2014-02
10. Basiaga, M., Jendruś, R., Walke, W., Paszenda, Z., Kaczmarek, M., Popczyk, M.: Influence of surface modification on properties of stainless steel used for implants. Arch. Metall. Mater. 60(4), 2965–2969 (2015)
11. Marciniak, J., Szewczenko, J., Kajzer, W.: Surface modification of implants for bone surgery. Arch. Metall. Mater. 60(3), 2123–2129 (2015)
12. Szewczenko, J., Marciniak, J., Kajzer, W., Kajzer, A.: Evaluation of corrosive resistance of titanium alloys used for medical implants. Arch. Metall. Mater. 61, 2 (2016). doi:10.1515/amm-2016-0118
13. Ziębowicz, A., Ziębowicz, B., Bączkowski, B.: Electrochemical behavior of materials used in dental implantological systems. Solid State Phenom. 227, 447–450 (2015)
14. Sobieska, S., Zimowska, B., Łagan, S.: Porównanie zwilżalności oraz swobodnej energii powierzchniowej biomateriałów i tkanki kostnej. Aktualne Problemy Biomechaniki 7, 153–156 (2013). (in Polish)
15. Batory, D., Gorzędowski, J., Kołodziejczyk, Ł., Szymański, W.: Modification of diamond-like carbon coatings by silver ion implantation. Eng. Biomater. 105, 9–10 (2011)
16. Paszkowski, M., Wieleba, W., Wróblewski, R.: Badania właściwości adhezyjnych stali oraz tworzyw sztucznych w kontekście zastosowania ich na węzły tarcia. Tribologia 5, 95–104 (2010). (in Polish)
17. Walke, W., Paszenda, Z., Pustelny, T., Opilski, Z., Drewniak, S., Kościelniak-Ziemniak, M., Basiaga, M.: Evaluation of physicochemical properties of SiO_2-coated stainless steel after sterilization. Mater. Sci. Eng. C 63, 155–163 (2016)
18. Xu, L.C.: Effect of surface wettability and contact time on protein adhesion to biomaterial surfaces. Biomaterials 28, 3273–3283 (2007)

Fretting Wear of NiTi - Shape-Memory Alloy

Marcin Klekotka and Jan Ryszard Dąbrowski$^{(\boxtimes)}$

Department of Materials and Biomedical Engineering,
Bialystok University of Technology, Wiejska 45 C, 15-351 Bialystok, Poland
{m.klekotka,j.dabrowski}@pb.edu.pl

Abstract. This study presents the results of tests of friction processes and fretting wear of NiTi shape-memory alloy, which is used in orthodontics and surgery. This research problem is significant because nickel ions released as a result of nitinol wear exhibit toxic action in the human body. Knowledge about wear mechanisms will allow for more effective prevention of processes leading to the destruction of elements of medical constructions and extend the time of their safe operation. Tests were performed on a pin-on-disc fretting tester under dry friction conditions and in a simulated oral cavity environment. Wear assessments were conducted on the basis of microscopy (SEM, TEM, CLM). Obtained results indicate that friction conditions have a significant impact on the mechanism of fretting wear, which is primarily related to oxidation and phase transformation of nitinol.

Keywords: Fretting · Nitinol · Saliva · Wear · Biomaterials

1 Introduction

Shape-memory alloys are among the group of smart materials and are finding ever broader and growing applications in medicine. Nickel-titanium alloys, with a near-equiatomic chemical composition, are used most commonly. Orthodontic wires and arches, as well as braces, intramedullary rods and implants for treatment of spinal defects, among other things, are made from these alloys. The shape-memory effect of nitinol is related to its thermo-elastic martensitic transformation, however, in medical applications, the phenomenon of superelasticity is most frequently used. This transformation is reversible, however exceeding the yield point of strain-induced martensite leads to loss of the material's superelastic properties [1–3].

Reports in the literature indicate that nitinol alloys are susceptible to tribological wear. This particularly pertains to adhesive grafts, which significantly limit the application of titanium alloys in friction pairs [4,5]. However, it must be noted that fretting wear mechanisms of nitinol have not sufficiently been described in the professional literature, and strain-induced phase transformations have a significant impact on wear kinetics [6]. The susceptibility of nickel-titanium alloys to fretting-corrosion processes is also a significant problem [7,8].

© Springer International Publishing AG 2017
M. Gzik et al. (eds.), *Innovations in Biomedical Engineering*, Advances in Intelligent
Systems and Computing 526, DOI 10.1007/978-3-319-47154-9_5

Due to its high nickel content, wear products of nitinol are particularly hazardous to the human body, which is why more shape-memory alloys with similar functional parameters are continuously being sought. Nickel is one of the most common allergens. 10 % of the population is allergic to this metal [9,10]. It has been demonstrated that nickel ions induce lipid peroxidation and inhibit blood platelet aggregation. This process can be held back by means of ascorbic acid. Nickel may also induce a series of carcinogenic processes, and chronic exposure to excessive nickel doses may also weaken innate immunity [11]. It seems that, in light of the above, the planned tests of friction and fretting wear of alloys of this type will bring cognitive and utilitarian value in the context of the application of these materials in medical constructions, particularly orthodontic appliances.

2   Material and Test Methodology

Fretting tests were performed using a friction tester designed and made at the Department of Materials and Biomedical Engineering of the Bialystok University of Technology, and a detailed description of this tester has been presented in an earlier publication [12].

A

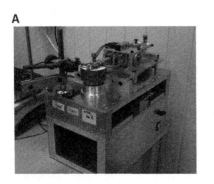

B

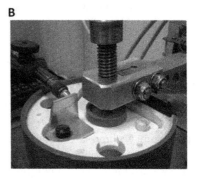

Fig. 1. Research station: A - general view, B - friction pair

Tests were conducted in a pin-on-disc system - Fig. 1. Elements of the kinematic pair were made from NiTi alloy with the following chemical composition: nickel (50.5 % at.), titanium (49.5 % at.). Pins of a cylindrical shape had a 1.1 mm contact surface, and the sample diameter amounted to 4 mm. Sample surfaces were polished mechanically until roughness on the order of $Ra = 0.4\mu m$ was achieved. To remove contaminants, pins and discs were immersed in ethanol and placed in an ultrasound bath for 10 min. After this period of time, samples were thoroughly rinsed with distilled water and dried. Discs were fastened on the tester's moving table, which performed reciprocating movements. The amplitude of displacement was on the order of 100 μm, frequency - 0.8 Hz, and average unit pressures that were set amounted to 5, 15 and 30 MPa. Friction was applied for one hour (2880 cycles) under dry friction conditions and in the environment of human saliva, respectively. Saliva was collected in fasting condition from a 28-year-old healthy man according to a previously developed collection methodology [13]. Each test was repeated 3 times for statistical purposes.

Observations of sample surfaces were conducted using a confocal microscope (CLM, Olympus Lext OLS4000) with 3D imaging capability and a scanning electron microscope (SEM, Hitachi S-3000N). Fretting wear products were observed using a transmission electron microscope (TEM, Tecnai G2 X-TWIN). The application of a confocal microscope made it possible to measure wear and evaluate volumes of lost material and material accumulated over the course of the friction process. Measurements were conducted according to a previously developed research methodology [14]. The chemical composition of the surfaces of friction traces was assessed using an EDS (energy dispersive spectroscopy) module in the scanning microscope.

3   Results and Discussion

Fretting tests were commenced by taking measurements of friction forces in selected friction pairs. This made it possible to determine changes of the coefficient of friction over time at the set unit pressures (Fig. 2).

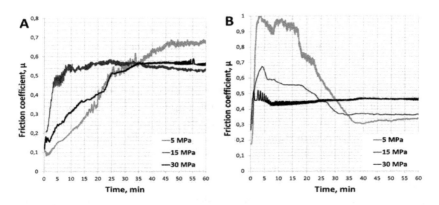

Fig. 2. Changes in coefficient of friction over time: A - under dry friction conditions, B - in the environment of saliva

Nickel-titanium alloys are a characteristic material capable of phase transformations as a result of applied stress (psuedoelasticity) or temperature changes. Data in the literature confirms that the application of strain to the alloy while it is in an austenitic state leads to its martensitic transformation, which is irreversible after the yield point of strain-induced martensite is exceeded [1]. The results presented in Fig. 2 show that, under dry friction conditions, the resistance to motion of kinematic pairs after one hour of friction is the greatest at low unit pressures (5 MPa). However, an inverse phenomenon can be observed in the environment of saliva. When interpreting test results, one should remember that friction is a complex process accompanied by many overlapping mechanisms. Besides phase transformations of nitinol, ingredients of saliva, particularly mucins, may also have an influence on friction. Oxidation processes of nickel and titanium should also be accounted for, as illustrated by the data presented in Fig. 3.

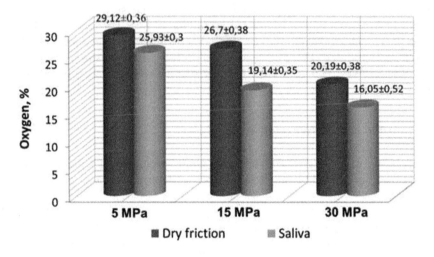

Fig. 3. Oxygen content in wear products

Conducted research indicates that fretting fosters the formation of oxides, and the amount of oxides has a significant impact on friction conditions. In the environment of saliva, where oxygen access was limited, the application of stresses leads to transformation of the soft parent phase (austenite) into the hard martensitic phase, which results in reduction of friction. However, additional structural studies must be carried out to confirm the correctness of this assumption.

Assessment of fretting wear is a complex process, which often takes on a stochastic character. Due to the low amplitude of displacements under fretting conditions, removal of wear products from the friction zone is difficult. Under such conditions, secondary wear may occur, in which formed products act as an abrasive and intensify wear. Due to two-way transport of material between friction surfaces (pin and disc), measurement of material losses is typically insufficient to reflect the actual state of samples. This is why it is indispensable to also account for the volume of accumulations of material permanently affixed to the surface. The results of these measurements have been presented in Fig. 4.

The results of these measurements confirm that susceptibility to adhesive grafts of nitinol increases as load increases. Human saliva is a lubricant that effectively prevents permanent deposition (accumulation) of material on the alloy's

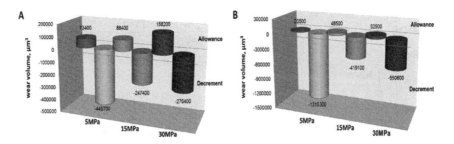

Fig. 4. Fretting wear of disks, accounting for losses and accumulations of material: A - under dry friction conditions, B - in the environment of saliva.

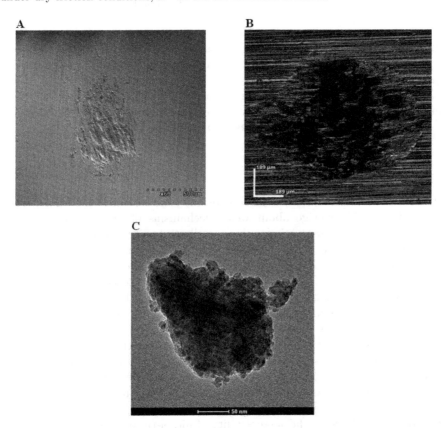

Fig. 5. Photographs of surfaces and products of fretting wear: A - dry friction conditions (SEM), B - in environment of saliva (CLM), C - wear nano-products (TEM)

surface, however, it still intensifies wear in terms of volume (losses), particularly at low unit pressures. This is presumably related to the fact that less energy is supplied to the contact zone, required for the martensitic transformation to occur (longer time of transformation). Figure 5 presents photographs of the

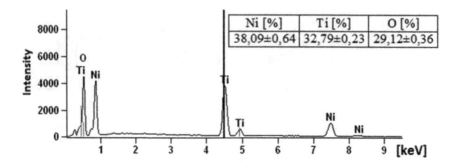

Fig. 6. Chemical composition of wear products on friction surface.

friction surface, with visible wear products. The presence of nanoparticles in the friction zone was confirmed (Fig. 5C) and was also observed in previously conducted tests of this type [15].

Analysis of the chemical composition of wear products (SEM, EDS) confirmed the presence of nickel, titanium and oxygen, which clearly indicates intensive oxidation of the alloy's ingredients during friction - Fig. 6.

4   Conclusions

Obtained test results demonstrated susceptibility to wear of nitinol under fretting conditions. Knowledge about wear mechanisms of biomaterials used in elements of medical constructions may contribute to their effective safeguarding against destruction, and thus extend the lifetime of medical constructions. Fretting processes are characterized by a low amplitude and high frequency of movement between contacting elements, which takes place in many medical constructions, particularly orthodontic appliances. Metal oxides are the most frequently occurring wear products. Their presence in the friction zone may lead to intensification of wear as a result of abrasion (so-called secondary wear), and high unit pressures are the cause of adhesive grafts onto the kinematic pair.

In the case of shape-memory alloys, their phase transformations must also be taken into consideration. As a result of energy supplied in the form of heat or applied stress, the martensitic transformation may occur, which usually leads to a change in the character of wear. Moreover, reports in the literature indicate a problem related to the susceptibility of nickel-titanium alloys to fretting-corrosion processes [8]. Further tests and analysis of these processes may bring measurable benefits, in terms of both knowledge and utility.

Acknowledgments. Studies were conducted within the framework of study no. S/WM/1/2014 and financed with funds for science from the Ministry of Science and Higher Education.

References

1. Morawiec, H., Lekston, Z.: Medical Implants with Shape Memory. Publishing House of the Silesian University of Technology, Gliwice (2016). (in polish)
2. Qian, L.M., Sun, Q.P., Zhou, Z.R.: Fretting wear behavior of superelastic nickel titanium shape memory alloy. Tribol. Lett. **18**(4), 463–475 (2005)
3. Bronzino, J.D., Peterson, D.R. (eds.): Biomedical Engineering Fundamentals, 4th edn. CRC Press, Boca Raton (2015)
4. Yan, L., Liu, Y., Liu, E.: Wear behavior of martensitic NiTi shape memory alloy under ball-on-disk sliding tests. Wear **66**, 219–224 (2013)
5. Ducheyne, P., Healy, K., Hutmacher, D.E., Grainger, D., Kirkpatrick, C.J.: Comprehensive biomaterials. Elsevier, Oxford (2011)
6. Qian, L., Zhou, Z., Sun, Q.: The role of phase transition in the fretting behavior of NiTi shape memory alloy. Wear **259**, 309–318 (2005)
7. Winston Revie, R. (ed.): Uhlig's Corrosion Handbook. Wiley, Pennington (2011)
8. Dong, H., Ju, X.: H. YYang, L. Qian, Z. Zhou, Effect of ceramic conversion tratments on the surface damage and nickel ion release of NiTi alloys under fretting corrosion conditions. Journal of Materials Science: Materials in Medicine **19**, 937–946 (2008)
9. Okazaki, Y., Gotoh, E.: Metal release from stainless steel, Co-Cr-Mo-Ni-Fe and Ni-Ti alloys in vascular implants. Corros. Sci. **50**, 3429–3438 (2008)
10. Yang, H., Qian, L., Zhou, Z., Ju, X., Dong, H.: Effect of surface treatment by ceramic conversion on the fretting behavior of NiTi shape memory alloy. Tribol. Lett. **25**(3), 215–224 (2007)
11. Valko, M., Morris, H., Cronin, M.T.D.: Metals, toxicity and oxidative stress. Curr. Med. Chem. **12**, 1161–1208 (2005)
12. Klekotka, M., Dąbrowski, J.R., Kalska-Szostko, B., Klekotka, U.: Studies of fretting processes in titanium implantation alloys from the Ti-Al.-V group
13. Andrysewicz, E., Dąbrowski, J.R., Leonow, G.: Methodical aspects of rheological study on saliva, Your Stomatologic Industry. Thematic Issue, pp. 10–15 (2008). (in polish)
14. Dąbrowski, J.R., Klekotka, M., Sidun, J.: Fretting and fretting corrosion of 316L implantation steel in the oral cavity environment. Eksploatacja i Niezawodnosc - Maintenance and Reliability **16**(3), 441–446 (2014)
15. Szymanski, K., Olszewski, W., Satula, D., Recko, K., Waliszewski, J., Kalska-Szostko, B., Dąbrowski, J.R., Sidun, J., Kulesza, E.: Characterization of fretting products between austenitic and martensitic stainless steels using Mossbauer and X-ray techniques. Wear **300**, 90–95 (2013)

Carbon Based Coatings with Improved Fracture and Wear Resistance

M. Kot[1(✉)], L. Major[2], J. Lackner[3], and W. Rakowski[1]

[1] AGH University of Science and Technology, 30 Mickiewicza Ave,
30-059 Cracow, Poland
kotmarc@agh.edu.pl
[2] Institute of Metallurgy and Materials Science, Polish Academy of Sciences,
25 Reymonta Street, 30-059 Krakow, Poland
[3] Joanneum Research Forschungsges mbH,
Institute of Surface Technologies and Photonics, Functional Surfaces,
Leobner Strasse 94, 8712 Niklasdorf, Austria

Abstract. The paper presents the results of mechanical and tribological tests of two kinds of carbon coatings with advanced microstructures - nanocomposite CrC/a-C:H and multilayer TiN/Ti/a-C:H. The introduction of barriers for dislocation motion and microcrack propagation as CrC nanograins in nanocomposite coating or Ti and TiN interlayers in multilayer led to coatings hardening and improved fracture and wear resistance in comparison to a single amorphous a-C:H coating. It was confirmed by wide range of mechanical tests. The mechanism of microcrack deflection and splitting on CrC nanograins and Ti layers was studied using spherical indentation tests and TEM observations of indent cross-sections.

Keywords: Carbon coatings · Nanocomposite coatings · Multilayers · Hardness · Fracture · Wear · Tribology

1 Introduction

The demands for tools, machine components and biological implants are continuously increasing. From tribological point of view they high wear resistance, low friction force and substrate protection are required. In this field thin coatings could be a solution, hence they appear in many branches of industry. In the area of bioengineering carbon based coatings deposited by vacuum technologies particular interest is the carbon coating are of great interest. The main reason for this is their excellent tribological properties and biocompatibility. Deposited on contacting elements of joint implants they could extend implant lifetime but in a case of artificial elements of cardiovascular system they prevent the direct contact of substrate with tissues and blood. Unfortunately, the main application problem of carbon coatings is their low fracture resistance, even lower than ceramic ones, which is extremely important when they are deposited on susceptible substrates like titanium alloys and polymers. Low stiffness such a substrates

© Springer International Publishing AG 2017
M. Gzik et al. (eds.), *Innovations in Biomedical Engineering*, Advances in Intelligent
Systems and Computing 526, DOI 10.1007/978-3-319-47154-9_6

results high deformations even at low external loads what leads to the same deformations of coatings and their fracture. Cracks can also appear at repeating tribological contact cause coating fragments chipping. When this debris remains in contact zone can significantly accelerate abrasive wear of the whole tribological system. Sufficient support by substrate allow to demonstrate high wear resistance of carbon coatings and a very low friction coefficient, even below 0.1 in dry sliding condition [1,2]. Among the carbon based coatings the most popular are hydrogenated a-C:H and nonhydrogenated a-C coatings [3,4]. Depends on microstructure they exhibit different mechanical and tribological properties. The main parameter that affect them is the ratio of sp2 (graphite type) to sp3 bonds (diamond type). The softer and crack resistant are coatings with high amount of sp2 bonds, while the sp3 reach coatings exhibit high hardness and wear resistance but are prone to fracture. Appropriate parameters of deposition process allow to obtain coatings with pre-planned sp2/sp3 ratio and required mechanical properties [5]. For biotribological applications carbon coatings should be hard but remain also crack resistant what provide high wear resistance. None of pure carbon coatings fulfill all of this demands. However the enhancement of fracture resistance could be obtained by the introduction of additional barriers to microcrack propagation into the microstructure of amorphous carbon coatings. It could be obtain in two different ideas, hence two kinds of coatings have been developed and presented in the literature - multilayers and nanocomposite coatings. First of them multilayers are composed on repeated many layers of two materials. These materials usually exhibit different properties e.g. one is hard second pliable. The bilayer (sum of the thickness of two following layers) is within few to hundreds nanometers range. Such thin layers results fine-grained microstructure what cause coating hardening. Further enhancement is due to the interfaces between [7] the following layers being the barriers for dislocations and cracks. The mechanism of strengthening and crack deflection in ceramic/metal multilayers was presented in previous papers for Cr/CrN and Ti/TiN [6,7]. Such a phenomena has been also found in a case of TiN/Ti/a-C:H coatings [8] where the appropriate selection of number and thickness of layers resulted 3 times and 2 times higher scratch and wear resistance respectively. The second idea to archive the fracture toughness enhancement of carbon coatings is introduction of nanometer size ceramic grains into the carbon matrix. Such a coatings are signed as nc-MX/a-Mtx, where nc-MX means hard particles of carbides or nitrides of transition metals embedded in an a-Mtx amorphous matrix [9,10]. Voevodin et al. [11] postulate that appropriate diameter of grains is 5–10 nm. While the 1–3 nm thick amorphous carbon layer should entirely surround them. Such a small grain size prevents the formation of dislocations hence the dominating deformation mechanism becomes the grain boundary sliding. Large amount of nanograins are also an effective barrier for crack propagation. Moreover the thin amorphous layers reduces the initial crack size, which demands a higher stress level to start brittle fracture.

The aims of the present work were:

- characterization of basic mechanical properties: nanohardness, Young modulus, adhesion to the substrate and wear resistance of TiN/Ti/a-C:H multilayer and nc-CrC/a-C:H nanocomposite coating deposited by hybrid magnetron sputtering on AISI 304 austenitic steel substrate,
- analysis of the effect of complex coating architecture on the rise of fracture and wear resistance.

2 Tested Coatings

The mechanical and tribological properties of coatings with advanced microstructures: nanocomposite CrC/a-C:H and multilayer TiN/Ti/a-C:H, were compared to properties of the reference hydrogenated a-C:H coating. Coatings were deposited in an industrially scaled sputtering machine (Leybold, Cologne, Germany) equipped with 4 rectangular $3'' \times 17''$ unbalanced magnetrons with -50 V bias. All coatings were deposited on AISI 304 austenitic steel substrates. Substrates were continuously rotated (4 rpm) in one axis on the sample cage. Prior to the deposition, the substrates were mirror-polished and ultrasonically cleaned in acetone and ethanol and then plasma cleaned and plasma activated in Ar and Ar+O2 plasma by applying a linear anode layer ion source (ALS), Veeco ALS 340. A reactive C2H2+Ar gas mixture at a total flow of 50 sccm, resulting in a pressure of 3×10^{-3} mbar was applied for deposition of a-C:H coating. During the deposition of CrC/a-C:H nanocomposite coating the pure Cr target (Seibersdorf, Austria) was used. The optimal 10 sccm C2H2 gas flow was applied based on results of coatings group presented in previous paper [10]. The second coating with advanced microstructure - multilayer contains combination of a-C:H, TiN and Ti layers with about 40, 30 and 7 nm thickness respectively. TiN layers were deposited in N2+Ar gas mixture, while Ti layers in a pure Ar atmosphere. The Ti source was titanium Grade 2 (Eurotitan) target. The effect of layers thickness in TiN/Ti/a-C:H coatings was presented in [8]. The total thickness of all coatings single, nanocomposite and nanocomposite, controlled by the deposition time after earlier calculation of deposition rates, was 1 μm. To improve the strength of coating-substrate interface ≈ 100 nm thick Cr or Ti adhesive layers was applied.

3 Experimental Part

The transmission electron microscopy (TEM), Philips CM20 (200 kV) and JEOL EX4000 (400 kV) microscopes were used to study coatings microstructure. Observations were conducted on thin foils prepared by a focus ion beam (FIB) technique. Basic mechanical properties like nanohardness and elasticity modulus were determined using CSM nanoindenter with a Berkovich geometry diamond at 2 mN maximum load [12]. Instrumented spherical indentation with a 20 μm diamond tip radius was also used to studied fracture resistance [13].

The first pop-ins on indentation curves was assumed as critical load leading to the formation of circular cracks. The mechanisms of deformation and the effects of Ti layers and CrC nanograins were studied by TEM analysis of thin foils performed at indent symmetry axis on coatings cross-sections. Furthermore the coatings adhesion to steel substrates was studied by scratch testing [14] with a standard conical Rockwell C indenter - $200 \neq m$ tip radius. The same scratch parameters, such as 5 mm length, 5 mm/min scratch speed and 0–30 N load range were adopted for all coatings. Tribological tests of the coating-substrate systems using a ball-on-disc tribometer [15], 6 mm diameter Al2O3 balls, 0.05 m/s sliding speed, 20000 cycles and Fn = 5 N load, allowed to determine wear resistance and coefficient of friction. The wear index was calculated from the profiles of wear scar, as:

$$\frac{V}{F_n s}$$

where: V - volume of removed material, s -length of the wear track.

4   Results and Discussion

Microscopic examination exhibited the amorphous microstructure of the single a-C:H carbon coating. Such a microstructure also exhibited carbon layers in the multilayer coating and the matrix of the nanocomposite coating. Figure 1 presents the TEM images of all coatings. In a case of TiN/Ti/a-C:H multilayer well defined interfaces between the following carbon and ceramic layers in were found. The ceramic TiN and metal Ti posse, typical for coatings deposited at low temperatures by PVD techniques, columnar microstructure. The pre-defined 7 nm thick Ti layers between the TiN and a-C:H ones, that should stop or even split nanocracks, are clearly seen. Detailed analysis such a multilayers were presented previously in [16]. Whereas HRTEM analysis of CrC/a-C:H nanocomposite coating exhibited the existence of 5–10 nm size Cr_2C nanoparticles what was confirmed by EDS quantitative analysis of these nanograins. The 65 % Cr atom amount was determined. The beneficial for good mechanical properties is the low thickness 1–3 nm of the carbon layers that separates the neighboring ceramic grains [11].

Nanoindentation results showed the positive effect of advanced microstructure on hardness and elasticity modulus. The nanohardness of CrC/a-C:H - 18 GPa and TiN/Ti/a-C:H - 17 GPa is over 2-times higher than for a single a-C:H coating - 7 GPa (Fig. 2a). The same tendency was found in the case of the elasticity modulus (Fig. 2b). Such a higher values of Young's modulus are extremely advantageous for coatings deposited on steel substrates with E = 210 GPa. Low mismatch of coating and substrate elasticity results the lower stress concentration in the coating-substrate interface and promote good coating to substrate adhesion.

This behavior was confirmed by scratch testing. Critical load led to a-C:H coating delamination and substrate exposure was only 5N (Fig. 3a), what excludes the application possibility in many biotribological systems. The low adhesion of carbon coatings is explained mainly by high state of residual stress

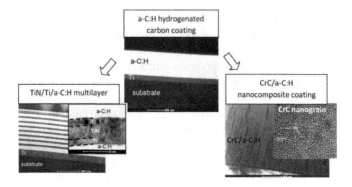

Fig. 1. Microstructure of a-C:H, TiN/a-C:H and CrC/a-C:H coatings - TEM and HRTEM images.

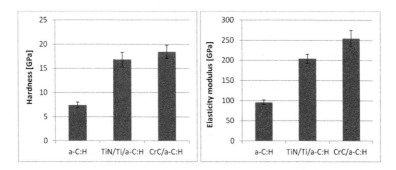

Fig. 2. Results of indentation curves: (a) nanohardness, (b) elasticity modulus

after the deposition process that may reach several gigapascals [17]. Meanwhile first adhesive failures as first minor chipping with the removal of small multilayer fragments from the scratch track was observed at 16 N load (Fig. 3b). Whereas up to maximum normal load 30 N adhesive cracks were not induced by an indenter on the surface of nanocomposite coating (Fig. 3c). A large improvement of adhesion to the substrate of both multilayer and nanocomposite coatings may result primarily from lower residual stress after the deposition process. Reduction of residual stress in CrC/a-C:H and TiC/DLC compared to pure carbon coating is presented in [17,18]. The rise in scratch resistance is also reported in the literature in the case of multilayers [7,19]. Coatings deposited on susceptible substrate should also exhibit high fracture toughness. Figure 4 presents the spherical indentation load-penetration curves. It is clearly seen that the higher stiffness results the lower penetration depth which was reduced from 2100 nm measured for a-C:H to 1200 nm for CrC/a-C:H coating. First pop-ins on indentation curves, corresponded to the crack formation in the coatings, were found at 160 and 260 mN for TiN/Ti/a-C:H and CrC/a-C:H coatings respectively, while for a-C:H coating first crack appeared at 110 mN.

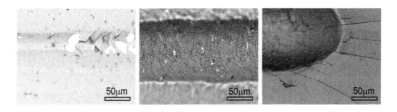

Fig. 3. Scratch tracks images: (a) - 5 N, (b) TiN/a-C:H - 16 N, (c) CrC/a-C:H - 30 N.

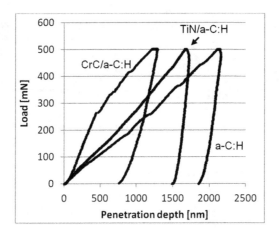

Fig. 4. Spherical indentation curves

From the symmetry axis of indents thin foils were performed for TEM analysis of crack propagation mechanism trough coatings thickness (Fig. 5). Crack in a-C:H coating nucleated at the coating surface and propagated firstly perpendicular to the surface as a result of tensile stress at the side of indent. At the middle of the coating thickness, crack was deflected due to the maximum shear stress in this area. Such a changes of crack direction it is caused A detailed analysis of contact mechanics and stress distribution in coating-substrate systems during spherical indentation was given in [13]. The crack on coating-substrate interface confirmed poor coating adhesion to the substrate found by scratch testing. Crack in multilayer was not propagated so easily despite the low fracture toughness of the ceramic TiN and carbon a-C:H layers.

The higher fracture resistance of TiN/Ti/a-C:H is a result of incorporation of thin Ti layers, which reduce the rigidity and facilitate the deformation of the coating, allows "sliding" of hard ceramic and carbon layers. Microcracks propagated trough TiN and a-C:H were deflected or closed by plastic deformation of Ti layers. Hence cracks have low energy and they cannot be noticed on indentation curve which is smooth with no popins. Such a crack closing was also observed in a ceramic/metal type multilayer and shown in the previous papers [7,20]. In a case of CrC/a-C:H coating crack surfaces exhibited irregular, a step-like

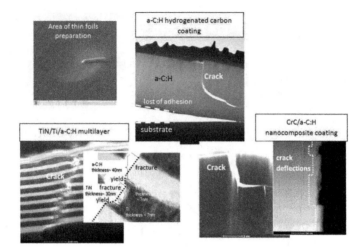

Fig. 5. TEM images of coatings cross-sections after spherical indentation

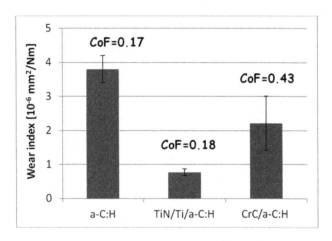

Fig. 6. Result of indentation tests - wear index and coefficient of friction (CoF)

character. Crack probably was splitting at hard nanograins and at the end was divided into two smaller cracks. This resulted a greater applied load to induce the crack propagation compared to a-C:H coating. Coatings with complex architecture showed significant enhancement of tribological properties what was also confirmed by ball-on-disc testing. The nanocomposite coating exhibited 40 % lower Wv wear index than the carbon coating, while for the multilayer coating wear resistance it is up to 5 times higher. In many applications the friction forces reduction is also crucial. For carbon coatings low coefficient of friction (CoF) is a result of graphitization of the wear debris and creation of a third body with very low shear strength in a friction zone [21]. In this studies CoF of a-C:H coating was 0.17, while for multilayer was only slightly higher CoF = 0.18, despite the large amount of ceramic TiN and metallic Ti phases for which tests performed at single coating showed CoF = 0.2 and 0.5, respectively. However, much higher CoF = 0.43 was measured for CrC/a-C:H nanocomposite coating. This could be a result of the presence of small hard nanograins in debris that can remove the lubricating graphite layer. The similar phenomena for CrCx/a-C:H coatings was found by Gassner et al. [22] (Fig. 6).

5   Conclusions

Introduction of barriers for easy crack propagation into carbon coatings can significantly improve their mechanical and tribological properties. This may allow to utilize carbon coating deposited by PVD techniques in areas where high fracture toughness and wear resistance are necessary. Two groups of coatings can fulfill such demands - multilayers and nanocomposite coatings. The conducted research program of mechanical and tribological testing of carbon based coatings with advanced microstructures permits the following conclusions:

- Hardness of the TiN/a-C:H multilayer and CrC/a-C:H nanocomposite coatings is over two times higher than hardness of the pure a-C:H carbon coating. The same trend was found for elasticity modulus.
- TiN/a-C:H and CrC/a-C:H coatings exhibited much better adhesion to steel substrates than a-C:H coating.
- Results of spherical indentation revealed improved fracture resistance of coatings with advanced microstructure. Compared to a-C:H coating, the critical load that led to coatings fracture was 50 and 100
- TEM studies of indents after spherical indentations showed that Ti layers in multilayer and CrC nanograins in nanocomposite coating cause crack deflection what disrupts their easy propagation.
- Wear index for the CrC/a-C:H coating is 40 % lower than for the a-C:H coating while the TiN/a-C:H multilayer exhibited 5 times higher wear resistance than single coatings.

References

1. Gahlin, R., Larsson, M., Hedenqvist, P.: ME-C: H coatings in motor vehicles. Wear **249**, 302–309 (2001)
2. Erdemir, A.: Genesis of superlow friction and wear in diamond like carbon films. Tribol. Int. **37**, 1005–1012 (2004)
3. Hauert, R.: An overview on the tribological behavior of diamond-like carbon in technical and medical applications. Tribol. Int. **37**, 991–1003 (2004)
4. Lu, X., Li, M., Tang, X., Lee, J.: Micromechanical properties of hydrogenated diamond-like carbon multilayers. Surf. Coat. Technol. **201**, 1679–1684 (2006)
5. Zhang, W., Tanaka, A., Xu, B.S., Koga, Y.: Study on the diamond-like carbon multilayer films for tribological application. Diam. Relat. Mater. **14**, 1361–1367 (2005)

6. Kot, M., Rakowski, W., Major, B., Major, L., Morgiel, J.: Effect of bilayer period on properties of Cr/CrN multilayer coatings produced by laser ablation. Surf. Coat. Technol. **202**, 3501–3506 (2008)

7. Was, G.S., Foecke, T.: Deformation and fracture in microlaminates. Thin Solid Films **286**, 1–31 (1996)

8. Kot, M., Major, L., Lackner, J.: The tribological phenomena of a new type of TiN/a-C: H multilayer coatings. Mater. Des. **51**, 280–286 (2013)

9. Czyzniewski, A.: Deposition and some properties of nanocrystalline WC and nanocomposite WC/a-C: H coatings. Thin Solid Films **433**, 180–185 (2003)

10. Kot, M., Major, L., Chronowska-Przywara, K., Lackner, J.M., Waldhauser, W., Rakowski, W.: The advantages of incorporating CrxC nanograins into an a-C: H matrix in tribological coatings. Mater. Des. **56**, 981–989 (2014)

11. Voevodin, A.A., Zabinski, J.S., Muratore, C.: Recent advances in hard, tough, and low friction nanocomposite coatings. Tsinghua Sci. Technol. **10**, 665–679 (2005)

12. ISO 14577–1. Metallic materials - instrumented indentation test for hardness, material parameters - Part 1: Test method

13. Kot, M., Major, L., Lackner, J., Rakowski, W.: Analysis of spherical indentations of coating-substrate systems: experiments and finite element modeling. Mater. Des. **43**, 99–111 (2013)

14. EN 1071–3. Advanced technical ceramics - methods of test for ceramic coatings - Part 3: determination of adhesion and other mechanical failure modes by a scratch test

15. ISO 20808: 2004. Fine ceramics (advanced ceramics, advanced technical ceramics) - determination of friction and wear characteristics of monolithic ceramics by ball-on-disc method

16. Major, L., Lackner, J.M., Kot, M., Janusz, M., Major, B.: Contribution of TiN/Ti/a-C: H multilayers architecture to biological and mechanical properties. Bull. Pol. Acad. Sci. Tech. Sci. **62**, 565–570 (2014)

17. Wang, P., Wang, X., Xu, T., Liu, W., Zhang, J.: Comparing internal stress in diamond like carbon films with different structure. Thin Solid Films **515**, 6899–6903 (2007)

18. Singh, V., Jiang, J.C., Meletis, E.I.: Cr-diamondlike carbon nanocomposite films: synthesis, characterization and properties. Thin Solid Films **489**, 150–158 (2005)

19. Bull, S.J., Jones, A.M.: Multilayer coatings for improved performance. Surf. Coat. Technol. **78**, 173–184 (1996)

20. Kot, M., Rakowski, W., Major, L., Lackner, J.: Load-bearing capacity of coating - substrate systems obtained from spherical indentation tests. Mater. Des. **46**, 751–757 (2013)

21. Liu, Y., Erdemir, A., Meletis, E.I.: An investigation of the relationship between graphitization and frictional behavior of DLC coatings. Surf. Coat. Technol. **86–87**, 564–568 (1996)

22. Gassner, G., Patscheider, J., Mayrhofer, P.H., Sturm, S., Scheu, C., Mitterer, C.: Tribological properties of nanocomposite CrCx/a-C: H thin films. Tribollogy Lett. **27**, 97–104 (2007)

Preparation and Characterization of a Novel Activated Laurocherry/Calcium Alginate Biomorphous Monolithic Composite and its Application in Methylene Blue Adsorption

Justyna Majewska$^{(\boxtimes)}$, Marta Krzesińska, and Bartłomiej J. Sawaryn

Department of Biosensors and Biomedical Signals Processing,
Faculty of Biomedical Engineering, Silesian University of Technology,
Roosevelta Street 40, 41800 Zabrze, Poland
justyna.majewska@polsl.pl

Abstract. The aim of the study was to develop the technology of obtaining biodegradable monolithic biomorphous activated carbon/calcium alginate (LWA/AW) adsorbent. The composite was prepared by chemical activation of cuboid samples which were cut from a laurocherry stem and further impregnation with calcium alginate. The polymer impregnation effect on the selected composite properties was investigated. The surface area and porous structure of the composite were characterized using low temperature nitrogen adsorption and helium pycnometry. The functional groups analysis was performed using infrared spectroscopy (FTIR). The iodine number and the adsorption capacity in the methylene blue (MB) removal from aqueous solution were also determined. The adsorbent was characterized by a high porosity on the level of 60 %, and developed specific surface area (S_{BET}=785 m^2/g). Preliminary studies showed that the resulting material is effective in dye removal from water. The efficiency of the methylene blue adsorption was found to be 95.7 %.

Keywords: Biomorphous composite · Adsorbent · Calcium alginate · Chemical activation · Surface area · Methylene blue

1 Introduction

Intensive industry development generates hazardous wastes that causes environmental pollution increases. One of such dangerous substances are dyes present in industrial waste water. These compounds, even in small amounts, may reduce the light penetration into the water and thus inhibit photosynthesis. Dyes, because of the complex structures, and the possibility of many substitution are hardly biodegradable. Furthermore, some of their metabolites are toxic, mutagenic and carcinogenic for living organisms, and therefore should be removed from the

© Springer International Publishing AG 2017
M. Gzik et al. (eds.), *Innovations in Biomedical Engineering*, Advances in Intelligent Systems and Computing 526, DOI 10.1007/978-3-319-47154-9_7

wastewater. Among several methods used for dye removal from aqueous solutions, adsorption has been most widely applied [1]. Adsorbents, because of high specific surface area and surface reactivity, remove impurities from water very well. Unfortunately, their production costs often are very high, therefore it is important to search for new, more effective, low cost adsorbents.

A noteworthy may prove to be a monolithic activated carbons derived from plants being agricultural waste. Plants are characterized by a hierarchical ordered, unidirectional open pores structure, that is retained after the carbonization process [2,3]. Such a structure has many advantages e.g. does not cause significant pressure drop during the passage through it different kinds of substances. Furthermore, such materials have much greater resistance to wear and can be easily placed in the mobile systems in vertical or horizontal positions without losing their shape [4]. Therefore, the monolithic carbon materials can be widely used in the enzymes immobilization, a high throughput bioreactor, a separation column with high flow rates, as catalyst supports, [5] and as adsorbents [6,7].

The properties of the monolithic carbon materials can be easily modified using chemical and physical activation or impregnation with various types of substances e.g. polymers [8,9]. This modification does not affect significantly open pores structure, but it can lead to improve their functional characteristics, e.g. increasing the adsorption capacity.

The objective of this study was to obtain novel monolithic, biomorphous adsorbent by chemical activation of shapes cut from laurocherry stem and further impregnation with biopolymer of high sorption capacity – calcium alginate, to achieve a monolithic composite adsorbent that was used for methylene blue adsorption from aqueous solution. The literature reports of composite materials based on calcium alginate and activated carbon [10,11]. However, so far, powdered activated carbon was immobilized in calcium alginate capsules. In the following work the monolithic, biomorphous activated carbon forms the composite matrix and the calcium alginate is the substance impregnating its surface.

It is worth noting that the activated carbons and activated carbon/biopolymer composites can be also successfully used in medicine e.g. for the organism purification [12].

2   Materials and Methods

2.1   Preparation of Carbon Adsorbent (LWA)

For the preparation of carbon adsorbents rectangular shapes cut from laurocherry stem were impregnated with 42 % phosphoric(V) acid and carbonized at 400 °C. The heating rate was 5 °C/min, and the holding time at the final temperature was 1.5 h. Derived samples were washed using distilled water and dried at 80 °C to constant weigh.

2.2   Preparation of Composite Adsorbent (LWA/AW)

The derived activated carbon materials were vacuum impregnated with 1 % sodium alginate solution and immersed in 3 % calcium chloride solution for 3 h. The resulting composites were dried at 70 °C till constant weight was reached.

2.3   Characterization of Adsorbents

2.3.1   The Open Porosity Determination
In order to determine the open porosity of the samples, apparent and true densities were used. The true density – the density of the material which is the average mass per unit volume, exclusive of all voids that are not fundamental part of the molecular packing arrangement – was measured using a helium gas displacement pycnometer. The apparent density was determined from the volume of a regular sample and its weight.

The open porosity (P%) was calculated using an expression:

$$P(\%) = \frac{\rho_{true} - \rho_{app}}{\rho_{true}} \cdot 100 \qquad (1)$$

where:

ρ_{true} – true density, g/cm^3,
ρ_{app} – apparent density, g/cm^3.

2.3.2   The Specific Surface Area
Low temperature adsorption isotherms of the matrix and the composites were determined using Autosorb IQ, Quantachrome. Before studies the samples were degassed under vacuum at 105 °C for 5 h. Adsorption isotherms were recorded using gas nitrogen adsorption for relative pressures ranging from 0.05 to about 0.99, at the liquid nitrogen temperature. The surface area was determined using Brunauerr, Emmett, Teller method (S_{BET}).

2.3.3   The Surface Chemistry Studies
In order to determine the functional groups expected in the developed materials, the samples were examined using FTIR spectroscopy (FTIR spectrometer Bruker Hyperion 2000). Powdered samples were mixed with potassium bromide in weight ratio of 1:20, placed in a measuring flask and put on the path of the beam of infrared light.

2.3.4   The Adsorption Activity Studies
The adsorption activity towards iodine was measured using monolithic samples. 4 mL of 5 % hydrochloric acid and 20 mL of 0.2 mL/L iodine solution were added to the sample and shaken vigorously for 4 min. After removing the monolithic sample, iodine solution was titrated with sodium thiosulfate (0.1 mol/L) in presence of starch.

The iodine number (IN) was calculated according to the following equation:

$$IN = \frac{(V_1 - V_2) \cdot C_1 \cdot 126.9}{m}$$ (2)

where:

V_1 – volume of $Na_2S_2O_3$ solution spent on titration of the iodine solution without sample, mL,

V_2 – volume of $Na_2S_2O_3$ solution spent on titration of the iodine solution with the sample, mL,

C_1 – $Na_2S_2O_3$ concentration, mol/L,

m – sample weight, g.

The monolithic samples were put into flask, next solution of methylene blue (MB) in water in proportion of 50 mL/120 mg/L was added and left for 70 h. In order to determine the equilibrium dye concentration in the solution after the adsorption a UV–VIS spectrophotometer Jasco manual V530 was used (wavelength equal 664 nm). The final concentration was calculate using following equation:

$$q_e = \frac{(C_0 - C_e) \cdot V}{m}$$ (3)

The percentage MB removal (R%) by the adsorbent was described by the following:

$$R(\%) = \frac{(C_0 - C_e)}{C_0} \cdot 100$$ (4)

where:

q_e – concentration at equilibrium, mg/g

C_0 – dye initial concentration, mg/L

C_e – the equilibrium concentration, mg/L

V – the dye solution volume used for the adsorption, L

m – sample weight, g.

3 Results and Discussion

3.1 Characterization of the Porous Structure

The open porosity, which is the percentage of empty space in the porous sample, was calculated using the values of apparent and true densities. The values of the true density of composite adsorbent as well as of activated carbon being the composite matrix are shown in Fig. 1(a). It is visible that calcium alginate thin film impregnation slightly decreases the activated carbon density (from 1.68 to 1.60 g/cm^3). Probably it is due to lower value of polymer density. Figure 1(b) depicts the influence of the polymer component on the adsorbent open porosity. It can be seen that polymer impregnation slightly reduce the porosity of the composite. Both the activated carbon and the composite adsorbent are characterized by high open porosity of order 60–64 %. Determined on the basis of true and apparent densities porosity (P) is the sum of the volume of all pores in the

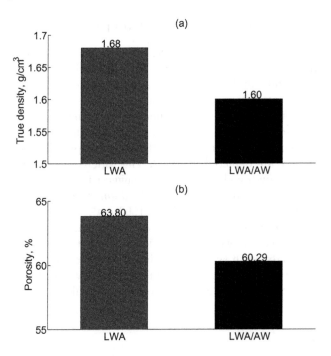

Fig. 1. The true density (a) and the open porosity (b) of the activated carbon (LWA) and the activated carbon/calcium alginate composite (LWA/AW)

material, but does not give information about the surface area of the samples. For a more detailed analysis of the received materials low temperature nitrogen adsorption was used. On the nitrogen adsorption isotherms basis the surface areas (S_{BET}) were determined. Table 1 shows a comparison of the S_{BET} surface area of the materials received. Both the matrix and the composite are characterized by developed surface area. The results show that matrix has slightly larger surface area than the composite. Probably during calcium alginate impregnation small part of open pores has been sealed, which is confirmed by open porosity determination results.

Table 1. Specific surface area (S_{BET}) values determined for the adsorbents studied. Notation: LWA – the activated carbon, LWA/AW – the activated carbon/calcium alginate composite

Surface area (S_{BET}), m^2/g	
LWA	901.7
LWA/AW	784.8

3.2 Determination of the Functional Groups

The material's surface chemical character, which is determined by kind of surface functional groups, is extremely important due to its applications. It may be modified by various kinds of substances (e.g. functionalization) or by thermal treatment (e.g. activation, carbonization). The most important are oxygen groups, which determine adsorption properties of the materials. The chemical nature of the surface of the activated carbon and its changes due to the presence of calcium alginate was tested by FTIR spectroscopy. The FTIR spectra of LWA and LWA/AW are depicted in Fig. 2. The wide band at 3600–3280 cm^{-1} corresponds to O–H (hydroxyl) groups which suggest the existence of a phenolic group. The absorption bands at 2890 and 2830 cm^{-1} showing the presence of alkyl groups. The band observed at about 1600 cm^{-1} could be caused by the vibration of C=O groups present in single or multiple aromatic rings contained in the carbon materials as well as vibration of C–O–O groups from alginate molecule. Interestingly, both spectra are almost identical. This is probably due to the fact that activated carbon and calcium alginate have the functional groups having an absorption band at the same wave number values.

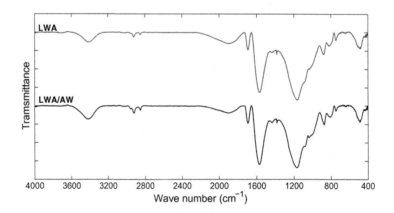

Fig. 2. The FTIR spectra of the LWA and the LWA/AW composite

3.3 Adsorption Properties

A key step in the study was determination of the influence of the calcium alginate presence on the adsorbent sorption capacity. For this purpose an iodine number (IN), i.e. a designated amount of iodine adsorbed by 1 g of the adsorbent, of the activated carbon and the composite was measured. The results are shown in Fig. 3. As it can be seen from this figure, the presence of calcium alginate in the composite significantly increases the iodine adsorption capacity from 53.4 to 125.6 mg/g. This value, in comparison with commercial adsorbents, is not high, so it can be concluded, that these materials have no competitive properties in

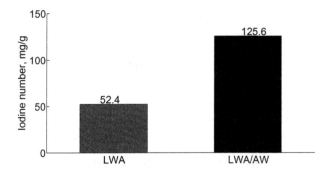

Fig. 3. Iodine number values determined for the adsorbents studied

Table 2. The adsorption capacity of methylene blue (MB) adsorbed on the activated carbon (LWA) and the composite (LWA/AW)

Sample	Adsorption capacity (mg/g)	MB removal (R%)
LWA	4.3	90.1
LWA/AW	5.1	95.7

removal of substances having a particle size of less than 1 nm (the diameter of the iodine molecule is equal to 0.9 nm). The adsorption properties of received materials (LWA and LWA/AW) were examined in the process of removing from water the substance of larger particles diameter (1.8 nm) – methylene blue dye. Data in Table 2 show that both materials are characterized by high (over 90 %) degree of the MB removal from water. It can be also noted that the coating of activated carbon surface with thin layer of polymer having a good adsorption properties – calcium alginate, increases the dye adsorption capacity of the composite.

4   Conclusions

Both monolithic biomorphous adsorbents performed using agricultural waste, i.e. laurocherry were found to be biodegradable and renewable materials characterized by high porosity of order of 60–64 % and developed surface area ($S_{BET} \sim$ 785–902 m^2/g). Preliminary studies showed that these monolithic materials are effective in the dye removal from an aqueous solution. Furthermore, surface coating of a monolithic activated carbon with calcium alginate, despite of a reduction in porosity and specific surface area, increased the efficiency of the dye adsorption properties of the materials from 90.1 to 95.7 %.

Acknowledgement. This study was financed by the Ministry of Education and Science (MES) (Poland), under Grant No. BKM/534/RIB4/2014.

References

1. Rangabhashiyam, S., Anu, N., Selvaraju, N.: Review: Sequestration of dye from textile industry wastewater using agricultural waste products as adsorbents. J. Environ. Chem. Eng. **1**, 629–641 (2013)
2. Byrne, C.E., Nagle, D.C.: Carbonization of wood for advanced materials applications. Carbon **35**, 259–266 (1997)
3. Krzesińska, M., Majewska, J.: Biomorphous carbon and carbon-polymer materials. Scientific Publishers Silesia, Katowice, Poland (2011). (in Polish), (ISBN 978-83-7164-678-2)
4. Valdes-Solis, T., Linders, M.J.G., Kapteijn, F., Maraban, G., Fuertes, A.B.: Adsorption and breakthrough performance of carbon-coated ceramic monoliths at low concentration of n-butane. Chem. Eng. Sci. **59**, 2791–2800 (2004)
5. Siyasukh, A., Maneeproma, P., Larpkiattawornd, S., Tonanona, N., Tanthapanichakoonb, W., Tamonc, H., Charinpanitkula, T.: Preparation of a carbon monolith with hierarchical porous structure by ultrasonic irradiation followed by carbonization, physical and chemical activation. Carbon **46**, 1309–1315 (2008)
6. Mohan, D., Pittman, C.U.: Arsenic removal from water/wastewater using adsorbents-A critical review. J. Hazard. Mater. **142**, 1–53 (2007)
7. Garcia-Bordeje, E., Lazaro, M.J., Moliner, R., Alvarez, P.M., Gomez-Serrano, V., Fierro, J.L.G.: Vanadium supported on carbon coated honeycomb monoliths for the selective catalytic reduction of NO at low temperatures: Influence of the oxidation pre-treatment. Carbon **44**, 407–417 (2006)
8. Budinova, T., Krzesińska, M., Tsyntsarski, B., Zachariasz, J., Petrova, B.: Activated carbon produced from bamboo pellets for removal of arsenic(III) ions from water. Bul. Chem. Comm. **40**, 166–172 (2008)
9. Krzesińska, M., Majewska, J.: The development and characterization of a novel chitosan/carbonised yucca(Yucca flaccida) bio-composite. Mater. Sci. Eng. C **30**, 273–276 (2010)
10. Hassan, A.F., Abdel-Mohsen, A.M., Elhadidy, H.: Adsorption of arsenic by activated carbon, calcium alginate and their composite beads. Int. J. Biol. Macromolec. **68**, 125–130 (2014)
11. Hassan, A.F., Abdel-Mohsen, A.M., Founda, M.M.G.: Comparative study of calcium alginate, activated carbon, and their composite beads on methylene blue adsorption. Carbohydr. Polym. **102**, 192–198 (2014)
12. Howell, C.A., Sandeman, S.R., Zheng, Y., Mikhalovsky, S.V., Nikolaev, V.G., Sakhno, L.A., Snezhkova, E.A.: New dextran coated activated carbons for medical use. Carbon **97**, 134–146 (2016)

Periimplantitis as the Cause of Separation the Prosthetic Bridge Based on Implant

Alicja Mondrzejewska[1], Anna Ziębowicz[2($\boxtimes$)], Bohdan Bączkowski[3($\boxtimes$)], and Marta Rybarska

[1] Institute of Medical Technology and Equipment ITAM,
Roosevelta 118, 41–800 Zabrze, Poland
[2] Faculty of Biomedical Engineering,
Department of Biomaterials and Medical Devices Engineering,
Silesian University of Technology, Roosevelta 40, 41–800 Zabrze, Poland
anna.ziebowicz@polsl.pl
[3] Department of Prosthetic Dentistry, Medical University of Warsaw,
Nowogrodzka 59, 02–006 Warsaw, Poland

Abstract. The paper discusses the basic problems of the possible complications after implant-prosthetic treatment, with particular emphasis on periimplantitis. Presented are the results of materials science expertise for prosthetic bridge based on the implant, lost by sixty year old female patient as a result of perigraft tissue inflammation. The results allowed to assess whether the separation of the prosthetic system – in addition to biological factors – was influenced by mechanical factors, such as damage to restoration structures.

Keywords: Computational geometry · Graph theory · Hamilton cycles

1 Introduction

The development of implant prosthetics over the past few decades has made that, starting from the experimental field of dentistry, it has become almost routine solution for the reconstruction of partial or complete lack of teeth. Evolution comprised here both the procedures applied, instrumentation, and implants themselves in – terms of design and material solutions. While the said method of treatment has gained great popularity, there are still some failures (around 10 %), leading to loss of stability of the implant-bone system, and in effect the implant separation. Scheme of the course of implant-prosthetic therapy is shown below – Fig. 1 [3,6].

Complications arising after the implant surgery are twofold: mechanical and biological (Fig. 2). The main causes of complications of a mechanical nature can include improper implant construction, structural defects of materials of which individual components are made, as well as unfavourable loading of the implant with occlusion forces. As regards the biological causes complications: they have their origin in a variety of factors, some of which being only cited

M. Gzik et al. (eds.), *Innovations in Biomedical Engineering*, Advances in Intelligent Systems and Computing 526, DOI 10.1007/978-3-319-47154-9_8

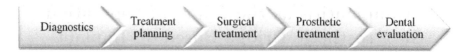

Fig. 1. Diagram of the course of the implant-prosthetic treatment [5]

below because of their plurality. Among others these include: systemic diseases (osteoporosis, diabetes), abnormal occlusion, inadequate design of the implant, poor oral hygiene, impaired wound healing after surgery, stimulants [1].

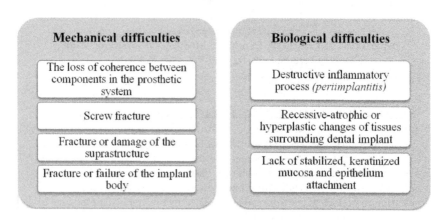

Fig. 2. Categorizing of difficulties occurring after implant-prosthetic treatment [4]

One of the most common causes of stability loss, and then separating the implant is an inflammation of the perigraft tissues (periimplantitis). The direct consequences of this phenomenon is the soft tissues atrophy of the gingiva and resorption of bone tissue. Periimplantitis reasons lie in imbalance of the equilibrium between the resident flora surrounding the implant and the immune system of the body, often intensified by the presence of occlusal disorders, systemic diseases, genetic and/or social conditions, such as poor oral hygiene, tobacco smoking, and even stress [1,2].

2   Materials and Methods

Materials science expertise has been applied to elements of the three-point prosthetic bridge fixed in the mouth of sixty years old female patient for a period of six years, lost in the course of periimplantitis. The bridge was anchored to the conical, self-drilling implant Alpha Bio SPI of nominal diameter 3.75 mm and a length of 10 mm, made of the alloy Ti6Al4V. The implant system consisted of an angle joint, screw and implant. Abutment of prosthetic crown was made of Ni–Cr–Mo alloy, whereas as a veneering layer was feldspathic ceramics GC Initial

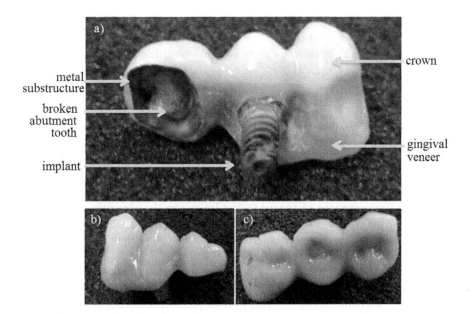

Fig. 3. Dental bridge after removal from the oral cavity of the female patient: (a) bottom view; (b) buccal view; (c) occlusal view

MC, determined by the manufacturer as being compatible with metal alloys having a coefficient of thermal linear expansion in the range of $13.8 \div 14.9\,\mu\text{m/m·K}$. Part imitating gum (Fig. 3) is made of acrylic. Based on an interview conducted by a dentist, it was determined that due to smoking tobacco patient is at risk group of biological complications.

In order to prepare the prosthetic restoration to carry out testing separated were the system components by using precision cutting device Struers Secotom–15. In the following steps performed were:

- microscopic observations using a stereoscopic microscope (Zeiss Discovery V8), scanning electron microscope, a light microscope (Zeiss Observer),
- electrochemical impedance spectroscopy,
- study of resistance to pitting and galvanic corrosion.

Electrochemical impedance spectroscopy was performed by the measuring system AutoLab PGSTAT 302N in the frequency range $10^{-3} \div 10^{4}\,\text{Hz}$. Measuring system was equipped with a module FRA2. The experiment was performed in Ringer's solution, which was to simulate the environment of perigraft tissues. Obtained results provided information on the electrochemical properties of the implant and enabled the assessment of the phenomena taking place on its surface.

The examinations of corrosion resistance have been carried out using a potentiostat PGP–201 of Radiometer Analytical SAS company. The evaluation of pitting corrosion resistance was carried out – as in the case of the EIS – for the titanium implant in an Ringer's solution. For the abutment and metal substructure, the evaluation of resistance to galvanic corrosion (Evans method) was performed, and as a study environment the solution of artificial saliva was selected.

3   Results

Based on preliminary observations using a stereoscopic microscope, it was found that the prosthetic system revealed signs of wear in the form of small cracks, and abrasions of the surface of ceramic crown. As a result of damages the exposure of the substructure material has occurred (Fig. 4a). There was also damage to the thread observed (Fig. 4c), probably caused by the destabilization of the implant and its movement in regard to the bone. On the abutment surface, the areas covered by corrosive changes were observed (Fig. 4d). It was also found that within the substructure of the crown based on the patient's own tooth the remnants of that pillar have retained (Fig. 4b).

After cleaning the implant surface, observations were made by using a scanning electron microscope. Despite carefully conducted process of removing impurities from the implant surface it failed to remove all biological residues (Fig. 5a). It was also noticed that the porous surface structure of the implant has deformed (Fig. 5b).

After preparation of metallographic specimens in accordance with obligatory methodology, observations were made of the constituent materials structures of

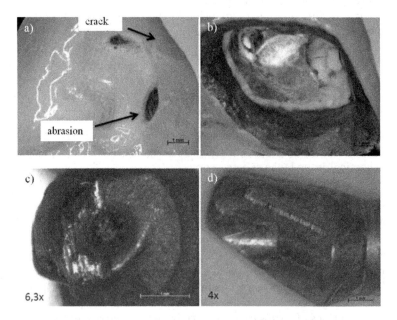

Fig. 4. Images from the stereomicroscope: (a) prosthetic crown; (b) tooth retained in substructure; (c) thread abrasion; (d) abutment with corrosive changes of the surface

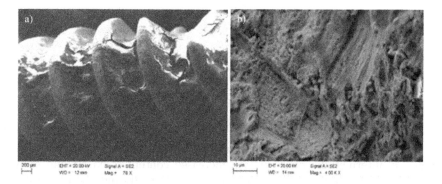

Fig. 5. SEM image of the surface of the implant in magnification: (a) 78x; (b) 4000x

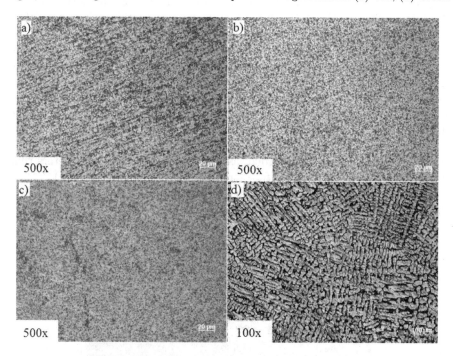

Fig. 6. The structures revealed in observations made by light microscope: (a) longitudinal section of the implant; (b) cross-sectional view of the implant; (c) longitudinal section of the abutment; (d) cross-sectional view of the substructure

the prosthetic system being examined. For this purpose a light microscope was used. The disclosed structures are depicted (Fig. 6) and described below.

On the basis of obtained images, it was found that the material of both the implant and abutment was characterized by fine-grained two-phase structure $\alpha+\beta$ (Fig. 6a–c), typical for the alloys Ti6Al4V. In the case of the substructure material, observed was the existence of dendritic structure being characteristic

Table 1. The results of impedance examinations

Material	R_s $[\Omega cm^2]$	C_{dl}		$R_{ct}[k\Omega cm^2]$
		$Y_{dl}[\Omega^{-1}cm^{-2}s^{-n}]$	n_{dl}	
Ti6Al4V	40.1	$2.535 \cdot 10^{-4}$	0.7568	14.25

for the components made by casting, not subjected to metal forming. On the
basis of observations and their comparison with the literature, revealed was the
presence of intermetallic phase γ with increased content of Ni–Cr and molybdenum enriched interdendritic areas [7]. In addition, during the observations
of microscopic cross-section of a prosthetic crown (Fig. 7) confirmed was the
existence of a layered construction of veneering layer – on the surface of the
substructure, it was clearly visible layer of opaquer (not translucent) with a
thickness of approx. 150 μm.

Literature sources also show the presence of the porous oxide layer on the
surface of the metal substructure, however, used magnifications do not create
the possibility of separating it from remaining structures of prosthetic crown.
The presence of this layer, produced by oxidation process (after streamed abrasive treatment of substructure surface), aims to increase the strength of the
connection between the ceramic veneering and substructure materialy [8].

As a result of impedance examinations EIS the spectra of Bode (Fig. 8a)
and Nyquist (Fig. 8b), were recorded, as well as characteristic parameters that
describe the properties of the surface structure of the implant (Table 1).

Nyquist diagram indicates the occurrence of characteristic impedance
response of thin oxide layers, which means that the implant surface has been

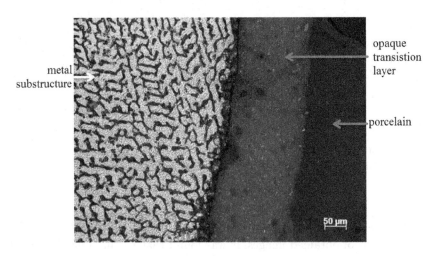

Fig. 7. Section through a prosthetic crown in 200x magnification (image from a light
microscope)

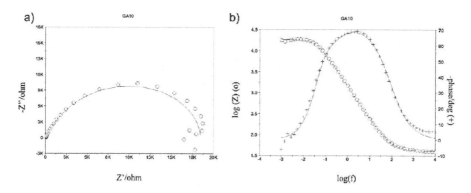

Fig. 8. Impedance spectra (a) Nyquist diagram (b) Bode diagram

passivated. On their basis, it was stated that the phase shift angle is approximately $70°$, whereas the slope of the $\log|Z|$ in the applied frequency range is close to value -1.

Before testing the resistance to pitting corrosion of the implant the opening potential was established, which amounted to $E_{ocp} = -91\,\text{mV}$. Then, starting from the value $E_{start} = E_{ocp} - 100$, using the rate of potential change of $1\,\text{mV/s}$, recorded was the anodic polarization curve (Fig. 9). Then the specific parameters were appointed: $E_{cor} = -148.9\,\text{mV}$, $R_p = 456.5\,\Omega\text{cm}^2$, $I_{cor} = 11.85\,\text{A/cm}^2$.

Resistance to galvanic corrosion of the abutment and crown started from the identification of opening potential. The values of these potentials are $-192\,\text{mV}$ for the abutment and $-378\,\text{mV}$ for the substructure. On the basis of this measurement, it was found that an electrode with a higher electronegativity (substructure) in the main study is to act as the anode while the abutment having smaller electronegativity – the role of the cathode. The area ratio of anode to

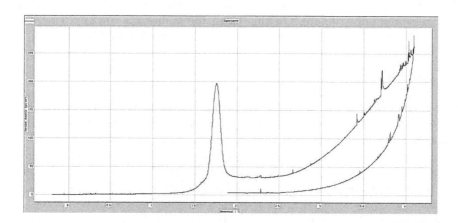

Fig. 9. Anodic polarization curve for implant of Ti6Al4V

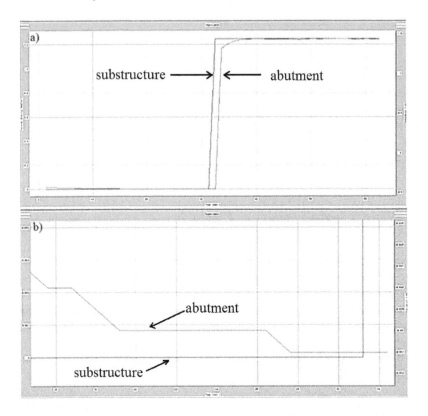

Fig. 10. Graphs of changes of the potential and current density in time (a) curves of polarization; (b) the point of intersection of the curves

cathode was set at 1:1. As a result of measurements recorded were the graphs (Fig. 10a) of changes course of the current density and potential in time for the abutment and substructure. On this basis, the values $i = 0.13 \, \mu\text{A}/\text{cm}^2$ oraz $E = -450 \, \text{mV}$ at the curves intersection has been established (Fig. 10b).

4   Conclusions

Microscopic observations allowed a preliminary assessment of exploitative damages within the prosthetic crown, which could be caused by abnormal occlusion, and therefore the occurrence of occlusal parafunctions and adverse overloading of the implant. The reason for the appearance of defects could also be in mismatched shape of prosthetic crown to the antagonistic teeth. As a result, it could lead to the emergence of micro-cracks and loss of integration of the implant with the bone.

It was also noted the presence of adverse corrosive changes on the surface of the substructure and abutment, which could – by penetration of metal ions into the surrounding tissues – to have an effect of perigraft structures irritation. This in turn could induce inflammation or exacerbate the adverse influence of other potential factors responsible for the occurrence of periimplantitis.

Observations with methods of light microscopy confirm that the materials used, despite the many years of being in the female patient's body, were characterized by structures typical for these specific material groups. It was also established that as a result of the periimplantitis course and loss of stability of the implant there has distorted the porous structure of the implant surface.

Characteristic of impedance spectra EIS and the results of assessment of resistance to pitting corrosion provide a basis to conclude that the Ti6Al4V implant has good corrosion resistance in assumed conditions. The basis of this reasoning is the phenomenon of transpassivation that occurred on the implant surface.

Evaluation of resistance to galvanic corrosion for the substructure-abutment system showed that despite the conditions conducive to the formation of a galvanic cell, the examined elements exhibit invulnerability to this type of corrosion. This is due to the low current density value. The environment of tissues and body fluids in the course of inflammation, however, changes its characteristics and becomes more aggressive (higher temperature, lower pH). Corrosion changes on the surface of the substructure and the abutment observed through a stereoscopic microscope can therefore be the result of the implant stay just in the inflammatory environment. However, relevant experience has not been performed in conditions simulating the tissue reaction changed by inflammation, so it is impossible to formulate a clear opinion about the cause of corrosion changes referred to above.

From the information obtained in dental interview it was determined that the female patient was at risk of biological complications due to habitual smoking resulting in increase of the number of anaerobic bacteria in the oral cavity and increase of the bacteria activity that cause inflammation of the periodontal tissues. Therefore, it was concluded that nicotine addiction could be a major causative factor initiating the periimplantitis. However, the attention should also be paid to information on the patient's age (60 years) which may indicate a reduced bone density or osteoporotic lesions of bone tissue.

References

1. Szaniawska, K., Rasiński, A., Kresa, I., Drężek, A., Duplaga, A., Łazarczyk, P., Płachta, M., Siuciak, K., Wilk, M., Wojtaszewska, M., Wojtowicz, A.: Periimplantitis - przegląd piśmiennictwa w oparciu o wybrane przypadki własne. [at:] Implants 4_2014
2. Pancerz-Łoś, M., Kmieć, Z., Bereznowski, Z., Witalis, A.: Miejscowe i ogólnoustrojowe konsekwencje peridontis i periimplantitis. Przegląd piśmiennictwa. [at:] Protetyka Stomatologiczna, LX, 1, 44–49 (2010)
3. Wysokińska-Miszczuk, J., Sitarski, O., Michalak, M.: Peri-implantitis - diagnostyka, leczenie, przykład kliniczny. [at:] Implantologia Stomatologiczna PSI Implant Dentistry 02/2012

4. Ziębowicz, A., Bączkowski, B.: Numerical analysis of the implant – abutment system. In: Piętka, E., Kawa, J. (eds.) ITIB 2012. LNCS, vol. 7339, pp. 341–350. Springer, Heidelberg (2012). doi:10.1007/978-3-642-31196-3_34
5. Spiechowicz, E.: Protetyka stomatologiczna podręcznik dla studentów stomatologii. Wydanie V unowocześnione, Wyd. Lekarskie PZWL, Warszawa, s. 130–185 (2004)
6. Pietruski, J.K., Pietruska, M.D.: Zastosowanie łączników indywidualnych wykonywanych w technologii CAD/CAM w implantoprotetyce. [at:] e-Dentico nr 1 (35)/2012
7. Castro, I.J., Echeverri, D., Garzón, H., Molina, A., Olave, G., Parra, M., Valencia, C.H.: Caracterizatión metalográfica de Barras para sobredentaduras, elaboradas por sobrecolado de polares para implantes dentales. [at:] Revista Facultad de Odontología Universidad de Antioquia - vol. 25, no. 1 - Segundo semestre (2013)
8. Zdziech, T.K.: Wpływ przygotowania powierzchni stopu chromowo-niklowego i chromowo-kobaltowego na charakter połączenia strukturalnego z ceramiką - Rozprawa na stopień doktora, Zakład Technik i Technologii Dentystycznych Uniwersytetu Medycznego w Poznaniu, Poznań, s. 3 (2014)

Microscopic Assessment of Damage to Miniplates for Mandible Osteosynthesis

Jarosław Sidun[1(✉)], Jan Borys[2], Jan Ryszard Dąbrowski[1],
and Żaneta Anna Mierzejewska[1]

[1] Mechanical Faculty, Białystok University of Technology, Wiejska 45c,
15-351 Białystok, Poland
{j.sidun,j.dabrowski}@pb.edu.pl, a.mierzejewska@doktoranci.pb.edu.pl
[2] Faculty of Medicine, Medical University of Białystok, J. Kilinskiego 1,
15-089 Białystok, Poland
jjbb7@wp.pl

Abstract. Degradation processes of implant materials have a significant effect on the reactions taking place around them. Processes related to mechanical wear, corrosion and tribological wear can be distinguished here. The phenomenon of fretting has a particularly significant impact on changes around the implant. Destruction of materials' surface layers by fretting occurs in biomedical implants. Oxide formation was observed in the friction zone. Wear products remain in the area of contact, inside the fretting corrosion pit, until they accumulate in excess and leave the area of contact. In fretting, oxidation may be a factor protecting against wear, when a wear-resistant oxide layer forms on metal surfaces at high temperatures. The presence of NaCl in the tissue environment intensifies the progression of fretting corrosion.

Keywords: Degradation processes · Plate fixations · Microscopy

1 Introduction

Setting and immobilizing bone fragments is an important therapeutic problem in facial bone fractures. In an insufficiently immobilized fracture, the gap widens and healing (union) is delayed. If fragments are shifted constantly, the healing process is severely disrupted. The introduction of stable osteosynthesis provides better stabilization of bone fragments, enables further functional treatment without the use of intermaxillary (maxillomandibular) fixation, and shortens the time of treatment. The application of micro- or mini-plates in treating facial bones is currently considered to be one of the most effective methods of maxillofacial surgery. Osteosynthesis by means of miniplates is recommended in all cases of mandibular fractures. These plates are made from titanium and its alloys.

As a result of tribological wear and/or corrosion wear processes, metallic implants may be an "emitter" of many chemical elements and compounds harmful to human health and cause illnesses defined as "metalloses". Marciniak's

© Springer International Publishing AG 2017
M. Gzik et al. (eds.), *Innovations in Biomedical Engineering*, Advances in Intelligent
Systems and Computing 526, DOI 10.1007/978-3-319-47154-9_9

research demonstrated that a connective tissue capsule is formed and osteolytic processes (bone atrophy) develop as a consequence of the development of bio-corrosion [10,14,17,18]. Peri-implant osteolysis is a complex biochemical process strictly linked to an implant's mechanical functioning [1]. Activation of osteoblast differentiation is stimulated by cytokines released by macrophages as a result of phagocytosis of hydroxyapatite and polymethylmethacrylate (PMMA) particles as well as of metal originating from the implant [1,9,10]. Reports in the literature show that wear products of metallic implants and chronic tissue inflammation are linked to the excessive presence of toxic elements. Parts of osteosyntheses are particularly susceptible to tribological and corrosion wear processes. The accu-mulation of particles and ions of metallic elements in surrounding tissues are the results of implant materials' degradation processes. It is observed in the case of both austenitic steels and titanium alloys, considered to be highly biocompatible. Reduction of the effects of tribological and corrosion wear of metallic implants is one of the main subjects of research conducted in many scientific centers [15,17]. A better understanding of the phenomena and mechanisms of tribological and corrosive destruction of materials at moving joints of systems serving to stabilize bone fractures will allow for assessment of the impact of environmental factors in the human body on these processes of materials' degradation. The presence of biofilm on metal surfaces may alter the mechanisms of and drastically accelerate corrosion processes. The effect that biofilm has on friction and wear processes of implant materials is also not without significance, as mentioned earlier. The influ-ence of saliva and biofilm on initiation of fatigue cracking of parts in osteosyn-theses must be explained. Aerobic microbes intensify the formation of cells of varying oxygenation, which fosters the development of crevice corrosion. In turn, the presence of anaerobic bacteria in the layer of biofilm aids the development of pitting corrosion of metals. Under such conditions, hydrogen may be released as a result of complex biochemical transformations, leading to unfavorable metal hydrogenation phenomena (hydrogen embrittlement). Data concerning intensive hydrogen absorption by implant titanium alloys in a biological environment can be found in professional literature. This leads to reduction of plasticity, changes of structure and grain size (refinement), and reduction of the fatigue strength of titanium implants. It should be noted that there is no data in the literature about tribological degradation of materials used in bone fixations, particularly in a biological environment [2,7,10,12,13].

After analyzing reports in the literature concerning interactions between implants and surrounding tissues, one can observe that problems linked to peri-implant reactions have not been unambiguously explained. The goal of this paper is to characterize the degradation processes taking place in plate fixations of the mandible.

2   Research Materials and Methodology

15 mandible fixation plates were tested after the treatment had been completed. Fixation plates was made of Ti6Al4V titanium alloy - Fig. 1. The system con-sisted of plates and inter-operating bolts that were present in the human body

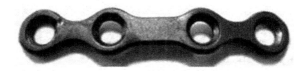

Fig. 1. View of mandible fixation plate tested as discussed below

for a period of about 3 months. Tests were conducted with the consent of the Local Ethical Committee for Animal Testing in Białystok.

Miniplates were observed from the perspective of surface wear, and their chemical composition was tested by means of an HITACHI S-3000N scanning electron microscope equipped with an NSS (Noran System Six) X-ray microanalyzer.

Analysis of the structure of the surface layer after fretting and fretting-corrosion was also conducted using an FIB (Focus Ion Beam system) microscope [5]. An Hitachi NB5000 double-beam scanning microscope equipped with a Ga+ ion source, with a maximum acceleration voltage of 40 keV and beam current up to 80 nA, was used in investigations.

The surface of the deformed conical seat was conducted using an 3D confocal laser microscope LEXT OLS 4000.

3   Research Results and Discussion

Ensuring the proper durability of implants in the environment of tissues is a very important engineering and clinical problem. The following figure among the dominant processes of biomaterials' degradation: corrosion, mechanical damage and tribological wear, particularly under conditions of so-called fretting [8]. Processes related to fretting, i.e. friction between two apparently permanently joined parts due to micro-displacements, are the most dangerous and the least understood [3,11]. These processes are intensified under the influence of an aggressive biological environment with significant participation of saliva or so-called biofilm.

The plate's surface, in its initial state, may undergo a change as early as during the technological process of its manufacturing due to local damage to the implant's passive layer. Plate wear in the form of scratches is also observed, leading to a change in hole shape. All conditions required for fretting to occur are met in a plate fixation of bone, and various wear mechanisms accompany fretting, particularly abrasive (fretting-wear), corrosive (fretting-corrosion) and fatigue (fretting-fatigue) mechanisms. The destructive action of fretting is intensified by loosening of bolts as well as by damage to the passive layer [4,6,16,18].

It should be emphasized that deformation of plate seats may lead to instability of the entire system. This is a very unfavorable phenomenon due to the probability of a reaction on the implant – tissue interface. Changes to the design of the fixation system and introduction of changes to its manufacturing process should be considered due to its susceptibility to fretting.

In the case of large deformations, greater plate wear is observed, meaning that wear products migrated to surrounding tissues. Wear products are very fine and can migrate via diffusion to many internal organs, such as: the lungs, kidneys, liver, brain and bone marrow.

However, the greatest threat is micro-crack initiation in bone plates when they are primarily, and unskillfully, modeled. This threat is very real when modeling is performed on a segment already weakened by holes. Initiated micro-cracks propagate very rapidly, resulting in the risk of further destruction of implants. Implant destruction is further facilitated by the stress state, which leads to accelerated development of corrosion in areas of stress concentration.

The results of a'posteriori investigations of parts of plate stabilizers used to make fixations indicate characteristic traces of damage. These traces include damage to the surface layer of coned seats, and to a lesser extent, damage to flat surfaces of plates.

Traces of abrasive wear, primarily due to micromachining, are formed during rotation of joining bolts and bone screws while their conical heads are pressed into their seats in plates. This unambiguously indicates the form of wear and the areas where it is present. Only the passive layer on surfaces undergoes abrasion. Wear processes develop with particularly intensity in areas of micro-contact between joining elements. Self-unscrewing of bone screws under the influence of low-frequency variable loads that a stabilizer is subject to during the period of its use, also cannot be ruled out as a cause of abrasive wear.

Damage of the second type is characteristic of corrosive destruction processes. It occurs at points of contact between interlocking parts (stress concentration). Corrosion pits have a decisive contribution to the process of surface layer destruction, and their sizes are much larger than in the case of mechanical wear. Corrosion pitting is the greatest in areas where scoring (abrasion) is present, which is typical. This means that the process of corrosive destruction is initiated and, to a large degree, activated by damage of the first type. It is precisely in these areas where the passive layer is destroyed and pitting corrosion develops. Moreover, tribo-corrosion (friction corrosion) processes, augmented by pitting corrosion, take place at points of contact. Tribo-corrosion is caused by mutual micro-displacements of contacting parts. Such displacements may occur as a result of insufficient tightening or loosening of joining bolts, and they may also be the result of elastic deformations of elements. Crevice corrosion does not have a decisive effect on the total size of corrosion losses, due to its slow rate of progression.

The conducted observations indicate that damage of the first type, probably occurring during the surgical procedure itself when the stabilizer was mounted, is the most frequently observed (Fig. 2).

Figure 3 presents damage of the second type. Visible fine wear particles may intensify secondary abrasive wear processes. Greater wear on elements of the stabilization system in the single-plate fixation is due to the nature of this fixation's operation. It is exposed, above all, to bending and torsion loads. The largest areas of wear are observed on interlocking surfaces of the plate seat and head of the last screw found in bone, which is caused by greater mobility.

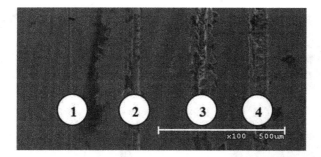

Fig. 2. Photograph of bolt surface with visible damage of the first type

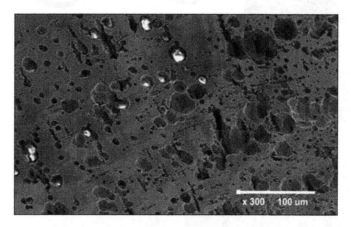

Fig. 3. Photograph of plate surface with damage of the second type

Examinations of plate surfaces under a microscope revealed visible corrosion pits formed as a result of the interaction of bodily fluids on the metallic material. Moreover, the presence of wear particles is visible on the plate's surface. These are metal oxides formed as a result of abrasion and/or adhesive interactions. The degree of wear and deformation of holes in the plate are shown in Fig. 4.

The development of corrosion is observed near holes as a result of the action of the aggressive environment. Numerous discolorations (Fig. 5a) and corrosion pits (Fig. 5b) are visible on the surface. Traces of abrasive wear can also be found near holes. In addition, deformation of hole shape is very frequently observed. Both processes occur when screws are screwed in and as the implant is used after that.

Over the course of observations of fixation elements under a microscope, much damage caused by fretting processes was visible. Fretting losses were formed on the surface of the screw as a result of micro-displacements accompanied by elastic deformations occurring between fixation elements. These are characteristic pits. In addition, discolorations formed on the screw surface that was in contact with surrounding tissue, and traces of pitting corrosion are visible. The action of

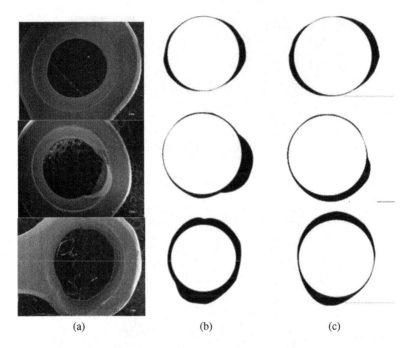

(a)   (b)   (c)

Fig. 4. Example results of investigations of screw seat deformations in fixing plates (a) initial image, (b) changed image for interior hole diameter (c) changed image for exterior hole diameter

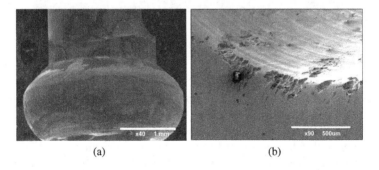

(a)   (b)

Fig. 5. Photograph of plate hole surface: (a) discolorations, (b) corrosion pits

the surrounding environment, of reduced pH, and the presence of ions, mainly chloride ions, were the factors initiating the development of pits.

Observations of plate seats revealed damage to the surface layer in the form of abrasive wear. The scratches and ridges visible on the presented photograph are indicative of this. The plastic deformation that can be observed most probably occurred during the mounting procedure. Figure 6 presents the results of plate assessment using a LEXT OLS 4000 3D confocal laser microscope. The central part of the plate, on which traces of wear are visible, was subject to assessment.

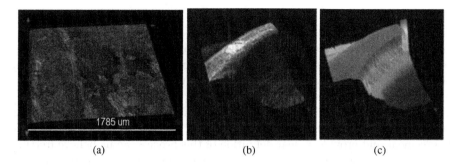

(a)   (b)   (c)

Fig. 6. 3D view: (a) of the corrosion pit analyzed above, (b), (c) of part of the conical seat in the miniplate

Traces of friction were imaged and measured, and the depth, width and slope of these traces were assessed, along with average values arising from the capability of measuring multiple profiles.

Figure 6b, c presents a part of the conical seat in a fixing miniplate after the period of its use. Both changes of the surface layer and changes in the seat itself are visible here. The surface of the conical seat was deformed and sustained losses due to corrosion as well as fretting. The complex phenomenon that is fretting corrosion took place here. This phenomenon is still not fully understood and is practically unknown in the context of osteosyntheses. Understanding it and describing wear mechanisms will make it possible to prevent much damage occurring in bone fixations. Furthermore, the presence of a morphological texture was observed at a depth of approx. 1.5 μ m (Fig. 7). This texture was formed by plastic deformation generated over the course of friction processes. The presence of a crack oriented parallel to the surface, marked with an arrow, was observed just under the sample's surface. The thickness of the material above the crack, depending on the point of observation, ranged from approx. 20 to approx. 100 nm.

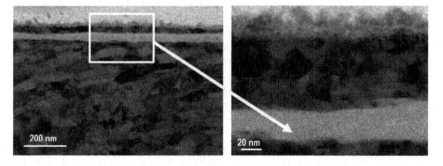

Fig. 7. Morphological texture along with layer formed as a result of tribo-corrosion processes at a depth of approx. 1.5 μ m

4 Summary

Various types of degradation processes are observed in facial bone fixations. Besides mechanical and corrosion damage, tribological damage can also be seen. The greatest wear processes are generated as a result of fretting. Fretting is a very complex process that results in various types of destruction, which have very significant consequences. Nearly a century has passed since the first reports of this type of destruction, but despite this fact, scientists still cannot come to an agreement and provide a clear definition of this process. Some believe fretting to be a type of wear or corrosion, while others believe it to be a type of friction occurring under specific conditions. In our opinion, it seems more justified to define fretting as a specific type of friction between two surfaces subjected to load and remaining in constant contact. To expound on the above, it is justified to distinguish the following component processes: fretting wear, fretting fatigue, fretting corrosion. The surface layer of elements may undergo fretting corrosion. Corrosion wear is linked to oxygen diffusion and grows along with load and friction path. In fretting, oxidation may be a factor protecting against wear, when a wear-resistant oxide layer forms on metal surfaces at high temperatures. The presence of NaCl in the tissue environment intensifies the progression of fretting corrosion.

Acknowledgements. This research was supported by Białystok University of Technology under Research Project S/WM/1/14 and financed from the funds for science MNiSW.

References

1. Archibeck, M., Jacobs, J., Roebuck, K., Glant, T.: The basic science of periprosthetic osteolysis. A current concepts review. J.B.J.S. 82-A, 1478–1489 (2000)
2. Duisabeau, L., Combrade, P., Forest, B.: Environmental effect on fretting of metallic materials for orthopedic implants. Wear **256**, 805–816 (2004)
3. Everitt, N.M., Ding, J., Bandak, G., Shipway, P.H., Leen, S.B., Williams, E.J.: Characterization of fretting-induced wear debris for Ti-6Al-4 V. Wear **267**, 283–291 (2009)
4. Gao, S., Cai, Z., Quan, X., Zhu, M., Yu, H.: Comparison between radial fretting and dual-motion fretting features of cortical bone. Wear **43**, 440–446 (2010)
5. Hatton, P.V., Brook, I.M.: The role of electron microscopy in the evaluation of biomaterials. European Microscopy and Analysis, 39–41 (1998)
6. Hebda, M., Wachał, A.: Trybologia. Wydawnictwa Naukowo-Techniczne Warszawa (1980). ISBN 83-204-0043-0, (in Polish)
7. Krischak, G.D., Gebhart, F., Mohr, W., Krivan, V., Ignatiuk, A., Bech, A., Wachter, N.J., Reuter, P., Arand, M., Kinzl, L., Claus, L.E.: Diffrence in metallic wear distribution released from commercially pure titanium compared with stainless steel plates. Arch. Orthop. Trauma Surg. **124**, 104–113 (2004)
8. Kulesza, E., Dąbrowski, J.R., Sidun, J., Neyman, A., Mizera, J.: Fretting wear of materials - methodological aspects of research. Acta Mech. at Automatica **6**(3), 58–61 (2012)

9. Kumar, S., Narayanan, T.S.N.S., Raman, S.G.S., Seshadri, S.K.: Evaluation of fretting corrosion behaviour of CP-Ti orthopaedic implant applications. Tribol. Int. **43**, 1245–1252 (2010)

10. Marciniak, J.: Biomateriały w chirurgii kostnej. Wydawnictwo Politechniki Śląskiej, Gliwice (2002)

11. Neyman, A.: Fretting w elementach maszyn, Gdańsk (2003). ISBN 83-7348-048-X

12. Sivakumar, M., Shanadurai, K.S.K., Rajeswari, S., Thulasiraman, V.: Failures in stainless steel orthopaedic implant devices: A survey. J. Mater. Sci. Lett. **14**, 351–354 (1995)

13. Winner, C., Gluch, H.: Aseptic loosening after CD instrumentation in the treatment of scoliosis: a report about eight cases. J. Spinal Disord. **11**, 440–443 (1998)

14. Voggenreiter, G., Leiting, S., Brauer, H., Leiting, P., Majetschak, M., Bardenheuer, M., Obertache, V.: Immuno - inflammatory tissue reaction to stainless - steel and titanum plates used for internal of long bones. Biomaterials **24**, 247–257 (2003)

15. Vadiraj, A., Kamaraj, M.: Effect of surface treatments on fretting fatigue damage of biomedical titanium alloys. Tribol. Int. **40**, 82–88 (2007)

16. Yu, H.Y., Quan, H.X., Cai, Z.B., Gao, S.S., Zhu, M.H.: Radial fretting behavior of cortical bone against titanium. Tribol. Lett. **31**, 69–76 (2008)

17. Zaffe, D., Bertoldi, C., Konsolo, U.: Accumulation of aluminium in lamer bone after implantation of titanium plater, Ti-6Al-4V screws, hydroxyapatite granules. Biomaterials **25**, 3837–3844 (2004)

18. Zhu, M.H., Zhou, Z.R.: On the mechanisms of various fretting wear modes. Tribol. Int. **44**, 1378–1388 (2011)

Characteristics of Surface Layers of Ti6Al4V Implants

Janusz Szewczenko[1]([✉]), Marcin Basiaga[2], Magdalena Grygiel-Pradelok[2], and Marcin Kaczmarek[2]

[1] Department of Biomechanics, Faculty of Biomedical Engineering, Silesian University of Technology, Zabrze, Poland
`janusz.szewczenko@polsl.pl`
[2] Department of Biomaterials and Medical Devices Engineering, Faculty of Biomedical Engineering, Silesian University of Technology, Zabrze, Poland

Abstract. The paper presents the results of influence of surface pretreatment of Ti6Al4V alloy, used for short-term implants in orthopedics, followed by anodic oxidation and steam sterilization on its physical and chemical properties. The pretreatment was a combination of: grinding, vibration machining, mechanical polishing, sandblasting and electrolytic polishing. Studies of surface topography, wettability, hardness and stress profiles of the substrate after various surface treatments were carried out. Furthermore, studies of pitting and crevice corrosion as well as ion release into a Ringer's solution after long-term exposure were also performed. The results show that the pretreatment preceding the anodic oxidation and steam sterilization affects the physical and chemical properties of the surface layer of Ti6Al4V alloy implants. Moreover, they indicate that the use of appropriate methods of pretreatment enable formation of a passive layer characterized by good osteoconductive properties.

Keywords: Ti6Al4V · Anodic oxidation · Osteoconductivity · Wettability · Hardness · Stresses in a layer

1 Introduction

Titanium alloys, next to an austenitic stainless steel, are the most often used metal biomaterials for parts of osteosynthesis systems [1–3]. Popularity of titanium alloy is connected with a high relative strength (Rm/ρ), good corrosion resistance in the environment of human body and a value of modulus of elasticity similar to the modulus of a bone. This enables to produce implants providing an elastic fixation of bone fragments [4–8].

In the initial period of application it was believed that titanium alloys are biologically inert. However, long-term clinical observations have shown that they can cause a peri-implant reaction in the implant-bone tissue interlayer. This is not only due to corrosion products containing alloying elements such as vanadium

© Springer International Publishing AG 2017
M. Gzik et al. (eds.), *Innovations in Biomedical Engineering*, Advances in Intelligent Systems and Computing 526, DOI 10.1007/978-3-319-47154-9_10

and aluminum but also of titanium. Nowadays the number of patients who have allergic reactions to titanium is increasing [9–11].

Adverse peri-implant reactions observed after implantation of titanium implants resulted in the need to modify their chemical composition or their surface layer. On the surface of implants of titanium alloys usually a passive layer is generated to ensure the increase of corrosion resistance under conditions of synergistic interaction of mechanical factors and environment of the organism. However, for implants used in osteosynthesis, methods of modifying the surface should also provide a surface layer exhibiting good osteoconductive properties. Such layer provides favorable conditions for ingrowth of newly formed bone tissue on the implant surface. This affects a quality of bone tissue-implant interface and fixation stability of bone fragments. Osteoconductive properties of surface layers of titanium alloys implants depends on their chemical composition, thickness of passive layer, surface roughness and wettability [12,13].

In order to modify the surface layer of titanium implants, mechanical processing, chemical and physical treatment may be used [14–17]. These methods allow the formation of a wide range of properties of the surface layer. However, due to the need of efficiency, repeatability and complex shape of implants used for osteosynthesis the most common method of modifying the surface is an anodic oxidation. It is preceded by other initial surface treatment, for example: grinding, vibration machining, mechanical polishing, sandblasting and electrolytic polishing.

In order to ensure osteoconductive properties of titanium alloy implants the anodic oxidation performed at medium voltages (40V–100V) is applied. The resulting passive layer consisted mainly of amorphous TiO_2 oxide with a small fraction of oxides of the alloying elements. The layers are homogeneous, having a thickness of several hundred nm, depending on the applied voltage [18,19]. They also reflect the topography of the substrate.

Despite numerous works on the influence of anodic oxidation parameters and the applied pretreatment on the corrosion resistance of titanium alloys [20–24], no comprehensive studies concerning corrosion resistance, degradation kinetics, physical and chemical properties as well as sterilization have been carried out.

2   Materials and Methods

Ti6Al4V alloy of chemical composition, microstructure and mechanical properties that meet the requirements of ISO 5832-3 was used in the studies. Samples were obtained from rods with diameters of 14 mm, 8 mm and 6 mm. Samples were subjected to preliminary surface treatment consisting of grinding (G), vibration machining (VM), mechanical polishing (MP), sandblasting (SB), and electrolytic polishing (EP). An anodic oxidation (AO) and steam sterilization (S) were applied as the final surface treatment. The grinding was carried out sequentially with the use of abrasive papers of 120, 320 and 600 grit. The vibration machinig was carried out with ceramic abrasive grains and a wetting agent. Electrolytic polishing was carried out in a bath based on chromic acid (E-395

POLIGRAT Company GmbH) at a current density of j $= 10 \div 30\,\mathrm{A/dm^2}$. The process of anodization was carried out using an electrolyte based on phosphoric acid and sulfuric acid (Color Company POLIGRAT Titan GmbH) at the voltage of 97 V. The steam sterilization was conducted at 407 K under a pressure of $2.1 \cdot 10^5$ Pa for 720 s.

Topography of the surface was performed by scanning electron microscope (SEM) Supra 35 ZEISS and atomic force microscopy (AFM) NTegra Spectra NT-MDT. In the semi-contact mode silicon probes VIT_P of resonance frequency equal to 400 kHz were used.

Measurements of hardness of the surface layer were carried out by the Oliver and Pharr method using a Vickers indenter. The hardness was measured at penetration depth in the range $500 \div 8000$ nm. The value of the loading force and the penetration depth of the indenter was recorded continuously during the entire cycle. The loading and unloading rate was equal to 3000 nm / min, and the loading time was equal to 15 sec. The measurements were conducted on the CSM open platform equipped with a micro-combi tester.

Residual stress measurements of the substrate was made using the $\sin^2\psi$ technique. The X'Pert Stress Plus program was applied. The ψ angles of the samples with reference to the original beam was varied in the range of 0° to 75°. The measurements were conducted for two orthogonal directions. Studies were performed using the X'Pert PRO Panalytical diffractometer using a strip detector Xcelerator. A cobalt lamp was used. The applied voltage was equal to 40 kV and current was equal to 30 mA.

To determine the **wettability** of the surface layers, contact angle measurements were performed using SURFTENS UNIVERSAL by OEG GmbH goniometer with the Surftens 4.3 software. The volume of the dispensed droplet of distilled water was 1 mm^3.

In studies of concentrations of **metal ions releasing** to the solution from the titanium alloy the Ringer's solution was used. Samples were held for 28 days in the solution of 0.1 dm^3 at the temperature of 37±1°C. The concentration of metal ions was determined by the JY 2000 spectrometer using ICP-AES (Inductively Coupled Plasma - Atomic Emission Spectrometry) method.

3   Results

Surface studies of Ti6Al4V samples after various surface treatments using the atomic force microscopy allowed determination of roughness parameters Ra and Sa (Table 1, Fig. 1). Values of determined parameters were dependent on the applied pretreatment preceding the anodic oxidation and steam sterilization. The highest values of surface roughness were recorded for the sample for which the pretreatment consisted of grinding, mechanical polishing, sandblasting and electropolishing (G/MP/SB/EP/AO/S) while the lowest valued for the samples after grinding, vibratory machining and electropolishing (G/VM/EP/AO/S). For the anodically oxidized and sterilized samples after the sandblasting (G/VM/MP-/SB/AO/S and G/MP/SB/AO/S), the measured surface roughness was similar.

Table 1. Roughness parameters and their standard deviations (in brackets) of the samples modified by various surface treatments

The method of surface modification	Ra, nm	Sa, nm
G/VM/MP/SB/AO/S	247(19)	260(10)
G/MP/SB/AO/S	254(21)	249(11)
G/MP/SB/EP/AO/S	310(25)	316(15)
G/VM/EP/AO/S	111(10)	117(10)

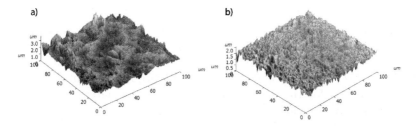

Fig. 1. Images of the Ti6Al4V samples after the applied surface treatments: (a) G/VM/MP/SB/AO/S, (b) G/VM/EP/AO/S, (AFM)

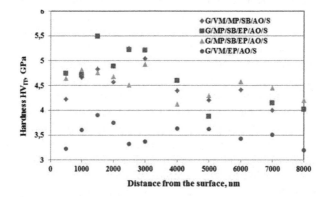

Fig. 2. Hardness distribution in the surface layer as a function of distance from the surface for the Ti6Al4V samples after various surface treatments

On the basis of the hardness measurements, hardness distribution of the surface layer formed after the various treatments was determined (Fig. 2). The hardness of the surface layers varied depending on the treatment applied before the anodic oxidation and the sterilization. The lowest hardness was measured for the surface layer, for which the pretreatment consisted of grinding, vibration machining, and electropolishing (G/VM/EP/AO/S), whereas the highest hardness was measurer for the anodized samples and sterilized directly after sandblasting (SB). The hardness of the untreated alloy was equal to 3.4 GPa.

Table 2. Compressive stresses and their standard deviations (in brackets) in the modified surface layers on the Ti6Al4V substrate

The method of surface modification	Stress, MPa
G/VM/MP/SB/AO/S	−774(21)
G/MP/SB/AO/S	−898(24)
G/MP/SB/EP/AO/S	−650(22)
G/VM/EP/AO/S	−550(45)

Studies of stresses in the surface layer showed the presence of compressive stresses of different values depending on the applied pretreatment (Table 2). Larger values of stresses were observed for the anodically oxidized samples after sandblasting (G/VM/MP/SB/AO/S and G/MP/SB/AO/S), while smaller values were measured for the anodically oxidized samples after electropolishing (G/MP/SB/EP/AO/S and G/VM/EP/AO/S).

Regardless of the method of modifying the surface layer of Ti6Al4V alloy, its surface was characterized by hydrophilic properties (Fig. 3). The value of the θ contact angle depends on the applied pretreatment. The highest wettability was measured for the layers formed in the process of anodic oxidation and sterilization preceded by grinding, vibratory machining, mechanical polishing, and sandblasting (G/VM/MP/SB/AO/S), while the lowest value was obtained after grinding, vibration machining, and electropolishing (G/VM/EP/AO/S).

After the exposure to the Ringer solution a concentration of released metal ions was determined. Ion concentration was calculated on the mass of the element released from the sample surface (μg/cm^2) (Table 3).

The mass density of the metal ions released into the Ringer's solution in 28 days from the samples depends on the applied method of surface treatment (Table 3). The lowest mass density was observed for the samples subjected to grinding, mechanical polishing and sandblasting (G/MP/SB/AO/S), while the highest value was recorded for the samples after grinding, vibration machining and mechanical polishing (G/VM/EP/AO/S). Moreover, for the electropolished

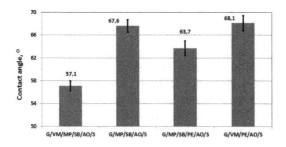

Fig. 3. Wettability angle (with standard deviation) of modified surface titanium alloy

Table 3. Surface mass density and their standard deviations (in brackets) of metal ions released to Ringer's solution from anodized Ti6Al4V alloy after various surface treatment

The method of surface modification	Surface mass density of metal ions, $\mu g/cm^2$			
	Ti	Al	V	Cr
G/VM/MP/SB/AO/S	14.98(43)	1.681(31)	0.343(78)	-
G/MP/SB/AO/S	10.62(15)	2.435(31)	0.0624(15)	-
G/MP/SB/EP/AO/S	14.51(90)	2.711(36)	0.208(68)	3.37(17)
G/VM/EP/AO/S	36.99(99)	16.056(26)	14.152(46)	0.078(10)

samples (EP), beside the presence of ions of alloying elements, chromium ions were observed.

4   Discusion

Analysis of the results indicates that the final physical and chemical properties of the surface layer formed on the Ti6Al4V alloy during the anodic oxidation and steam sterilization depend on the applied pretreatments. The pretreatment not only affected the geometric structure of the surface of the samples Table 1) but also the color thereof as a consequence of varying the thickness of the passive layer. The layers obtained from the anodic oxidation preceded by sandblasting are characterized by a lower intensity of color and less brightening compared to those obtained after the electropolishing. The electropolishing also affects the increase of surface roughness after sandblasting (Table 1).

Differences in hardness of the surface layers, depending on the applied pretreatment, demonstrate varying degrees of their strengthening (Fig. 2). The greatest strengthening was observed for the anodically oxidized and sterilized after sandblasting. The applied electropolishing after the sandblasting slightly reduced the degree of strengthening of the surface layer. Compressive stresses and hardness have the same influence on strengthening as the applied pretreatment (Fig. 2, Table 2).

An important feature of short-term implants used for osteosynthesis should be good osteoconductive properties of their surface. These properties are influenced by the surface topography, and its wettability. For anodized titanium the best osteoconductive properties are observed for surfaces for which the roughness parameter Ra $< 0.3\mu m$ [12,24] and the contact angle is in the ranges $20 \div 55°$ and $55 \div 70$ [25,26].

Analysis of the obtained results indicates the surface layers formed on the Ti6Al4V substrate with the proposed pretreatments prior to the anodic oxidation and steam sterilization are characterized by roughness (Ra $= 111\,nm - 310\,nm$ - Table 1) and surface wettability ($\theta = 57.1° - 68.1°$ - Fig. 3), which should ensure them good osteoconductive properties.

The main factor determining the suitability of metal biomaterials for implants is a good corrosion resistance in body fluids. Analysis of the results of pitting corrosion resistance, regardless of the applied method of surface treatment prior to the anodic oxidation and sterilization, showed a positive effect of passivation up to the potential of +2000 mV [27]. This value, according to the requirements of the PN-EN ISO 10993-15 standard, is a maximum value for which potentio-dynamic tests of implants should be carried out.

After holding the samples in the Ringer solution for 28 days the presence of Ti, Al, V ions was observed (Table 3). The concentration of metal ions depends on the applied pretreatment. The use of sandblasting effects beneficially, reducing the amount of metal ions releasing to the solution. In contrast, electropolishing exerts a negative effect in terms of penetration into a solution of chromium ions.

5 Conclusion

Analysis of the results indicates that properties of the passive layer formed on the Ti6Al4V substrate by anodic oxidation, and steam sterilization can be tailored by the appropriate pretreatment. Hardening of the surface layer occurred as the result of the sandblasting before the anodic oxidation benefits the properties of the layer. As a result of the pretreatment consisting of grinding, mechanical polishing, sandblasting, and the final anodic oxidation and steam sterilization the obtain surface layers are characterized by resistance to pitting and crevice corrosion, limited ion release into the tissue environment, and good osteoconductive properties.

References

1. Frosch, K.H., Sturmer, K.M.: Metallic biomaterials in skeletal repair. Eur. J. Trauma **32**, 149–159 (2006)
2. Anselme, K.: Biomaterials and interface with bone. Osteoporos. Int. **22**, 2037–2042 (2011)
3. Basiaga, M., Jendrus, R., Walke, W., Paszenda, Z., Kaczmarek, M., Popczyk, P.: Influence of surface modification on properties of stainless steel used for implants. Arch. Metall. Mater. **60**(4), 2965–2969 (2015)
4. Kiel, M., Marciniak, J., Basiaga, M., Szewczenko, J.: Numerical analysis of spine stabilizers on lumbar part of spine. ITiB Adv. Intell. Syst. Comput. **69**, 447–456 (2010)
5. Kajzer, W., Kajzer, A., Gzik-Zroska, B., Wolański, W., Janicka, I., Dzielicki, J.: Comparison of numerical and experimental analysis of plates used in treatment of anterior surface deformity of chest. In: Piętka, E., Kawa, J. (eds.) ITIB 2012. LNCS, vol. 7339, pp. 319–330. Springer, Heidelberg (2012). doi:10.1007/978-3-642-31196-3_32
6. Geetha, M., Singh, A.K., Asokamani, R., Gogia, A.K.: Ti based biomaterials, the ultimate choice for orthopaedic implants a review. Prog. Mater. Sci. **54**, 397–425 (2009)

7. Marciniak, J., Szewczenko, J., Walke, W., Basiaga, M., Kiel, M., Manka, I.: Biomechanical analysis of lumbar spine stabilization by means of transpedicular stabilizer. ITiB Adv. Soft Comput. **47**, 529–536 (2008)
8. Pochrzast, M., Basiaga, M., Marciniak, J., Kaczmarek, M.: Biomechanical analysis of limited-contact plate used for osteosynthesis. Acta. Bioeng. Biomech. **16**(1), 99–105 (2014)
9. Makuch, K., Koczorowski, R.: Biocompatibility of titanium and its alloys used in dentistry. Dent. Med. Probl. **47**, 81–88 (2010). (in Polish)
10. Ziębowicz, A., Bączkowski, B.: Numerical analysis of the implant – abutment system. In: Piętka, E., Kawa, J. (eds.) ITIB 2012. LNCS, vol. 7339, pp. 341–350. Springer, Heidelberg (2012). doi:10.1007/978-3-642-31196-3_34
11. Rusinek, B., Stobiecka, A., Obtulowicz, K.: Titanium allergy and implants. Alerg. Immunol. **5**, 5–7 (2008). (in Polish)
12. Yamamoto, D., Kawai, I., Kuroda, K., Ichino, R., Okido, M., Seki, A.: Osteoconductivity and hydrophilicity of TiO2 coatings on Ti substrates prepared by different oxidizing processes. Bioinorg Chem Appl, Article ID 495218 (2012)
13. Park, J.W., Jang, J.H., Lee, C.S., Hanawa, T.: Osteoconductivity of hydrophilic microstructured titanium implants with phosphate ion chemistry. Acta. Biomater. **5**, 2311–2321 (2009)
14. Sobieszczyk, S.: Surface modifications of Ti and its alloys. Nat. Adv. Sci. Inst. Se. **10**, 29–42 (2010)
15. Basiaga, M., Walke, W., Paszenda, Z., Kajzer, A.: The effect of EO and steam sterilization on mechanical and electrochemical properties of titanium grade 4. Mater. Tehnol. **50**(1), 153–158 (2016)
16. Marciniak, J., Szewczenko, J., Kajzer, W.: Surface modification of implants for bone surgery. Arch. Metall. Mater. **60**(3B), 2123–2129 (2015)
17. Szewczenko, J., Pochrzast, M., Walke, W.: Evaluation of electrochemical properties of modified Ti-6Al-4V ELI alloy. Przegl. Elektrotechniczny **87**(12b), 177–180 (2011)
18. Krasicka-Cydzik, E.: Anodic layer formation on titanium and its alloys for biomedical applications, titanium alloys. In: Nurul Amin, A.K.M. (Ed.) Towards Achieving Enhanced Properties for Diversified Applications (2012)
19. Szewczenko, J., Jaglarz, J., Basiaga, M., Kurzyk, J., Skoczek, E., Paszenda, Z.: Topography and thickness of passive layers on anodically oxidized Ti6Al4V alloys. Przegl. Elektrotechniczny **88**(12B), 228–231 (2012)
20. Diamanti, M.V., Del Curto, B., Pedeferri, M.: Anodic oxidation of titanium: from technical aspects to biomedical applications. J. Appl. Biomater. Biomech. **9**, 55–69 (2011)
21. Fojt, J.: Ti-6Al-4V alloy surface modification for medical applications. Appl. Surf. Sci. **262**, 163–167 (2012)
22. Karambakhsh, A., Afshar, A., Malekinejad, P.: Corrosion resistance and color properties of anodized Ti-6Al-4V. J. Mater. Eng. Perform. **21**, 121–127 (2012)
23. Barranco, V., Onofre, E., Escudero, M.L., Garcia-Alonso, M.C.: Characterization of roughness and pitting corrosion of surfaces modified by blasting and thermal oxidation. Surf. Coat. Tech. **204**, 3783–3793 (2010)
24. Zhang, D., Cheng, H., Wang, Y., Ning, C.: Effect of different acid treatment on surface characteristics of titanium alloy. Mater. Sci. Forum. **694**, 490–496 (2011)
25. Yamamoto, D., Kuroda, K., Ichino, R., Okido, M.: Hydrophilicity and Osteoconductivity of Ti Anodized in Various Aqueous Solutions. Honolulu PRiME, Abstract 2054 (2012)

26. Yamamoto, D., Iida, T., Arii, K., Kuroda, K., Ichino, R., Okido, M., Seki, A.: Surface hydrophilicity and osteoconductivity of anodized Ti in aqueous solutions with various solute ions. Mater. Trans. **53**, 1956–1961 (2012)
27. Szewczenko, J.: Formation of physical and chemical properties of surface layer on titanium alloys used for implants for traumatology and orthopaedics. Ed. Silesian Technical University, Gliwice (2014)

The Influence of the Mechanical Properties of a-C:H Based Thin Coatings on Blood-Material Interaction

Klaudia Trembecka-Wojciga[1]([✉]), Roman Major[1], Piotr Wilczek[2],
Jurgen M. Lackner[3], Ewa Jasek-Gajda[4], and Bogusław Major[1]

[1] Institute of Metallurgy and Materials Science, Polish Academy of Sciences,
25 Reymonta Street, 30-059 Crakow, Poland
r.major@imim.pl

[2] Bioengineering Laboratory, Heart Prosthesis Institute, Wolnosci 345A,
41-800 Zabrze, Poland

[3] Joanneum Research Forschungsges MbH,
Institute of Surface Technologies and Photonics,
Functional Surfaces, Leobner Strasse 94, 8712 Niklasdorf, Austria

[4] Department of Histology, Jagiellonian University Medical College,
Kopernika 7, 31-034 Cracow, Poland

Abstract. An interaction of blood with artificial materials is an important aspect in designing cardiovascular tissue analogues. The processes occurs on liquid/solid interface depends both on structural and mechanical properties of biomaterials. Main goal of the work was to develop novel blood contacting materials in the form of thin coatings with anti-thrombogenic properties by reduction of shear stress improving sufficient washing of biofunctional-adapted surfaces. Preliminary studies and simulations led us to carbon based thin coatings considered as silicon doped amorphous carbon. The rigidity of the surface design of materials dedicated for the biomedical purpose is of particular importance. The paper presents an analysis of the impact of material stiffness and mechanical for interaction with blood cells. Material analysis of in the context of the mechanical properties showed changes in stiffness depending on the thickness of the coating. The Young modulus and hardness of materials were examined by indentation test using Berkovich indenter geometry. Cell-material interactions were assessed using the cellular components of blood. Shear stress on the between the cell-and material were considered taking into account red blood cells and platelets concentrates.

Keywords: Hemocompatybility · Shear stresses · Blood-material interaction

1 Introduction

In blood-material interfacial the outermost layer of biomaterial is the most crucial for hemocompatibility properties of implant. Thus, an intensive research

© Springer International Publishing AG 2017
M. Gzik et al. (eds.), *Innovations in Biomedical Engineering*, Advances in Intelligent
Systems and Computing 526, DOI 10.1007/978-3-319-47154-9_11

has been focused on surface modification by controlling their physico - chemical properties [1]. There is growing interest in application of carbon based materials, in particular diamond like carbon (DLC) due to its bio-haemocompatible nature [2]. Carbon- based coatings exhibit attractive tribological, electrical, chemical and optical properties for blood contacting materials [3]. Many studies show that ultrathin a-C:H and a-C:H:Si films can be used to improve the surface features necessary for improved biocompatibility both metals and polymers [4]. Krishnan et al. [5] showed that DLC coating on titanium substrate exhibit a lower platelet adhesion in comparison to non-modified titanium. The blood compatibility of DLC coating depends on the deposition conditions which was confirmed by Alanazi et al. [6]. They have also proved that surface wettability and chemical composition is independent of film thickness. DLC coatings show very well adherent properties as well as the ability to protect biological implants against corrosion or serve as diffusion barriers [7]. Thus, DLC coatings have found many potential biological application for intra-coronary stents [8], prosthetic heart valves [9] or rotary blood pump [10]. Over the past decades evolution in the field of biomaterial engineering has shifted from developing materials that were merely tolerated by the body to creating those that elicit a specific response. When it comes to blood-material interaction it is necessary to design fully atrombogenic surface which do not adverse interact with any blood components [11,12]. This represents a really complex task due to a variety of processes occurring within this interface including plasma protein adsorption, cell adhesion, and activation followed by thrombus formation [1]. Interaction of blood cells with artificial surfaces plays a major role in host response and determine the material hemocompatybility [13]. Shear stresses as a consequence of blood flow can also improve cell activation and aggregation. Blood cascade activation can lead to a serious consequences including formation of blood clots followed by unhindered in blood flows and resulting in implant failure [14]. Thus, the blood -material interaction under physiological conditions is critical when designing new materials for blood interface. This interactions can be influenced by factor such as surface charge, hydrophobicity, topography and material strength. The work is focused on the in vitro interaction of red blood cells and platelets with artificial surfaces under physiological conditions. a-C:H and Si-DLC coatings with different thickness were deposited on the surface of silicon wafers by magnetron sputtering. The coatings adhesion strength, Young modulus, hardness and wettability were analysed. The protein adsorption from fatal bovine serum solution were performed in order to analyse surfaces affinity to albumin. Cell-materials interaction were analysed using dedicated radial flow chamber which gives ability to apply different values of shear stresses. Mechanical interaction between substrates and platelets/erythrocytes were analyzed. In the frame of the work, the radial detachment chamber was described in details.

2   Materials and Methods

2.1   Coatings Preparation

The silicon wafer (diameter 14 cm) were modified by ultrathin carbon based thin films using magnetron sputtering in direct current (DC), unbalanced mode. For the work the following thin coatings were prepared: a-C:H 100 nm, Si-DLC 500 nm, Si-DLC 300 nm, Si-DLC 200 nm, Si-DLC 125 nm and Si-DLC 15 nm thick. Carbon targets (the latter for Diamond Like Carbon-DLC) were used to deposit films on silicon wafer substrates at room temperature in an argon atmosphere. To ensure homogenous film thickness over the entire coated surfaces, substrates were rotated during deposition at a speed of 5.4 cm s^{-1} through the plasma plumes. A detailed description of the deposition arrangement is given elsewhere [15].

2.2   Radial Flow Chamber

Cell-material interactions were analysed using dedicated radial flow chamber (Fig. 1A). For analysis red blood cells concentrate and platelets concentrate were used irrespectively. The radial flow chamber allows to apply different values of shear forces in cell-material interface. The detachment of the cells from the surface depends on the value of applied shear forces (Fs) and adhesion forces (Fa), which determine the strength of cell adhesion (Fig. 1B). When the Fs is less or equal to Fa, cell detachment is not observed (Fig. 1Ba). In other cases, cells are removed from surface one by one (Fig. 1Bb) or randomly (Fig. 1Bc). In radial flow chamber, hydrodynamic stresses are applied on material surface by liquid flow along the radius of disc-shape sample (Fig. 1C). A workspace of chamber consists of a liquid reservoir with stand in a central location. A sample was placed on stand when liquid (phosphate buffered saline (PBS, pH 7.4)) level was below its surface. Concentrate of human erythrocytes and platelets (diluted 4000x by using a phosphate buffered saline (PBS, pH 7.4) was uniformly applied to the surface of the tested materials. The covered samples by cell solution were left for a 10 min in order to cells adhesion to the surface. After that time, the PBS level in reservoir was raised until the draft of the sample. On the top of sample, disc-shape tripod was placed leaving a 150 μm gap. A constant volumetric flow of PBS was pumped through the whole in center of the tripod and flows radially to the disc-shape sample edges. The distance between the surface of the investigated material and the flow chamber had the strong influence on the value of the shear stress. It was set on the level of 250 μm. The flow rate was constant during the entire experiment and depended individually on the tested material. In the center of the radial flow chamber, in the place of injection of the elution medium, the direction of flow of the liquid is perpendicular to the surface of the sample located under the chamber. At this point, the likelihood of the cell detachment is the lowest. At the edge of the hole the direction of flow of elution medium changed from perpendicular to parallel to the surface analyzed. At this point,

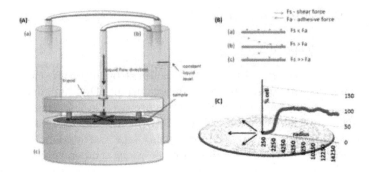

Fig. 1. Schematic illustration of radial flow test; (A) Radial flow chamber assembly (Aa) working reservoir (Ab) stress determining reservoir (Ac) radial flow chamber with sample; (B) Influence of shear forces into cell detachments (Ba) no cell detachment, (Bb) detachment one by one, (Bc) selective cell remove from substrate; (C) Distribution of shear forces on the sample and exemplary of cell detachment from surface. The arrows represent the liquid flows. The graph shows standard example of the percentage of cells on surface along radius (Color figure online)

the likelihood of cell detachment is the greatest. The applied shear stress can be calculated using Eq. (1).

$$\sigma = \frac{3D\eta}{\pi r e^2} \tag{1}$$

where D is the flow rate, which depends on the material, η is the dynamic viscosity of the fluid $(10\,g/(cm^*s))$, and e is the distance between the disk and the plate set at $150\,\mu m$ for this experiment.

3   Results and Discussion

3.1   Cell Detachment

The percentage of adhered erythrocytes and platelets in the function of applied stresses is presented in Figs. 2 and 3, respectively. The values of shear stresses were calculated using equation (1). Generally, the strength of cell-material inter-action depends on the coating composition, thickness as well as on cell type. The differences in erythrocytes and platelets affinity to substrates were observed. The platelets-material interaction reaches plateau at higher stresses than for erythrocytes except SI-DLC 300 nm film. Si-DLC 300 nm exhibit strong affinity to both, platelets and erythrocytes. The 85,5 % of attached erythrocytes were removed from the Si-DLC sample after exposure to 73 Pa. Comparing to other samples, at plateau the smallest number of detached cells at the highest value of applied stresses was observed. Si-DLC 500 nm, Si-DLC 200 nm and Si-DLC 15 nm films show weak affinity to erythrocytes but strong to platelets. For Si-DLC 15 nm coating, cell detachment at plateau is about 90 % for erythrocytes but only 70 % for platelets. For platelet-material interaction, Si-DLC 15 nm function reach plateau at stress equal to 60 Pa which is the highest value comparing to other samples. Comparing to other coatings, a-C:H 100 nm sample shows weak interactions with both, erythrocytes and platelets. About 90 % of attached cells were removed from the surface of a-C:H 100 nm film by applying the shear forces in the range of 20–25 Pa. For Si-DLC 125 nm film differences in materials interaction with erythrocytes and platelets are very gentle.

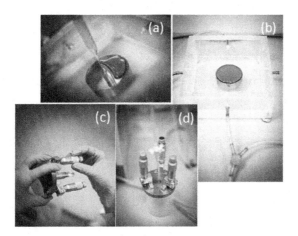

Fig. 2. The percentage of adhered erythrocytes to the surfaces in the function of applied shear stresses

In Figs. 2 and 3, 50 % of detached cells determine critical stresses in which the probability of cell detachment or their remain on the surfaces is the same. The values of critical stresses for each coating is presented on Table 1. In most cases critical stresses for erythrocytes are higher than for platelets except Si-DLC 300 nm and Si-DLC 15 nm. Generally, applying stresses between 4 Pa to 12 Pa remove half of adhered cells from surfaces. For all coatings detachment rates, which represent the number of detached cells per minute were presented in the function of applied stresses for erythrocytes (Fig. 4) and for platelets (Fig. 5). Exponential trends lines were adjusted to measurement points. The exponential function was extrapolated to 0 shear stress in order to determine the detachment rate under conditions where there is no shear force generated by flow applied. The values of the spontaneous shear rate are presented in (Table 1). For all materials the values of spontaneous detachment rate of platelets are much higher than derachment rate of erythrocytes.

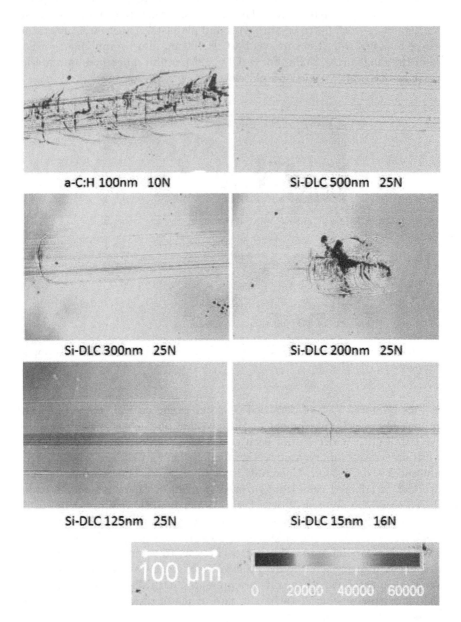

Fig. 3. The percentage of adhered platelets to the surfaces in the function of applied shear stresses.

Table 1. Critical shear stresses and spontaneous cell detachment rate for platelets and erythrocytes.

Material	Critical stress [Pa]		Spontaneous detachment rate [1/min]	
	Erythrocytes	Platelets	Erythrocytes	Platelets
a-C:H 100 nm	5.62	3.88	0.25	4.95
Si-DLC 500 nm	6.37	3.86	0.23	4.33
Si-DLC 300 nm	9.13	11.24	0.11	0.52
Si-DLC 200 nm	6.59	5.68	0.24	0.51
Si-DLC 125 nm	7.39	4.98	0.12	2.04
Si-DLC 15 nm	7,96	9.01	0.19	1.49

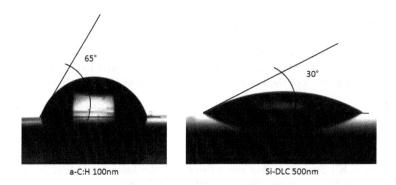

Fig. 4. Detachment rate in the function of applied stress for erythrocytes.

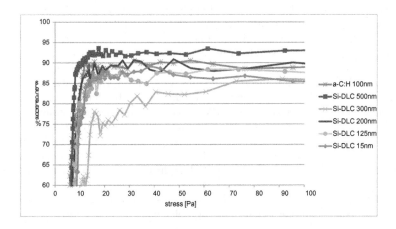

Fig. 5. Detachment rate in the function of applied stress for platelets.

4   Conclusions

Progress in developing materials for blood interfaces have been an area of active research over the last two decades. Thrombus formation as an effect of blood-biomaterial interaction represent one of the greatest risk factor of cardiovascular implant failure. Blood cells-material interaction is a key factor which has direct influence on surface hemocompatybility. Based on achieved results the following conclusions can be made: The surface modification by ultra-thin coatings deposition impacts on the interaction of materials with blood components

- The surface modification by ultra-thin coatings deposition impacts on the interaction of materials with blood components
- The interaction of Si-DLC coatings with platelets differs than for erythrocytes. Only Si-DLC 300 nm film exhibit strong interaction with both, platelets and erythrocytes (Table 1).

Acknowlegement. The research was financially supported by the Project no. 2014/13/B/ST8/04287 "Bio-inspired thin film materials with the controlled contribution of the residual stress in terms of the restoration of stem cells microenvironment" of the Polish National Centre of Science. Part of the research has been done in the frame of statutory funds of the Institute of Metallurgy and Materials Science PAS, the task Z-2.

References

1. Chittur, K.K.: Surface techniques to examine the biomaterial-host interface: an introduction to the papers. Biomater **19**, 301–305 (1998)
2. Hauert, R.: DLC films in biomedical applications. In: Erdemir, D.C., Springer-Verlag, A. (eds.) Tribology of Diamond-like Carbon Films Fundamentals and Applications, pp. 494–509. Springer, heidelberg (2008)
3. Dearnaley, G., Arps, J.H.: Biomedical applications of diamond-like carbon (DLC) coatings: a review. Surf. Coat. Tech. **200**, 2518–2524 (2005)
4. Lackner, J.M., Meindl, C., Wolf, C., Fian, A., Kittinger, C., Kot, M., Major, L., Czibula, C., Teichert, C., Waldhauser, W., Weinberg, A.M., FrÃühlich, E.: Gas permeation, mechanical behavior and cytocompatibility of ultrathin pure and doped diamond-like carbon and silicon oxide films. Coatings **3**(4), 268–300 (2013)
5. Krishnan, V., Krishnan, A., Remya, R., Ravikumar, K.K., Nair, S.A., Shibli, S.M.: Development and evaluation of two PVD-coated b-titanium orthodontic archwires for fluoride-induced corrosion protection. Acta. Biomater. **7**, 1913–1927 (2011)
6. Alanazi, A., Nojiri, C., Kido, T., Noguchi, T., Ohgoe, Y., Matsuda, T., Hirakuri, K., Funakubo, A., Sakai, K., Fukui, Y.: Engineering analysis of diamond-like carbon coated polymeric materials for biomedical applications. Artif. Organs. **24**(8), 624–627 (2000)
7. Lettington, A.H.: Applications of diamond films and related materials. In: Tzeng, Y., et al. (eds.) Materials Science Monographs, vol. 73, p. 703. Elsevier, New York (1991)

8. Kim, J.H., Shin, J.H., Shin, D.H., Moon, M.W., Park, K., Kim, T.H., Shin, K.M., Won, Y.H., Han, D.K., Lee, K.R.: Comparison of diamond-like carbon-coated nitinol stents with or without polyethylene glycol grafting and uncoated nitinol stents in a canine iliac artery model. Br. J. Radiol. **84**(999), 210–215 (2011)

9. Zheng, C., Ran, J., Yin, G., Lei, W.: In: Tzeng, Y., et al. (eds.) Applications of Diamond Films and Related Materials. Materials Science Monographs, p. 711. Elsevier, New York (1991)

10. Alanzi, A., Nojiri, C., Noguchi, T., Ohgoe, Y., Matsuda, T., Hirakuri, K., Funakubo, A., Sakai, K., Fukui, Y.: Engineering analysis of diamondâĂŘLike carbon coated polymeric materials for biomedical applications. Artif. Organs. **24**(8), 624–627 (2000)

11. Sanak, M., Jakieła, B., Wegrzyn, W.: Assessment of hemocompatibility of materials with arterial blood flow by platelet functional tests. B. Pol. Acad. Sci. Tech. **58**(2), 317–322 (2010)

12. Anderson, J.M., Rodriguez, A., Chang, D.T.: Foreign body reaction to biomaterials. Semin. Immunol. **2**, 86–100 (2008)

13. Williams, D.F.: A model for biocompatibility and its evaluation. J. Biomed. Eng. **11**, 185–191 (1989)

14. Amara, U., Rittirsch, D., Flierl, M., Bruckner, U., Klos, A., Gebhard, F., Lambris, J.D., Huber-Lang, M.: Interaction between the coagulation and complement system. Adv. Exp. Med. Biol. **632**, 71–79 (2008)

15. Lackner, J.M., Waldhauser, W., Major, R., Major, B., Bruckert, F.: Hemocompatible, pulsed laser deposited coatings on polymers. Biomed. Tech. **55**, 57–64 (2010)

Modelling and Simulations
in Biomechanics

Trends in Biomechanical Finite Element Breast Deformation Modelling

Marta Danch-Wierzchowska[1]($\boxtimes$), Kamil Gorczewski[2], Damian Borys[1], and Andrzej Swierniak[1]

[1] Institute of Automatic Control, Silesian University of Technology,
Akademicka 16, 44-100 Gliwice, Poland
`marta.danch-wierzchowska@polsl.pl`
[2] Department of PET Diagnostics, Maria Sklodowska-Curie Memorial Cancer Center
and Institute of Oncology, Gliwice Branch, Wybrzeze AK 15, 44-100 Gliwice, Poland

Abstract. Breast tissue deformation has recently gained interest in various medical application. The recovery of large deformation caused by gravity or compression loads and image registration is non-trivial task. The need arise to estimate large breast deformation, which can mimic natural body movement caused by examinations or surgery. Finite element methods (FEM) have been widely applied in this field. In this work we present the current breast deformation modelling trend. The meaningful applications and essentials examinations are described. The modelling software and basic techniques are presented.

Keywords: Breast deformation · FEM · Breast modelling

1 Introduction

Breast cancer is the most frequent women's cancer around the world and is the second most frequent among all human cancers. Consequently, diagnosis needs to be precise and fast, whereas treatment needs to be as personalised as possible. Considering specific anatomy of the female breast any examination or intervention results in breast deformation. Due to that, on every resulting image set the tumour in question is placed in different area. There are several methods, which were created to allow fusion of images obtained in different modalities. One can discriminate three types of deformation models: geometric transformation based on physical models, geometric transformation derived from interpolation theory and knowledge-based geometric transformation [32]. In case of breast deformation modelling both types of geometric transformation are mainly used for rigid and small non-rigid deformation (i.e. respiratory movements) [27]. To model big non-rigid deformation (i.e. mammography compression or prone to supine movement) knowledge-based transformation inspired by biomechanical models is used. The main motivation of biomechanical models usage is that more information enables reliable estimation of complex deformation [21]. Usually Finite Element

© Springer International Publishing AG 2017
M. Gzik et al. (eds.), *Innovations in Biomedical Engineering*, Advances in Intelligent
Systems and Computing 526, DOI 10.1007/978-3-319-47154-9_12

Method (FEM) is used to model biomechanical properties of tissue [32]. FEM is a numerical technique, which allows approximate solving of partial differential equations (PDE). Solving PDE for complex structures is reached by decomposing object domain into smaller elements which limits degrees of freedom of the object and simplified computations.

This paper presents briefly main ideas and techniques in FEM breast deformation modelling.

2   Finite Element Modelling of Breast Deformation

2.1   Model Simplification

Breast modelling relates strictly to its anatomical structure. Female breast consist of glandular lobules, adipose, milk ducts, connective tissues and skin. It is impossible to model glandular lobules and milk ducts as separate layers, since it is almost impossible to differentiate them on the MRI. Due to that, these are both usually treated as one fibroglandular tissue. Between breast tissue and chest wall, there is pectoralis muscle, which also determines the breast shape and movement.

2.2   Modelling Applications

There are several applications of biomechanical breast modelling. Almost all of them are related to breast cancer diagnostics and treatment. The oldest praxis is a mammography simulation which presents the breast deformation caused by the plates compression [14,24]. Another, more recent, application is breast deformation caused by the gravitational force. Such simulation is commonly used when different breasts shapes comparison is needed [15]. Breast shape simulation in different patient positions is used while treatment planning and to locate tumour during medical procedures, e.g. a biopsy procedure [2].

The breast cancer related simulations are used to predict the breast deformation in order to predict tumour location [3]. Examination performed in different patient position using equipment causing deformation needs to be converted into one space. Known practice is comparison between breast MRI and mammograms [35]. The modelling task is to get mammograms into MRI space. Fusion of different examinations helps with more accurate diagnosis [1]. There are also visualizations performed to simulate breast reconstruction after mastectomy [36]. The same praxis is used during a standard plastic surgery, which may not be related with the breast cancer [10]. FEM deformation modelling is also used to test movement of breast implant materials [11].

2.3   Model Input Data

The model usually is created using data from *in-vivo* acquisitions with modalities as described in following subsections [12,19]. However, in some cases it is more optimal to use known geometry and data conditions. A phantom measurements are very useful to obtain that aim [22].

2.3.1 Mammography

Mammography technique uses low-energy X-rays to contrast very low differences in electron densities between breast tissues. It has very high resolution in comparison to others modalities, but it requires high doses of radiation. High sensitivity and low risk on inducing cancer in women population after age of 50 makes it a perfect tool for screening [4]. The mammograms are taken while the breast is compressed for stabilization and better image quality. In most cases craniocaudal (CC) view and mediolateral oblique (MLO) images of the breast are taken. Any suspected regions of higher density are localised for biopsy and tissue identification.

2.3.2 Magnetic Resonance Imaging

The Magnetic Resonance Imaging (MRI) uses differences in proton's magnetization relaxation times to create contrast in images. MRI can create anatomical images of proton (water) concentrations and relaxation times. Additionally, MRI can create functional images like metabolite imaging, diffusion imaging and blood oxidation imaging. It can also measure flows of blood. During the examination a patient is in prone position with breasts placed in signal receiving coils. Breasts are not fixated. It is very safe technique because the MRI do not use the ionizing radiation. The possibility of multiple contrasts acquisitions, both anatomical and functional, plays a key role of MRI breast cancer detection.

2.3.3 Positron Emission Tomography and Computer Tomography

Positron emission tomography with computed tomography (PET) is a functional imaging modality. A radio-tracer is injected to patient and it binds according to its metabolic path. In breast cancer a Flurodeoxyglucose is administered. This radio-traces accumulates in all cells that use energy and the uptake is proportional to energy consumption. This method is very sensitive due to selective uptake, but it lacks of specificity. Higher uptake of glucose may localize, beside the cancer, inflammations, mechanical injuries and all other physiological processes that temporally elevate the glucose consumption. In breast cancer, the PET is used for metastasis localisation and for therapy effectiveness evaluation. Since the breast cancer is localised, the PET examinations during the chemotherapy can monitor the effects on-line and allows for treatment adjustments [33]. The patient is scanned in supine position with arms above the head and the breasts are not fixated.

2.3.4 3D Scanning

3D Scanning is a 3D, non-invasive surface imaging method. 3D scanning allows to acquire spatial coordinates of surface points with relative high resolution. 3D scanning provides useful information about shape [30]. It is commonly used to pre- and postoperatively evaluate breast shape [7]. Recent work presents also 3D scanning as a tool used for breast surface deformation simulation and correspondence finding. However, commercially available system do not take into account the biomechanical behavior of the tissue [10].

2.4 Modelling Software

To create breast model and deform it, several programs can be used. All of them are based on similar modelling techniques mentioned in further sections. The software used can be divided into two types. The first group consists of general purpose modeling software, like ANSYS [12,35], Abacus [40], MSC.Marc [31], which in particular case allow to create a breast deformation model. The second group consists of dedicated algorithms created in research facilities, specifically for breast modelling [3,16]. There are also papers which present solutions based on both own algorithms and commercial software [19,28].

2.5 Modelling Techniques

In breast deformation problem, one can specify a few issues that need to be addressed. According to breast deformation modelling medical images obtained during mammography, MRI or PET-CT examinations constitute basis for the domain creation.

2.5.1 Types of Mesh

To approximate breast shape created from medical images two mesh types are chosen. The most common is tetrahedral mesh [10,12,24,31], i.e. each element is a polygon composed from four triangular faces. Tetrahedron could be 4-nodes or 10-nodes. Another, less often used, is hexahedral mesh, i.e. each element is a polygon composed from six faces [3]. Similar to tetrahedrons there are more than one type of hexahedrons. One can discriminate between 8-nodes, 20-nodes and 27-nodes hexahedrons. Mesh element type determines it's shape function, which characterizes nodes dependencies and some of the material properties. Depending on the shape function one can obtain different computation precision. The more complex shape function of the element, the more precise the result, but also longer computational time. In practice, the simplest 4-nodes tetrahedron and 8-nodes hexahedrons meshes are used.

2.5.2 Types of Tissues Considered in Modelling

Whole model, also called object or geometry consist of layers, which represent individual tissue types. In general, breast models consist of fat, muscle and glandular tissues, tumour and skin. However, there are set of models, which do not consider separate part for skin. Fat tissue with modified parameters is treated as external model boundary [14,19]. There are also models, in which fat and fibroglandular tissues are one part with averaged parameters [9,16].

2.5.3   Types of Boundary Conditions

Boundary conditions describe models boundary behaviour. When concerning mammography simulation, the reaction between breast and compression plates needs to be described. The contact is modelled as frictionless [14], rough - no sliding [19] or as frictional, with estimated friction coefficient [22] e.g. set on values 0.2 [31] or 0.5 % [35]. In every type of model, back side of the breast needs to be considered. Created model ends on thorax wall [12,24,35], which movement can be also simulate [9]. Representation of the tissues boundaries are modelled as rigid - shared nodes between fat and glandular [19], surface based motion constrained for chest wall movement [8], frictionless - free sliding between chest wall and muscles [15] or constrained to zero-displacement - fixed chest wall [31] with Dirichlet boundary conditions [17].

2.5.4   Types of Tissue Constitutive Models

The simplest way to model breast deformations is to treat the whole object as isotropic, linear elastic, homogeneous, incompressible body - Poisson ratio close to 0.5 (eg. 0.4995) [35]. However to represent specific breast movement, there are several types of models, which represent the tissue behaviour in more reliable way. Most popular way to describe stress-strain relationship for fat and glandular tissues is the hyperelastic neo-Hokean constitutive model [14,18], isotropic with right Cauchy-Green deformation tensor [10,22]. There are also anisotropic [24], quasi-incompresible [13] and polynomial quadratic hyperelastic [35] models.

2.5.5   Model Parameters

In breast deformation modelling three main parameters are taken into account: Young modulus, which defines the relationship between stress and strain in a material, Poisson ratio, which is the negative ratio of transverse to axial strain and material density. The first two material parameters are usually set as constant [24] or optimised during simulations [12], with constant initial value, upper and lower limits [14]. Material density differs from real measured values, to water density for every model part.

Fat material parameters have more influence on deformation results than fibroglandular material parameters. 10 % fat parameter change results in 10 % change in deformation. 10 % fibroglandular parameters change results in 1 % change in deformation [24]. According to deformation modelling small tumour parameters has negligible impact on breast deformation. Its stiffness should be 10 times greater, than surrounding tissue, to imply deformation change ca. 5 %. Such difference do not occur in nature [24]. However, there are significant stiffness differences measured for malignant and benign tumours, which influences breast deformation [23]. Moreover spiculated tumour generate stress increase at a local level [39].

One of the reliability testing method is verification of calculated von-Mises stress values [17]. Another method is comparing resulting model with real MRI or mammograms [15,35] or with landmarks applied on patient skin [25].

2.6   Modelling Difficulties

Despite different models development there appear some limitations that cause inaccuracies of the created models. The main issue is accurate tissue parameter estimation. Biomechanical properties of breast tissues have been measured *ex vivo* [29,38]. However living tissues have different properties that those, extracted from body, void of blood circulation. Moreover existing *in vivo* measuring methods (i.e. elastography) do not provide information precise enough to estimate big deformation [20]. Another issue is accurate mesh selection. Different types of mesh elements and different mesh node density gives different results [28] and in some cases the FE mesh requires manual intervention [14] as well as image segmentation [15,24]. Further difficulty provides boundary conditions setting, especially on chest wall side, where the model ends but the real body consistency needs to be preserved [34]. Still unsolved modelling issue remains patient-specific fully-automation, which is essential in clinical practice.

3   Conclusions

This paper provides an overview of FEM practices applicable to breast deformation modelling. Common breast deformation practices have been outlined. The most popular models and techniques have been described and key difficulties for future development have been specified. Authors are currently working on own deformation model, which would enable patient-specific fusion of PET-CT and MR images in supine position. Our preliminary results and conclusions were presented in [5,6].

Acknowledgements. This work was supported by the National Science Centre (NCN) under Grant No. 2011/03/B/ST6/04384 (AS), the Polish National Center of Research and Development grant no. STRATEGMED2/267398/4/NCBR/2015 (DB,KG) and the Institute of Automatic Control under Grant No. BKM/506/RAU1/2016/t.7 (MDW).

References

1. De Abreu, F.B., Wells, W.A., Tsongalis, G.J.: The emerging role of the molecular diagnostics laboratory in breast cancer personalized medicine. Am. J. Pathol. **183**(4), 1075–1083 (2013)
2. Azar, F.S., Metaxas, D.N., Schnall, M.D.: A finite element model of the breast for predicting mechanical deformations during biopsy procedures. In: Proceedings of the IEEE Workshop on Mathematical Methods in Biomedical Image Analysis, pp. 38–45 (2000)
3. Azar, F.S., Metaxas, D.N., Schnall, M.D.: Methods for modelling predicting mechanical deformations of the breast under external perturbations. Med. Image Anal. **6**, 1–27 (2002)
4. Bleyer, A., Welch, G.: Effect of Three decades of screening mammography on breast-cancer incidence. N. Engl. J. Med. **367**, 1998–2005 (2012)

5. Danch-Wierzchowska, M., Borys, D., Swierniak, A.: Breast deformation modeling based on MRI images, preliminary results. Inf. Technol. Med. **472**, 227–234 (2016)
6. Danch-Wierzchowska, M., Borys, D., Bobek-Billewicz, B., Jarzab, M., Swierniak, A.: Simplification of breast deformation modelling to support breast cancer treatment planning. Preliminary Results Biomed. Eng. **36**(4), 531–536 (2016)
7. Dehghani, H., Doyley, M.M., Pogue, B.W., Jiang, S., Geng, J., Paulsen, K.D.: Breast deformation modelling for image reconstruction in near infrared optical tomography. Phys. Med. Biol. **49**(7), 1131–1145 (2004)
8. Eiben, B., Vavourakis, V., Hipwell, J.H., Kabus, S., Buelow, T., Lorenz, C., Mertzanidou, T., Reis, S., Williams, N.R., Keshtgar, M., Hawkes, D.J.: Symmetric biomechanically guided prone-to-supine breast image registration. Ann. Biomed. Eng. **44**(1), 154–173 (2016)
9. Gamage, T.P.B., Boyes, R., Rajagopal, V., Nielsen, P.M.F., Nash, M.P.: Modelling prone to supine breast deformation under gravity loading using heterogeneous finite element models. In: Computational Biomechanics for Medicine, pp. 29–38 (2012)
10. Georgii, J., Eder, M., BÄijrger, K., Klotz, S., Ferstl, F., Kovacs, L., Westermann, R.: A computational tool for preoperative breast augmentation planning in aesthetic plastic surgery. IEEE J. Biomed. Health Inform. **18**(3), 907-19 (2014)
11. Haddad, S.M., Omidi, E., Flynn, L.E., Samani, A.: Comparative biomechanical study of using decellularized human adipose tissues for post-mastectomy and post-lumpectomy breast reconstruction. J. Mech. Behav. Biomed. Mater. **57**, 235–245 (2016)
12. Han, L., Hipwell, J., Taylor, Z., Tanner, C., Ourselin, S., Hawkes, D.J.: Fast deformation simulation of breasts using GPU-based dynamic explicit finite element method. Digit. Mammo. **6136**, 728–735 (2010)
13. Han, L., Hipwell, J., Mertzanidou, T., Carter, T., Modat, M., Ourselin, S., Hawkes, D.: A hybrid FEM-based method for aligning prone and supine images for image guided breast surgery. In: 2011 IEEE International Symposium on Biomedical Imaging, From Nano to Macro, pp. 1239–1242 (2011)
14. Han, L., Hipwell, J., Tanner, C., Taylor, Z., Mertzanidou, T., Cardoso, J., Ourselin, S., Hawkes, D.: Development of patient specific biomechanical models for predicting large breast deformation. Phys. Med. Biol. **57**, 455–472 (2012)
15. Han, L., Hipwell, J.H., Eiben, B., Barratt, D., Modat, M., Ourselin, S., Hawkes, D.J.: A nonlinear biomechanical model based registration method for aligning prone and supine MR breast images. IEEE Trans. Med. Imaging **33**(3), 682–694 (2014)
16. Harz, M., Georgii, J., Schilling, K., Hahn, H.K.: Towards navigated breast surgery using efficient breast deformation simulation. In: Proceedings of Workshop on Breast Image Analysis, pp. 137–144 (2011)
17. Harz, M.T., Georgii, J., Schilling, K., Hahn, H.K.: Real-time breast defomation using non-linear tissue properties. In: Lecture Notes in Informatics, vol. 192 (2011)
18. Hopp, T., Baltzer, P., Dietzel, M., Kaiser, W.A., Ruiter, N.V.: 2D/3D image fusion of X-ray mammograms with breast MRI: visualizing dynamic contrast enhancement in mammograms. Int. J. Comput. Assist. Radiol. Surg. **7**(3), 339–348 (2012)
19. Hopp, T., Dietzel, M., Baltzer, P.A., Kreisel, P., Kaiser, W.A., Gemmeke, H., Ruiter, N.V.: Automatic multimodal 2D/3D breast image registration using biomechanical FEM models and intensity-based optimization. Med. Image Anal. **17**(2), 209–218 (2013)
20. Insana, M.F., Liu, J., Sridhar, M., Pellot-Barakat, C.: Ultrasonic Mechanical Relaxation Imaging and the Material Science of Breast Cancer IEEE Ultrasonics Symposium (2005)

21. Lee, A.W.C., Schnabel, J.A., Rajagopal, V., Nielsen, P.M.F., Nash, M.P.: Breast image registration by combining finite elements and free-form deformations. In: Martí, J., Oliver, A., Freixenet, J., Martí, R. (eds.) IWDM 2010. LNCS, vol. 6136, pp. 736–743. Springer, Heidelberg (2010). doi:10.1007/978-3-642-13666-5_99

22. Lee, A.W., Rajagopal, V., Babarenda Gamage, T.P., Doyle, A.J., Nielsen, P.B., Nash, M.P.: Breast lesion co-localisation between X-ray and MR images using finite element modelling. Med. Image Anal. **17**(8), 1256–1264 (2013)

23. Lorenzen, J., Sinkus, R., Lorenzen, M., Dargatz, M., Leussler, C., Räüschmann, P., Adam, G.: MR elastography of the breast: preliminary clinical results. Rofo. **174**(7), 830–834 (2002)

24. Pathmanathan, P., Gavaghan, D.J., Whiteley, J.P., Chapman, S.J., Brady, J.M.: Predicting tumor location by modeling the deformation of the breast. IEEE Trans. Biomed. Eng. **55**(10), 2471–2480 (2008)

25. del Palomar, A.P., Calvo, B., Herrero, J., Lãşpez, J., Doblarãl', M.: A finite element model to accurately predict real deformations of the breast. Med. Eng. Phys. **30**(9), 1089–1097 (2008)

26. Ramiao, N., Martins, P., Fernandes, A.A.: Biomechanical properties of breast tissue. In: ENBENG 2013, pp. 1–6 (2013)

27. Rueckert, D., Sonoda, L.I., Hayes, C., Hill, D.L., Leach, M.O., Hawkes, D.J.: Non-rigid registration using free-form deformations: application to breast MR images. IEEE Trans. Med. Imaging **18**(8), 712–721 (1999)

28. Samani, A., Bishop, J., Yaffe, M.J., Plewes, D.B.: Biomechanical 3-D finite element modeling of the human breast using MRI data. IEEE Trans. Med. Imaging **20**(4), 271–279 (2001)

29. Samani, A., Zubovits, J., Plewes, D.: Elastic moduli of normal and pathological human breast tissues: an inversion-technique-based investigation of 169 samples. Phys. Med. Biol. **52**(6), 1565–1576 (2007)

30. Seo, H., Cordier, F., Hong, K.: A breast modeler based on analysis of breast scans. Comput. Anima. Virtual Worlds **18**(2), 141–151 (2007)

31. Shih, T.C., Chen, J.H., Lium, D., Nie, K., Sun, L., Lin, M., Chang, D., Nalcioglu, O., Su, M.Y.: Computational simulation of breast compression based on segmented breast and fibroglandular tissues on magnetic resonance images. Phys. Med. Biol. **55**(14), 4153–4168 (2010)

32. Sotiras, A., Davatzikos, C., Paragios, N.: Deformable medical image registration: a survey. IEEE Trans. Med. Imaging **32**(7), 1153–1190 (2013)

33. Dose, S.J., Bader, M., Jenicke, L., Hemminger, G., JÃd'nicke, F., Avril, N.: Early prediction of response to chemotherapy in metastatic breast cancer using sequential 18F-FDG PET. J. Nucl. Med. **46**(7), 1144–1150 (2005)

34. Tanner, C., Schnabel, J., Smith, A.C., Sonoda, L., Hill, D., Hawkes, D., Degenhard, A., Hayes, C., Leach, M., Hose, D.: The comparison of biomechanical breast models: initial results. In: ANSYSConvergence, Pittsburgh, PA, US, April 2002

35. Tanner, C., Hipwell, J.H., Hawkes, D.J., Szekely, G.: Breast shapes on real and simulated mammograms. Digit. Mammo. **6136**, 540–547 (2010)

36. Thanoon, D., Garbey, M., Kim, N., Bass, B.: A computational framework for breast surgery: application to breast conserving therapy. In: Computational Surgery and Dual Training, 5, pp. 249–266 (2009)

37. Wang, L., Filippatos, K., Friman, O., Hahn, H.K.: Fully automated segmentation of the pectoralis muscle boundary in breast MR images. In: Medical Imaging, Computer-Aided Diagnosis, p. 796309 (2011)

38. Wellman, P.S., Howe, R.D., Dalton, E., Kern, K.A.: Breast tissue stiffness in compression is correlated to histological diagnosis. J. Biomech. p. 4017745 (1999)

39. Wessel, C., Schnabel, J.A., Brady, M.: Towards a more realistic biomechanical modelling of breast malignant tumours. Phys. Med. Biol. **57**(3), 631–648 (2012)
40. Wessel, C., Schnabel, J.A., Brady, M.: Realistic biomechanical model of a cancerous breast for the registration of prone to supine deformations. EMBC **2013**, 7249–7252 (2013)

Inertial Sensors and Wavelets Analysis as a Tool for Pathological Gait Identification

Sebastian Glowinski[✉], Andrzej Blazejewski, and Tomasz Krzyzynski

Technical University of Koszalin, Sniadeckich 2, 75-453 Koszalin, Poland
`sebastian.glowinski@tu.koszalin.pl`
`http://wtie.tu.koszalin.pl`

Abstract. The human gait analysis by using wavelets transform of signal obtained from six inertial ProMove mini sensors is proposed in this work. The angular velocity data measured by the gyro sensors were used to estimate the translational acceleration in the gait analysis. As a result, the flexion - extension of joint angles of the knees were calculated for healthy people and with impaired locomotion system. After measurements we propose to use one of wavelet transform (wavelet type) in order to analyze the signals, indicate a characteristic feature and compare them.

Keywords: Human gait · Inertial sensors · Wavelet analysis

1 Introduction

Gait analysis is a clinical tool for obtaining quantitative information of the gait of a person to diagnose walking disabilities [5,6]. Common methods of gait analysis include using cameras to track the position of body by using reflective markers. Although this conventional system has been utilized successfully in many research fields, such as sport and clinics, it is limited to the laboratory work space required by the camera [7]. An alternative is to use acceleration and angular velocity data measured from inertial sensors attached to the body. Miniature inertial sensors are steadily gaining interest because of their limited power consumption, low cost and good user compliance when they are embedded in wearable sensor systems or portable devices [2]. Currently several applications in human motion analysis may benefit from miniature inertial sensors [1,12]. Human body motions are captured and measured, next inertial data from IMUs are transmitted to computer via Bluetooth. Then data are processing because this method does not directly measure position. A major challenge is to translate these data into meaningful three dimensional positional data, such as the joint angles of hip, knee and ankle. The differences between lower limbs can be used for evaluating symmetric gait or some of disorders.

© Springer International Publishing AG 2017
M. Gzik et al. (eds.), *Innovations in Biomedical Engineering*, Advances in Intelligent Systems and Computing 526, DOI 10.1007/978-3-319-47154-9_13

2   Wireless Sensing System

The sensing system is composed of six body area wireless inertial sensor nodes based on ProMove mini platform [13]. The system creates the bridge between inertial measurements units and wireless sensor networks. It is embedding in one device the following: 10 degrees-of-freedom inertial sensors: ± 2 to 16 g accelerometer, $\pm 250°/s$ to $2000°/s$ gyroscope with resolution $0.007°/s$ and $\pm 250°/s$ range and magnetic field intensity (compass), 2 GB flash memory in each sensor, low-power RF transceiver in the 2.4 GHz license-free band. Inertia gateway as a central hub for synchronized data collection <100 ns. Battery life 4 h in full streaming mode.

The ergonomic design of ProMove-mini allows for easy strap attachment and body mount. Each sensor unit is 51-46-15 mm with weight 20 g (including battery). The Inertia Studio software enables real-time visualization of sensor data, as well as over-the-air reconfiguration of the sensors and wireless parameters. All data retrieved by the Inertia Studio software is logged for post-analysis. As shown in the Fig. 1, the ProMove mini sensors are placed on the part of body along the right and left leg on the thigh, shank and foot. In global coordinate system (green color) the x-axis is the walking direction, y-axis lateral direction and z-axis opposite direction of gravity. For each sensor the orientation is calculated relative to Earth reference frame in terms of roll, pitch and yaw angles. By combining the orientation of each node, we obtain the joint angles.

By using four quaternion parameters q_0, q_1, q_2, q_3 obtained from the investigations carried out in this work, we calculated the Euler angles of each node as follows

$$\theta = \arcsin\left(2(q_0 q_2 - q_3 q_1)\right) \tag{1}$$

where θ means rotation about y-axis.

3   Experiment

The main objective of our experiments is to validate the knee angle in sagittal plane and wavelet analysis of human gait. To achieve these objectives, we focus in the experiments on the following tasks:

- prepare the patient for testing (interview about the illnesses locomotor) and connect the gateway to the computer and sensor parameter settings (sampling 200 Hz);
- mount the sensor as shown in Fig. 1, turn sensors on and verify that data is received from all of them;
- standing starting position for the examination of the patient;
- resetting the button resets the algorithm used for calculating the orientation. After resetting, it is necessary hold the nodes still for a few seconds to stabilize their orientation;
- start recording (patient goes) and stop recording;

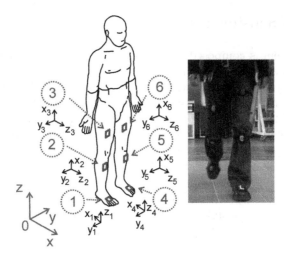

Fig. 1. The human model and coordinate systems. The x, y, z coordinates represent the global coordinate system, the x_s, y_s, z_s represents the sensor coordinate system (a), subject wearing the ProMove mini nodes (b)

- collect all the raw data from all sensors to a central computer via the USB (by using wireless system at the highest possible data rate there is packet loss). Therefore packet loss can be avoided by enabling flash logging and download-ing the logs after the experiment (via USB cable is faster);
- process the data on the computer and marking the beginning of each of the left and right step and calculation of the knee angles for the left and right leg as the arithmetic mean of several steps;
- data transformation into gait cycle and plots and wavelet analysis.

In the Fig. 2 the knee average flexion of left and right leg a health person in sagittal plane it is shown. The man 44 years old, 176 cm height and 76 kg weight. The angles were calculated by divided data into steps. Each step was interpolated, because there was different number of samples. The mean angle of right and left knee was transformed to the cycle. It is noted a slight difference between angles in loading response and swing (approx. 3°). In the left leg in stance phase there was noticed the characteristic change in flexion angle in 13–15 % of cycle, whereas in the right leg this phenomenon does not occur.

The 42 years male patient complaining of paralysis of the left foot limb. A study of MR spine lumbosacral. The smoothing lumbar lordosis and multi-level changes distort the intervertebral joints were determined. The symptoms of degenerative disc disease L4/L5/S1 with central protrusion disc m-k L5/S1 entailing root compression, and the center-left-sided disc protrusion m-k L4/L5 adjacent to the left L5 nerve root in the spinal canal. The conclusion was: The symptoms of lumbar disc L4/L5/S1, the more the left hand side at L4-L5 (Fig. 3). The disc herniation caused stretching and inflammation of an overlying nerve root. It also caused the leg pain, numbness and tingling and weakness in the

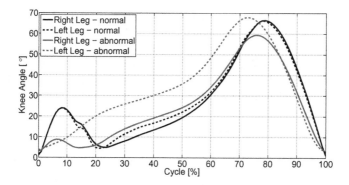

Fig. 2. Knee angles during a normal and abnormal gait

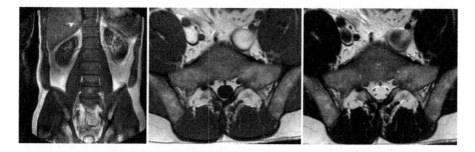

Fig. 3. The patient spine magnetic resonance-data from own sources

distribution of the nerve root. In the Fig. 2 red curves show knee angles in case of abnormal gait. The disc herniation caused stretching and inflammation of an overlying nerve root. It also caused the leg pain, numbness and tingling and weakness in the distribution of the nerve root.

4   Wavelet Analysis

The sensors transfer an acceleration signals, among others. The signals consist of three components related to three directions of Cartesian coordinate system of each sensor. The sum of the components is taken into consideration as analyzed signal, which describes the movement of the part of a leg. The signal includes acceleration of gravity. Because the human gait is characterized by periodicities and simultaneously some characteristic periods may occur in specific time periods, the wavelet tool is chosen. The advantage afforded by wavelets is the ability to perform local analysis. Because wavelets are localized in time and scale, wavelet coefficients are able to localize characteristic changes or differences in analyzed signals [3,4]. By shifting parameters of wavelets, they can be applied as a focus directed to interesting signal area described by time and scale related to frequencies.

Here it is introduced an algorithm combining discrete Fourier transform (DFT) and continuous wavelet transform (CWT). It applies DFT of the signal in first step and next the same transform of the analyzing wavelet at the appropriate angular frequencies in order to obtain directly comparable scales. In the next step the algorithm takes the product of the signal DFT and the wavelet DFT over all scales found. Eventually, it inverts the DFT to obtain the CWT coefficients. This procedure easy allows to convert wavelets scales to frequencies, precisely to so-called pseudo-frequencies. These pseudo-frequencies represent, not the exact frequencies, but some frequency ranges. But the most useful in the case of wavelets analysis is an ability of filtering and in the same time reconstruction of signal in the chosen range of scales. The Morlet wavelet is the analyzing wavelet in the using algorithm [8,9,11]. The conducted analysis shows some particular features of the human gait, which are not possible to observed in raw signal. Look out for important symptoms of human gait may be difficult as well in raw signal. The example of analysis of one step during a gait health person, for the sensors number 2 and 5 placed on right and left leg, is shown in Fig. 4.

In the Fig. 4a, b it is shown the analyzed signal and the signal after reconstruction by using inverse wavelet transform. These analyses are conducted in the case of normal gait i.e. during health person walk. In the upper row of figures one can see at first measured and next reconstructed signals (red curves), respectively for right and left leg. Both signals look like to be the same, which indicates that the wavelet transform does not cause any loss of information when it is conducted in properly width range of scales. Additionally in first figures for each leg in the upper row, blue curves show the signal which is reconstructed for chosen, limited range of scales. These limited range is considered as the part of the signal represents main feature of each leg movement during one step. In these figures (Fig. 4a, b) in the middle row, in first figures in case of each leg, there are absolute scales values (modulus) of wavelet coefficients shown. This kind of analysis, in a form of bands seen in these figures, may deliver details about components of a gait characterized by constant periodicity (frequencies), having variation similar to harmonic functions, for instance sine function. In the next figures there are shown real parts of wavelet coefficients, which precisely shown the periodicity. In the side legends of these figures the values of coefficients change from positive maximal to negative minimal values in the clearly seen areas in these particular figures. The area approximately between 0.24 and 0.49 scales values along whole time axis indicates constant pace of human gait. The character and variation of this pace, confirm the harmonic components, which is clearly seen in sides figures at the appropriate scales level. The other area is in the range of lower scales, at scale levels approximately below 0.24 value. First area up to about 0.25 ms is related to steps periods, when the human foot, at first moment a heel and next a mid-foot, take a contact with a floor and next it is lifted above. This period of step is represented in first 20 % of pace cycle, shown in Fig. 2 and characterized by appropriate knee angle changes. Next looking along the time axis at these figures, there is the another region that shows a moments, when a body weight

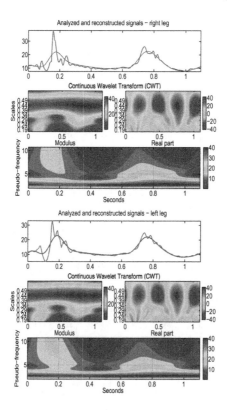

Fig. 4. The analyzed signal and reconstructed signal after inverse wavelets transform of a person right (a) and left (b) leg. Continuous wavelet transform of the analyzed signal obtained by using Morlet wavelet of parameter 4, where modulus, real part and modulus vs. pseudo-frequencies of wavelet coefficients are shown in case of normal gait.

is moved on other leg, what allows person step forward. In the Fig. 2. it is characterized by relatively large knee angle changes. It is seen in the figures, in the case of normal gait, that the pace is nearly harmonic. The main part of energy, which a man need to move, is relatively evenly distributed during the step and change harmonically during this step. The symmetry of the steps is also evident in these figures. Additionally, lower figures show the same wavelet transform as the figure presents absolute values (modulus) of wavelet coefficients but after recalculation to pseudo-frequencies. For comparison, in the Fig. 5 there is presented the case of abnormal gait obtained from a person with disease recorded and reported in the form of spine magnetic resonance, shown in Fig. 3. In real this disease appears as a human left leg limping. In the Fig. 5 there are recorded signal and analyzed by using the same wavelets with the same parameters as in case of normal gait. Comparing the analysis in both figures (Figs. 4 and 5) it is possible to observe the asymmetry of a gait in Fig. 5. In this case the significant

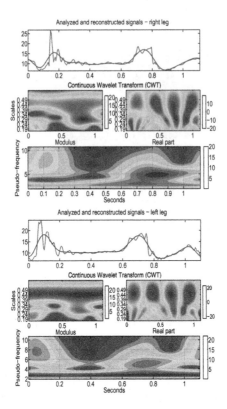

Fig. 5. The analyzed signal and reconstructed signal after inverse wavelets transform of a person right (a) and left (b) leg. Continuous wavelet transform of the analyzed signal obtained by using Morlet wavelet of parameter 4, where modulus, real part and modulus versus pseudo-frequencies of wavelet coefficients are shown below in case of abnormal gait.

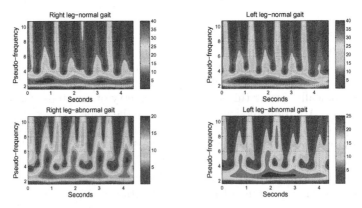

Fig. 6. Continuous wavelet transform of the analyzed signal obtained by using Morlet wavelet of parameter 4, modulus versus pseudo-frequencies of wavelet coefficients are shown in case of normal and abnormal gait for several step.

differences occur in scales low value range. In comparison to Fig. 4 i.e. the normal gait, the abnormality occurs in Fig. 5 as the areas in time range from 0 s to 0.2 s and from 0.6 s to 0.9 s in both legs. In the first time's range the sum of acceleration components and in the same way force characterized by pseudo-frequency between 6–10 Hz and in the second time range by pseudo-frequency between 4–6 Hz represents this abnormality. The next difference is clearly seen in values of wavelets coefficients in harmonic band of normal and abnormal gait signal. The normal gait is nearly harmonic and main amount of force is imposed on that period. In the case of normal gait the values of wavelet coefficients in harmonic band for both legs equal 40, while in the case of abnormal gait equal approximately 15 for right leg and 25 for left leg. It seems that some part of energy is "wasted" on unwanted movement. That mention above is confirmed in case of several steps analyzed in sequence shown in Fig. 6. It is still seen fro that analysis that normal gait is harmonic, which is the effect opposite to abnormal gait. In each step in case of person with disease is the additional force or move component in higher frequency than harmonic component.

5 Discussion

We presented the design of a portable wireless sensor network that can be used for real-time monitoring of lower-limb kinematics during gait. Due to the importance of the joint kinematics to assess the gait technique, we focus on measuring the knee joint angle. We performed experiments with a health and person and with patient with a lumbar disc. Firstly, the MR was performed and after diagnosis the experiment was done. The solution proposed is not constrained to obtain lower limb angles only. It can be used for analyzing human abnormal locomotion. In this work the wavelet transform is applied for chosen signal represented by acceleration. On the one hand it gives a information about the force introduce during the gait and other hand the wavelet transformation of this signal gives a energy concentration during the gait and possibility to focus on chosen part of signal simultaneously in time and frequency domain. These feature may be a useful tool to compare the specific details and differences in human gait. Next the analysis give the possibility to recognize a specific feature of abnormality in human gait caused by specific diseases. The many more analysis are possible using wavelets. In the paper we propose the methodology, which helps to recognize specific feature of human gait, that can be useful in health diagnostic or sport individual training programs creation.

References

1. Bamberg, S.J.M., Benbasat, A.Y., Scarborough, D.M., Krebs, D.E., Paradiso, J.A.: Gait analysis using a shoe-integrated wireless sensor system. IEEE Trans. Inf. Technol. Biomed. **12**, 413–423 (2008)
2. Chen, X.: Human Motion Analysis with Wearable Inertial Sensors. University of Tennessee, Doctoral Dissertation, Knoxville (2013)

3. Daubechies, I.: Ten Lectures on Wavelets Philadelphia. Society for Industrial and Applied Mathematics (SIAM), Philadelphia (1992)
4. Farage, M.: Wavelet transforms and their application to turbulence. Ann. Rev. Fluid. Mech. **24**, 395–457 (1992)
5. Glowinski, S., Krzyzynski, T.: An inverse kinematic algorithm for human leg. J. Theor. Appl. Mech. **54**(1), 53–61 (2016)
6. Glowinski, S., Krzyzynski, T., Pecolt, S., Maciejewski, I.: Design of motion trajectory of an arm exoskeleton. Arch. Appl. Mech. **85**, 75–87 (2015)
7. Liu, T., Inoue, Y., Shibata, K., Shiojima, K., Han, M.M.: Triaxial joint moment estimation using a wearable three-dimensional gait analysis system. Measurement **47**, 125–129 (2014)
8. Mallat, S.: A Wavelet Tour of Signal Processing. Academic Press, San Diego, CA (1998)
9. Sun, W.: Convergence of Morlet's Reconstruction Formula. Preprint (2010)
10. Tadano, S., Takeda, R., Miyagawa, H.: Three dimensional gait analysis using wearable acceleration and gyro sensors based on quaternion calculations. Sensors **13**, 9321–9343 (2013)
11. Torrence, C., Compo, G.P.: A practical guide to wavelet analysis. Bull. Am. Meteorol. Soc. **79**, 61–78 (1998)
12. Zhu, R., Zhou, Z.A.: A real-time articulated human motion tracking using tri-axis inertial/magnetic sensors package. IEEE Trans. Neural Syst. Rehabil. Eng. **12**, 295–302 (2004)
13. ProMove wireless inertial sensing platform. http://www.inertia-technology.com/promovemini

Interactive System of Enginering Support of Upper Limb Diagnosis

Marek Gzik[1], Piotr Wodarski[2], Jacek Jurkojć[2], Robert Michnik[3], and Andrzej Bieniek[4(✉)]

[1] Department of Biomechatronics, Silesian University of Technology,
ul. Roosevelta 40 p. 118a, 41-800 Zabrze, Poland
`mgzik@polsl.pl`
[2] Department of Biomechatronics, Silesian University of Technology,
ul. Roosevelta 40 p. 125, 41-800 Zabrze, Poland
`{pwodarski,jjurkojc}@polsl.pl`
[3] Department of Biomechatronics, Silesian University of Technology,
ul. Roosevelta 40 p. 119, 41-800 Zabrze, Poland
`rmichnik@polsl.pl`
[4] Department of Biomechatronics, Silesian University of Technology,
ul. Roosevelta 40 p. 114, 41-800 Zabrze, Poland
`abieniek@polsl.pl`

Abstract. System of engineering support of upper limb diagnosis was developed and verified as a part of the research. Virtual Cave 3D, System VRTouchDevice and inertial motion analysis system MVNBiomech were used to build this system. In cooperation with the physiotherapist 2 applications were developed to motivate to do exercises during which kinematic parameters of the examined people were registered. The prepared system was positively verified by correlating waveforms angles in joints for a physiotherapist with the waveforms of people who exercise in the developed system.

Keywords: Upper limb · Diagnostic · Technology of virtual reality · System Cave 3D · Virtual Cave 3D

1 Introduction

The use of computer graphics in the process of engineering support of diagnosis and therapy can be used to treat many ailments associated with abnormal or limited functions of the nervous system, skeletal and muscle system or impairments of cognitive and sensory functions [1–3]. Modern IT tools allow to effect many senses at the same time through specially designed, and consulted with doctors and physiotherapists, stimuli and scenarios applications in the world of two-dimensional and three-dimensional graphics. An increased activity of selected parts of the brain, obtained by suitably prepared visual stimulation [6], was also confirmed on the basis of the EEG measurement. This knowledge is used in researches on stimulating parts of the brain responsible for social reactions

© Springer International Publishing AG 2017
M. Gzik et al. (eds.), *Innovations in Biomedical Engineering*, Advances in Intelligent Systems and Computing 526, DOI 10.1007/978-3-319-47154-9_14

and learning [7] as well as maintaining an upright posture [4,5]. This technology is also used in the process of overcoming fears associated with the course of the therapeutic process and to increase motivation to exercise. This technology has attracted interest of patients, and by its interactivity, allows real-time correction of exercise. The literature review provides us with information on the effectiveness of systems based on Virtual Reality Technology in the field of: a supplement of traditional therapeutic methods, the positive impact of the use of virtual rehabilitation systems for posture control, improvement of the efficiency of visual processing, increase mobility and improve physical performance [1–3,7]. Still, there are no systems that would provide information useful in the diagnosis while simultaneously doing exercises.

2   Purpose of Research

The aim of the research is to develop and verify system of engineering support of the diagnosis of upper limb using Virtual Reality Technology.

3   Designing Interactive System of Engineering Support of Upper Limb Diagnosis

The construction of the diagnostics support system was based on the spatial image projection system called the Virtual Cave 3D together with interacting systems "MVNBiomech" and "VRTouchDevice." The system is modular, so it is possible to connect more devices to enrich its function. The developed solution is a tool that can be dedicated to the rehabilitation and diagnosis of many diseases depending upon the used applications and the hardware modules connected with motion tracking and feedback.

3.1   The Hardware

Cave system consists of a space bounded by four canvas screens (left, right, front and floor) on which the image is displayed, synchronized between neighbouring areas. Therefore the available exercise space is a cube with sides of about 3 m. Three-dimensional image is displayed by four projectors for each wall separately, in addition in some screens the projection is directed at the mirror, which enables a reduction of the size of the room and the extension of the projection way. The image is projected on the rear part of the translucent wall. An integral part of the Cave system is also an optical system for motion analysis DTrack2. It allows to automatically track the position of the glasses in the space delimited by the walls. Its construction account for four cameras working in infrared technology, positioned on the upper corners of the image, and computer with the software, responsible for the acquisition and processing of data from the cameras. Change of the image projection takes place in time to change of the markers position placed on the 3D glasses so that the user

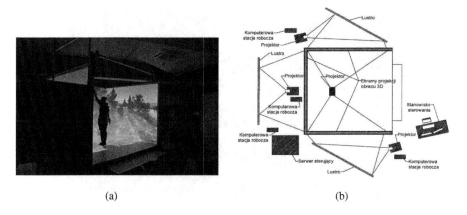

(a)   (b)

Fig. 1. Construction of the system of engineering support of upper limb diagnosis.

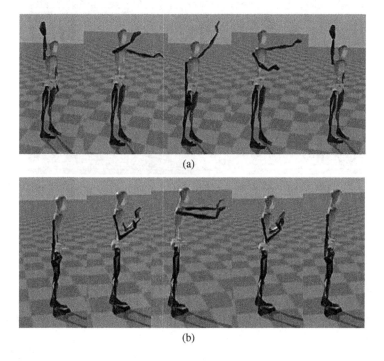

Fig. 2. Selected sequences of movements.

wearing the glasses has the feeling of being in the world of computer graphics. Optical tracking system also provides information about spatial position of a hand of an examined person thanks to locating the markers on the apparatus "VRTouchDevice". Cave part of the system associated with synchronization and image projection is shown in Fig. 1.

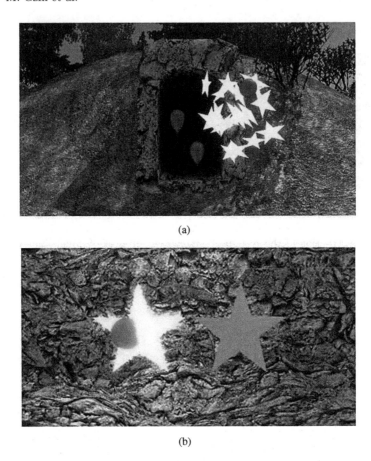

(a)

(b)

Fig. 3. Scenario diagnostic applications.

3.2   Measured Units

Measurement of kinematic quantity was based on inertial suit for motion analysis MVNBiomech produced by the company Xsens. During the research temporal change of the size of the angles for each of the joints in the upper limbs was registered.

3.3   Interactive Diagnostic Applications

Basing on the project recommendations and following consultation with therapists from the Department of Neurological Rehabilitation in Sosnowiec, in order to develop a diagnostic application scenario, motor function were selected. Two sequences of movement were selected from the rehabilitation exercises performed by patients in everyday clinical therapy and from exercises aimed at the diagnosis of muscle activity in the upper limbs referring to the tasks of large graphomotor abilities. The first sequence of movements consists of alternating lifting and lowering the hands as shown in Fig. 2(a). The second sequence involves lifting the hand in a movement which simulates pushing the object as shown in Fig. 2(b). Selected movement sequences formed the basis for the development of diagnostic scenario of interactive games based on two graphic scenes.

The first scenery, whose models prepared and distributed are presented in Fig. 3(a), is in a form of the diagnostic game. The task of the game is to knock down the approaching balloons in a given combination with ones hands. The distance between the balloons is prepared in such a way as to continuously encourage the patient to perform the first, pre-selected locomotive activity. The second scene, the layout of which is shown in Fig. 3(b), allows diagnostic game in the form of clapping hands or so-called "bouncing hands" motivating to perform the second sequence of movements. At the moment when a person, who does the exercises, places his/her hands on the items in the form of stars located in front of her at shoulder height, it will cause application interaction in the form of illumination of the upper limbs of fairy-tale characters. This effect is the reward, and information about the proper execution of this part of the exercise.

4   Receivers of the System

The recipient of the developed diagnostic systems are people with physical disabilities in the upper limbs, combined with other neurological diseases such as: dysfunction of interhemispheric integration or intellectual disability of deeper level.

5   Methodology of Verification of the System of Engineering Support of Upper Limb Diagnosis

In order to verify the developed system experimental studies were carried out in the presence of a physiotherapist performing complex sequences outside the system and with a group of 5 people (3 men and 2 women) exercising in the developed system. The measurements were performed three times for each of the selected physical activities for physiotherapists with the use of the system MVNBiomech by Xsens company for motion analysis. Then with the same system for motion analysis the kinematic scale of people exercising in the developed system was registered, taking into account three repetitions of the complex sequences of movement. The results obtained from measurements of the angle values of the joints of the upper limbs were presented graphically, then a comparison of the angle waveforms was made with the use of the correlation coefficients. For averaged waveforms for the examined patients Pearson correlation coefficient was calculated with the averaged course for a physiotherapist for each of the analysed movements in the joints of the upper limbs.

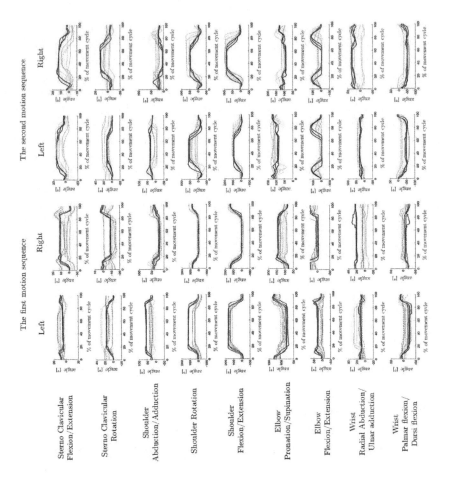

Fig. 4. The results of basic waveforms trajectory of joint angles during performing the first and second sequences of movement. The bold (red) line shows the results of a physiotherapist practicing outside the system, the other waveforms are the values for the examined patients exercising in this system. (Color figure online)

6   Results of the Verification

The results of the research for a physiotherapist performing exercises, on the basis of which the scenarios for applications were developed, were compared with the results for healthy people who exercised in the developed system. The comparison of results serves as a visual assessment of the shapes of joint movement trajectory performed by a healthy person, in relation to the established pattern. The results of angular values are shown in Fig. 4.

Absolute values of calculated average correlation coefficients are presented in Table 1.

Table 1. The absolute values of correlation coefficients for averaged charts for subjects with a averaged waveform for physiotherapists.

	The first motion sequence									
	Left					Right				
	p1	p2	p3	p4	p5	p1	p2	p3	p4	p5
Sterno clavicular flexion/extension	**0.85**	0.19	**0.84**	**0.86**	**0.76**	**0.81**	**0.88**	**0.87**	**0.59**	0.3
Sterno clavicular rotation	**0.99**	**0.6**	**0.88**	**0.98**	**0.68**	**0.89**	**0.85**	**0.84**	**0.98**	**0.6**
Shoulder abduction/adduction	**0.67**	**0.62**	**0.73**	**0.59**	**0.76**	**0.95**	**0.94**	**0.86**	**0.92**	**0.9**
Shoulder rotation	**0.99**	**0.96**	**0.93**	**0.96**	**0.96**	**0.99**	**0.97**	**0.92**	**0.99**	**0.98**
Shoulder flexion/extension	**0.99**	**0.95**	**0.97**	**0.99**	**0.95**	**0.99**	**0.98**	**0.95**	**0.99**	**0.96**
Elbow pronation/supination	**0.99**	0.47	**0.94**	**0.95**	**0.65**	**0.92**	0.36	**0.96**	**0.89**	**0.97**
Elbow flexion/extension	**0.52**	**0.68**	**0.64**	**0.5**	0.36	**0.93**	**0.95**	**0.81**	0.43	0.43
Wrist radial abduction/ulnar adduction	0.15	0.23	0.31	0.23	0.26	0.12	0.28	0.34	0.48	0.42
Wrist palmar flexion/dorsi flexion	**0.91**	**0.69**	**0.91**	**0.94**	**0.77**	**0.83**	**0.74**	**0.79**	**0.86**	**0.67**
	The second motion sequence									
	Left					Right				
	p1	p2	p3	p4	p5	p1	p2	p3	p4	p5
Sterno clavicular flexion/extension	**0.96**	**0.82**	**0.84**	**0.84**	**0.87**	**0.94**	**0.77**	**0.78**	**0.9**	**0.77**
Sterno clavicular rotation	**0.99**	**0.6**	**0.88**	**0.98**	**0.68**	**0.89**	**0.85**	**0.84**	**0.98**	**0.6**
Shoulder abduction/adduction	**0.71**	0.18	0.19	0.47	0.4	0.49	**0.6**	0.19	**0.51**	0.49
Shoulder rotation	**0.8**	**0.94**	**0.77**	**0.66**	**0.9**	**0.9**	**0.96**	**0.88**	**0.8**	**0.61**
Shoulder flexion/extension	**0.87**	**0.96**	**0.88**	**0.76**	**0.94**	**0.89**	**0.98**	**0.95**	**0.86**	**0.83**
Elbow pronation/supination	0.44	**0.83**	0.19	0.41	0.22	0.4	0.17	0.11	0.4	0.12
Elbow flexion/extension	**0.67**	**0.51**	**0.84**	**0.55**	**0.64**	**0.68**	0.32	**0.92**	**0.62**	**0.6**
Wrist radial abduction/ulnar adduction	**0.7**	**0.6**	**0.58**	**0.72**	**0.51**	0.3	0.31	**0.67**	0.32	**0.51**
Wrist palmar flexion/dorsi flexion	**0.91**	**0.8**	**0.58**	**0.91**	**0.66**	**0.84**	**0.82**	**0.51**	**0.76**	**0.51**

The values for correlation higher than 0.5 were bolded.

7   Discussion of the Results

Comparison of the angle waveforms for healthy people who exercise in this system with angle waveforms for those working with a physiotherapist indicate similarities in the shapes of obtained angle trajectory for most of the measured movements. It can also be indicated that angular values measured for healthy people, in some parts of the charts, differ by more than a dozen or so percentage points compared to the value achieved by a physiotherapist.

A more objective method to compare waveforms for patients with waveforms for the physiotherapist is the correlation tool between the curves. Basing on the analysis of the correlation coefficients one may draw a conclusion that trajectories measured for the physiotherapist have a similar shape as the trajectories for people exercising in the developed system as far as significant movements in the joints are concerned. As important movements for the first sequence of movements, after consultation with a physiotherapist, flexion/extension and rotation in the shoulder joint were indicated. For the second motion sequence flexion/extension and rotation in the shoulder joint, flexion/extension in the elbow and wrist were indicated as significant movements. The waveforms for these movements are highly correlated, with the exception of patient p2 for flexion/extension at the elbow, and the difference may be due to the smaller range of movement and its shift in time.

8   Conclusions

Comparative analysis of the results obtained by a physiotherapist with the results for healthy people, and the consultation of the registered results with the physiotherapist performing exercises, allows to accept the designed system as motivating to perform selected physical activities. A satisfactory recurrence was achieved with minor differences, which according to experts, do not affect the effectiveness of conducted diagnosis and therapy with the use of the developed system. The obtained results allow to evaluate the possibility of using the developed applications in the diagnostic and therapeutic processes.

References

1. Adamovich, S.V., Fluet, G.G., Tunik, E., Merians, A.S.: Sensorimotor training in virtual reality: a review. NeuroRehabilitation **25**, 29–44 (2009). doi:10.3233/NRE-2009-0497
2. Burstin, A., Brown, R.: Virtual environments for real treatments. Pol. Ann. Med. **17**(1), 101–111 (2010)
3. Cikajlo, I., Matjaćić, Z.: Advantages of visual reality technology in rehabilitation of people with neuromuscular disorders. In: Recent Advances in Biomedical Engineering, pp. 301–320 (2009). ISBN 978-953-307-004-9
4. Michnik, R., Jurkojć, J., Wodarski, P., Gzik, M., Bieniek, A.: The influence of the scenery and the amplitude of visual disturbances in the virtual reality on the maintaining the balance. Arch. Budo **10**(1), 133–140 (2014)

5. Michnik, R., Jurkojć, J., Wodarski, P., Gzik, M., Jochymczyk-Woźniak, K., Bieniek, A.: The influence of frequency of visual disorders on stabilographic parameters. Acta of Bioeng. Biomech. **18**(1), 25–33 (2016)
6. Slobounov, S.M., Teela, E., Newella, K.M.: Modulation of cortical activity in response to visually induced postural perturbation: combined VR and EEG study. Neurosci. Lett. **547**, 6–9 (2013). Elsevier
7. Schilbach, L., Wohlschlaeger, A.M., Kraemer, N.C., Newen, A., Shah, N.J., Fink, G.R., Vogeley, K.: Being with virtual others: neural correlates of social interaction. Neuropsychologia **44**, 718–730 (2006). Elsevier

Application of Dynamic Hip Screw System in Treatment of Intertrochanteric Fracture

Wojciech Kajzer[1(✉)], Grzegorz Prajsnar[2], Anita Kajzer[1], Łukasz Rodak[2],
Jan Marciniak[1], Michał Mielnik[2], Jacek Semenowicz[2], Jacek Hermanson[2],
and Bogdan Koczy[2]

[1] Department of Biomaterials and Medical Devices Engineering,
Faculty of Biomedical Engineering, Silesian University of Technology,
ul. Roosevelta 40, 44-800 Zabrze, Poland
wojciech.kajzer@polsl.pl
[2] Janusz Daab Provincial Hospital of Orthopaedics
and Traumatology in Piekary Śląskie, ul. Bytomska 62,
41-940 Piekary, Śląskie, Poland
gprajsnar@gmail.com

Abstract. The paper presents the results of clinical trials using dynamic hip screw (DHS) for the treatment of fractures of the proximal femur and the results of numerical simulation of the model of femoral fixation using stabilizer DHS for the fixations most commonly occurring in clinical cases. The simulation results constituted the basis for the selection of mechanical properties and allowed to define the zones most vulnerable to mechanical failure of both the implant and bone tissue. Furthermore, designated zones of maximum stress enable the identification and assessment of corrosion processes in the areas of the damaged surface layer of the metal biomaterial.

Keywords: Dynamic hip screw · DHS · Finite element analysis · Treatment of proximal femoral fracture · Treatment of intertrochanteric fracture · Osteoporosis

1 Introduction

Majority of proximal femur fractures occur among the elderly as a result of low-energy trauma - e.g. fall from own height (fall from stending height or less). Less fractures of this type is caused by high energy trauma or neoplastic lesions. In Poland, every year, there are around 16–20 thousand inter- or pertrochanteric fractures. Most of the cases involve older patients with more severe osteoporosis than in the case of femoral neck fractures [1,2]. According to the literature, over 50 years old the incidence of fractures of the proximal femur doubles every 6 years. Because of the concomitant osteoporosis fractures are more likely to occur among women than men. Fracture of the proximal femur is one of the

© Springer International Publishing AG 2017
M. Gzik et al. (eds.), *Innovations in Biomedical Engineering*, Advances in Intelligent
Systems and Computing 526, DOI 10.1007/978-3-319-47154-9_15

most dangerous complications of osteoporosis. It is associated with high mortality (fracture of the femoral neck - approximately 8–11 %), what is more leads to temporary or permanent loss of independence. Risk factors of proximal femur fractures include: age, sex, alcohol abuse, rheumatoid arthritis, impaired ability to walk, impaired brain function, dementia, use of psychotropic drugs and peripheral neuropathies [1–6]. The aim of the surgical treatment of trochanteric fractures is stable fixation, restoration of limb function and as soon as possible walking, which protects against general and local complications [1,2]. One of the methods used for osteosynthesis of proximal femur fractures, including the treatment of femoral neck fractures and intertrochanteric fractures is DHS (Dynamic Hip Screw) also known as Sliding Screw Fixation. DHS method includes three components: appropriate lenght lag screw (inserted into the neck of the femur) which is connected with sideplate and cortical screws (fixated into the proximal femoral shaft corticales). It is recommended to insert lag screw in longitudinal axis of femoral neck approx. 10 mm below bony surface of the femoral head. Rotational stabilization is achieved by introducing lag screw into sideplate (with special internal antirotational notch). Mechanism of dynamic osteosynthesis is a result of possible movement of lag screw into sleeve of sideplate. To carry out such a procedure it is necessary to have adequate instruments and variety of implants (screws and plates) of different geometry and size [1,2]. Biomechanical numerical analysis preceding implantation of the stabilizing system performed to determine the state of displacements and stresses occurring in the implant during the stabilization and in bones, and on the implant - bone interface is important due to the selection of biomechanical characteristics of the stabilizer and metal biomaterial, and modification of the surface layer structure of applied implants [7–13]. On the basis of the literature review, it may be said that the authors [14–19] attempt at the numerical analysis of the system: femur - dynamic hip screw system (DHS). In each case, the simulated fracture was an intertrochanteric fracture. The results of their analyses are based on the models of various degrees of simplification: from very simple models in which the plate is fixed with four screws [16] (made as one element), to sophisticated models with up to eight screws presented as separate elements [19]. However, in all of the cases, there is a simplification that the bolts are not threaded and the diameter of the cortical screws and thread geometry are not taken into consideration. The analyses resulted in determining the values of displacements, von Misses strains and stresses. Taking into consideration the simplifications applied by other authors, the study involved the biomechanical analysis using finite element method supplemented by clinical observations. DHS screw of thread diameter equal to $G = 12.5$ mm (standard DHS screw used for cancellous healthy bone), and standard cortical screws of $BS = 4.5$ mm diameter were used. The analysis was performed for the most frequent DHS fixations with the use of the plate intended for use with three cortical screws.

2 Materials and Methods

2.1 Clinical Studies

422 patients between years 2009–1013 were treated because of intertrochanteric fracture in the Janusz Daab Provincial Hospital of Orthopaedics and Traumatology in Piekary Śląskie. Clinical and radiological outcomes were analyzed. 369 patients were treated with open reduction and internal fixation with DHS method. Patients group consists of 272 (73.7 %) women and 97 (26.3 %) men. The average age of all treated patients was 78.4 years (mean age of women - 73 ± 26 years, men - 60 ± 37 years. The structure of patients gender, age, circumstances of the injury, time, method and results of treatment were analyzed.

2.2 FEM Analysis

Numerical simulation of loading of the femoral fixation model, with the use of dynamic hip screw DHS, was performed in Ansys Workbench 15 environment. The fixation of intertrochanteric femoral fractures of the type I according to the classification of trochanteric fractures of femur by Evans and Jensen modifications was analyzed [20]. Preliminary tests included evaluation of a non-fractured femur. The generated finite element mesh (element type SOLID 187) was characterized by the skewness parameter of mean value equal to 0.4 ± 0.2 providing its good match to the geometry of the analyzed system. The geometric model of the femur was prepared in the Mimics Innovation Suite software based on CT images with the following parameters: The size of the pixel in the lateral plane: 0.684 mm, The imaging field width: 171.68 mm, Distance between sections: 1.5 mm, The number of sections: 331. In order to segment bones, thresholding operation was performed with the lower threshold value of $226HU$ and upper threshold value of $1613HU$. It included both the cortical and the cancellous part of the femur. In the numerical analysis the DHS system was analyzed. The geometry of the system has been commonly used in the Provincial Hospital of Orthopaedics and Traumatology in Piekary Śląskie. The fixation was performed using the DHS plate of neck length of $Ls = 38$ mm, plate length of $L = 105$ mm and the angle $135°$. DHS screws with a thread diameter $G = 12.5$ mm and three cortical screws of diameter $BS = 4.5$ mm were used. The width of the fracture gap was $d = 0.2$ mm. A callus forming in the gap was simulated. In order to perform numerical calculations, the mechanical properties shown in Table 1 were assumed.

On the basis of the developed geometric models, numerical models were prepared. Because of the complex shapes and in particular the threads of the cortical screws and the irregular geometry of the bone, in order to reduce the number of finite elements and speed up the calculations a simplification omitting the threads in the cortical screws, as in works [14–19] was done. However, the thread of the DHS screw was taken into account in the analyses. The following were assumed for the needs of the analysis:

Table 1. Mechanical properties assumed in the numerical analysis

Element of a computing system		Mechanical properties				
		E	v	R_c	$R_{p0.2}$	R_m
Femur	Stem [21]	17900	0.3	180	–	–
	Head [18]	17000	0.3	–	–	–
	Trabecular bone [21]	10500	0.3	–	–	–
	Early stage of fracture healing [18,19]	3	0.4	–	–	–
Cr–Ni–Mo steel [22]		200000	0.3	–	690	1300

E - Young's modulus MPa, v - Poisson's ratio, R_c - Ultimate compressive strength MPa, $R_{p0.2}$ - Yield strenght MPa, R_m - Ultimate tensile strength MPa

- distal part of femur was immobilized by depriving the nodes situated along the plane of all the freedom degrees,
- the bone was loaded following Będziński model [23].

The values of forces assumed for the test corresponded to peak values reached when carrying a load with one limb by a walking person of 70 kg bodyweight - Table 2.

Table 2. Values and direction of forces assumed in the numerical calculations relative to the coordinate system

B, N			C, N			D, N		
x	y	z	x	y	z	x	y	z
0	−912	−247	10.5	0	27	0	604	247

B - force acting on the femoral head, C - ilio-tibial band reaction, D - muscle reaction force (gluteal band)

Furthermore, friction between the thread of the DHS bolt and the cancellous bone in the femoral head was assumed. An asymmetric friction coefficient of $\eta = 0.3$ [15,17] was assumed. The contacting surfaces were described as automatically adjusting to one another, and the calculations were made with Augmented Lagrange equations. Friction contact and geometry correction corresponding to M4 thread geometry were also applied between the compressive bolt and the DHS bolt. In the remaining contact areas between the elements of the DHS system and the model femur, a standard bonded contact was applied in order to simulate the connections between the cortical screws and the bone, and between the DHS plate and the bone. The stresses and strains obtained in the analysis are the values reduced in accordance with the Huber–Hencky–von Misses theory.

3   Results and Discussion

3.1   Clinical Studies

Hip fractures occurred as a result of fall from own height (standing height or less) in 325 (88.1 %) patients; as a result of other circumstances in 41 (11.1 %) patients, including fall from a higher altitude, e.g. ladders, chairs, stairs, roof, scaffolding, etc. 3 (0.8 %) patients had a traffic accident. 309 (83.7 %) reported to the hospital immediately after the injury, 30 (8.13 %) patients reported within 48 h after injury, 30 (8.13 %) more than 48 h after injury. In the Emergency Room after diagnosis in 237 (64.2 %) patients proximal tibial skeletal traction was applied, 132 (35.8 %) patients did not have skeletal traction. In 70 (19 %) patients underwent surgery immediately after admission, 59 (16 %) patients had surgery on the next day. 240 (65 %) patients had surgery later due to additional general conditions, other diseases or need to perform additional tests and consultations. Among analyzed cases 12.5 mm diameter DHS lag screw was used. The shortest lag screw length used was 60 mm, the longest - 135 mm (average - 94.24 mm). Side-plate used for surgery had angle of 135∘, 2 to 12 hole (average 3.75) with cortical screws 4.5 mm diameter and a length adapted to the anatomical characteristics of the femur. In 4 (1,1 %) cases 2 holes plate was used, 3-hole - in 174 cases (47.2 %), 4-hole - 133 (36 %), 5-hole - 13 (3.5 %), 6-hole - 14 (3.8 %), 8-hole - 4 (1.1 %), 10-hole - 5 (1.4 %), 12-hole - 1 (0.3 %). Compression screw was used in 287 cases (77.8 %). Additional stabilization devices were necessary in 28 (7.6 %) patients (metal loops, spongy and cortical screws). 176 (47.7 %) patients who underwent surgical treatment in outpatient clinic control showed complete radiographic bone union. This group consisted of 129 women (47.4 %) and 47 men (48.5 %). 94 (25.5 %) patients did not report at all for clinical control after surgery. In the group of patients treated with 2-hole plate bone union was achieved in 2 (50 %) cases, 3-hole - 78 (44.8 %), 4-hole - 69 (51.9 %), 5-hole - 8 (61.5 %), 6-hole - 4 (28.6 %), 8-hole - 3 (75 %), 10-hole - 4 (80 %), 12-hole - 1 (100 %).

3.2   FEM Analysis

The results of the analysis of the displacements, von Misses strains and equivalent stress for all femur - DHS system models are presented in Table 3 and Fig. 1.

In the presented work taking into account the results of the clinical evaluation of the DHS stabilizer the numerical analysis of the DHS system with three cortical screws with a diameter of 4.5 mm was performed. The DHS stabilizer was placed in the femur in accordance with the recommendations of the implantation technique. Placement of the implant corresponded to the one used in the Provincial Hospital of Orthopaedics and Traumatology in Piekary Śląskie and at the same time was in accordance with the works [15,17]. Calculations were carried out for bone models both non-fractured and with the intertrochanteric fracture. For the non-fractured model of the femur, wherein the implant was not used, a displacement of the proximal section of the femur $L = 6.5$ mm was

Table 3. The results of the numerical analysis for the models

No	Models	Results for whole model			von Misses stress for individual parts of models, MPa						
		L	ε	σ	σ_{fs}	σ_{fh}	σ_{fhc}	σ_{DHS}	σ_{coms}	σ_{DHSp}	σ_{cs}
1	Femur	6.50	0.19	34.20	–	–	–	–	–	–	–
2	Femur - DHS	7.9	0.49	401	85	9	14	315	154	306	401

L - displacement, ε - von Misses strain, σ - von Misses stress, σ_{fs} - femur steam, σ_{fs} - femur head, σ_{fhc} - femur head - cancellous bone, σ_{DHS} - DHS screw, σ_{coms} - compression screw, σ_{DHSp} - DHS plate, σ_{cs} - cortical screws

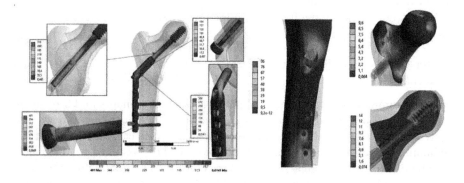

Fig. 1. Stress distribution in DHS system and femur elements, MPa

observed, which resulted in stresses in the cortical bone equal to $\sigma = 34$ MPa. The values of displacements of the femur - DHS stabilizer system were higher than those obtained for the non-fractured bone and were equal to $L = 7.9$ mm. Reduction in stiffness of bone after use of the DHS with three cortical screws can contribute to a reduction of treatment efficiency (44.8 % of full bone union according to clinical trials) compared to stabilization using more cortical screws for example 5 - 61.5 % efficiency. The results indicate that in the analyzed model, the maximum stress do not exceed the yield strength of the metal biomaterial - Table 3. Furthermore, the strength of both cortical and cancellous bone was not exceeded as well. The maximum stresses in the parts of the stabilizer were observed in the contact zones between the DHS screw and the neck of the DHS plate and cortical screw slots of the DHS plate. Furthermore, in the cortical screws an accumulation of stress in the transition zone between the shaft to the head was observed - Fig. 1. Taking into account the results of the analysis can be concluded that for the implant made of the austenitic stainless steel results obtained by authors [14–19,24] are similar, and on this basis threats related to the application of the DHS system in intertrochanteric femur fractures can be concluded. Maximum stress areas are vulnerable to mechanical failure of the implant, leading to its destruction. At the same time damage of passive layer in the contact zones may lead to initiation of corrosion processes. These zones will be exposed to the initiation and development of crevice, pitting and fatigue corrosion [24].

4 Conclusion

On the basis of the performed treatment analyses of intertrochanteric fractures stabilized with the DHS system in the Provincial Hospital of Orthopaedics and Traumatology in Piekary Śląskie in 2009–2013 it can be concluded that:

- pertrochanteric fractures occur more often among older females and are a result of low Energy trauma,
- DHS system is the most often used implant for trochanteric fractures stabilization in the hospital,
- DHS osteosynthesis is an effective method of treatment,
- better results of DHS surgical treatment were observed among men than women.

Moreover, summarizing the numerical analysis of displacements and stresses in the elements of the DHS dynamic hip stabilizer, in particular taking into account the stresses in the femoral shaft and cancellous bone, one can conclude that the maximum stress in the analyzed models do not exceed the assumed yield strength of the biomaterial $R_{p0.2} = 690\,\mathrm{MPa}$ and the established compression strength of bone $R_c = 180\,\mathrm{MPa}$. The analysis allows the determination of potentially dangerous areas, vulnerable to damage due to overload. Furthermore, the analysis identifies the areas of initiation and development of crevice, pitting and fatigue corrosion.

Acknowledgements. The work has been financed from research Project No. $BK - 262/RIB2/2014$.

References

1. Canale, T.S., Beaty, J.H.: Campbellś Operative Orthopaedics, 12nd edn. Chapter 1: 58–59, Chapter 55: 2725–2776 (2013)
2. Standard, J.P., Schmidt, A.H., Kregor, P.O.: Leczenie operacyjne obrażeń narządu ruchu. wyd.1, 2010, tom.3, rozdział 23 (in Polish)
3. Kenzora, J.E., McCarthy, R.E., Lowell, O.D., Sledge, C.B.: Hip fracture mortality: relation to age, treatment preoperative illness, time of surgery and complications. Clin. Orthop. Relat. Res. **186**, 45–56 (1984)
4. Ring, P.A.: Treatment of trochanteric fractures of the femur. Br. Med. J. **1**(5331), 654–656 (1963)
5. McNeill, D.H.: Hip fractures: influence of delay in surgery on mortality. Wis. Med. J. **74**(12), 129–138 (1975)
6. Griffiths, R., Alper, J., Beckingsale, A., Goldhill, D., Heyburn, G., Holloway, J., Leaper, E., Parker, M., Ridgway, S., White, S., Wiese, M., Wilson, I.: Management of proximal femoral fractures 2011 Association of Anaesthetists of Great Britain and Ireland. Anaesthesia **67**(1), 85–98 (2012)

7. Özkan, A., Atmaca, H., Mutlu, İ., Çelik, T., Uğur, L., Kiioğlu, Y.: Stress distribution comparisons of foot bones in patient with tibia vara: a finite element study. Acta Bioeng. Biomech. **15**(4), 67–72 (2013). doi:10.5277/abb130409

8. Świeczko-Żurek, B., Serbiński, W., Szumlański, A.: Analisys of the failure of fixator used in bone surgery. Adv. Mater. Sci. **8**(2), 84–88 (2008)

9. Ziębowicz, A., Bączkowski, B.: Numerical analysis of the implant – abutment system. In: Piętka, E., Kawa, J. (eds.) ITIB 2012. LNCS, vol. 7339, pp. 341–350. Springer, Heidelberg (2012)

10. Kajzer, W., Kajzer, A., Gzik-Zroska, B., Wolański, W., Janicka, I., Dzielicki, J.: Comparison of numerical and experimental analysis of plates used in treatment of anterior surface deformity of chest. In: Piętka, E., Kawa, J. (eds.) ITIB 2012. LNCS, vol. 7339, pp. 319–330. Springer, Heidelberg (2012). doi:10.1007/978-3-642-31196-3_32

11. Szewczenko, J., Pochrząst, M., Walke, W.: Evaluation of electrochemical properties of modified Ti–6Al–4V ELI alloy. Przeglad Elektrotechniczny **87**(12b), 177–180 (2011)

12. Basiaga, M., Jendruś, R., Walke, W., Paszenda, Z., Kaczmarek, M., Popczyk, M.: Influence of surface modification on properties of stainless steel used for implants. Arch. Metall. Mater. **60**(4), 2965–2969 (2015)

13. Walke, W., Paszenda, Z., Basiaga, M., Karasinski, P., Kaczmarek, M.: EIS study of SiO_2 oxide film on 316L stainless steel for cardiac implants. In: Piętka, E.,; Kawa, J., Wieclawek, W. (eds.) Information Technologies in Biomedicine, vol. 4. Book Series: Advances in Intelligent Systems and Computing, vol. 284, pp. 403–410 (2014)

14. Hrubina, M., Skotak, M., Behounek, J.: Complications of dynamic hip screw treatment for proximal femoral factures. Acta Chir. Orthop. Traumatol. Cachoslovaca **77**, 140–142 (2010)

15. Horák, Z., Hrubina, M., Dzupa, V.: Biomechanical analyses of proximal femur osteosynthesis by DHS system. Bull. Appl. Mech. **7**(27), 60–65 (2011)

16. Taheri, N.S., Blicblau, A.S., Singh, M.: Effect of different load conditions on a DHS implanted human femur. Int. J. Eng Technol. **1**(1), 141–146 (2012)

17. Hrubina, M., Horák, Z., Bartoška, R., Navrátil, L., Rosina, J.: Computational modeling in the prediction of Dynamic Hip Screw failure in proximal femoral fractures. J. Appl. Biomed. **11**, 143–151 (2013)

18. Rooppakhun, S., Chantarapanich, N., Chernchujit, B., Mahaisavariya, B., Sucharitpwatskul, S., Sitthiseripratip, K.: Mechanical evaluation of dynamic hip screwfor trochanteric fracture. Int. Sch. Sci. Res. Innov. **4**(9), 576–579 (2010)

19. Siamnuai, K., Rooppakhun, S.: Influence of plate length on the mechanical performance of dynamic hip screw. IACSIT Press, 23 Singapore (2012)

20. Bednarenko, M.: Classification systems for trochaneric fractures of the femur. Kwart. Ortop. **1**, 1–9 (2011)

21. Keaveny, T.M., Morgan, E.F., Yeh, O.C.: Bone mechanics. Standard book of biomedical engineering and design. Chapter 8 (2004)

22. Standard: ISO 5832-1: Implants for surgery - Metallic materials - Part 1: Wrought stainless steel

23. Będziński, R.: Biomechanika Inżynierska. Zagadnienia Wybrane. Oficyna Wydawnicza Politechniki Wrocławskiej (1997) (in Polish)

24. Szewczenko, J., Marciniak, J., Kajzer, W., Kajzer, A.: Evaluation of corrosive resistance of titanium alloys used for medical implants. Arch. Metall. Mater. **61**(2), 695–700 (2016). doi:10.1515/amm-2016-0118

Statistical Analysis of Cranial Measurements - Determination of Indices for Assessing Skull Shape in Patients with Isolated Craniosynostosis

Edyta Kawlewska[1]([✉]), Wojciech Wolański[1], Dawid Larysz[2], Bożena Gzik-Zroska[3], Kamil Joszko[1], Marek Gzik[1], and Katarzyna Gruszczyńska[4]

[1] Department of Biomechatronics, Faculty of Biomedical Engineering, Silesian University of Technology, Zabrze, Poland
edyta.kawlewska@polsl.pl
[2] Department of Radiotherapy, Maria Sklodowska-Curie Memorial Cancer Center and Institute of Oncology, Gliwice, Poland
[3] Department of Biomaterials and Medical Devices Engineering, Faculty of Biomedical Engineering, Silesian University of Technology, Zabrze, Poland
[4] Department of Radiology and Nuclear Medicine, School of Medicine in Katowice, Medical University of Silesia, Katowice, Poland

Abstract. This paper presents a morphological analysis of the skull shape in infants under one year of age. Three-dimensional measurements were performed on models generated from images in Mimics software. Subsequently, a multivariate statistical analysis of the measured dimensions was performed to determine key indicators of the skull shape. Eventually it was developed the norms of skull indices for children up to one year of age. Regular values of these indices were compared with abnormal values measured in patients with isolated craniosynostosis. With the use of these indices it is possible to perform a quantitative evaluation of head deformity.

Keywords: Skull · Craniosynostosis · Craniometry · Morphometry · Infant · Statistical analysis · Index · Norm

1 Introduction

Infant skull is composed of several major bones that are held together by fibrous material called sutures. In the first two years of life the skull growth is significant and its course can run properly only with non-ossified sutures. However, sometimes one or more cranial sutures are prematurely fused. Consequently, the growth is impaired and deformations occur [15,17]. This disease, called craniosynostosis, may result in very dangerous complications such as the increase of intracranial and intraorbital pressure and incorrect growth of the brain [6] Fig. 1.

Congenital craniosynostosis can be isolated or connected with more complicated genetic defects, such as Apert or Crouzon syndromes. There are four main types of craniosynostosis [2]:

© Springer International Publishing AG 2017
M. Gzik et al. (eds.), *Innovations in Biomedical Engineering*, Advances in Intelligent Systems and Computing 526, DOI 10.1007/978-3-319-47154-9_16

- scaphocephaly - sagittal suture synostosis,
- trigonocephaly - metopic suture synostosis,
- brachycephaly:
  - anterior - bilateral coronal suture synostosis,
  - posterior - bilateral lambdoid suture synostosis,
- plagiocephaly:
  - anterior - unilateral coronal suture synostosis,
  - posterior - unilateral lambdoid suture synostosis.

Most infants born with craniosynostosis will need surgery to repair their skull deformity and enable the proper growth of brain.

It is important, that there may be reasons other than synostosis that the child's head is misshapen, so only X-rays or CT scanning are the methods enabling the diagnosis and confirmation of the craniosynostosis.

Medical imaging such as CT scanning allows generating 3-dimensional models of selected structures. On the basis of these models it is possible to perform the quantitative analysis of geometry. Also there is a possibility to plan the surgical correction individually for each patient [4,5,8,14–17]. The craniometry based on CT images is known and used to evaluate the regular growth of the skull or skull asymmetry [1,3,7,9–14]. In this work the researchers performed complex cranial measurements based on the CT images and multivariate statistical analysis in order to obtain the skull indicators determining the deformation in craniosynostosis.

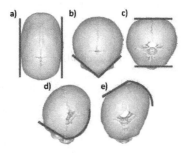

Fig. 1. Types of craniosynostosis (highlighted lines present the characteristic shape of deformation): (a) sagittal synostosis, (b) metopic synostosis, (c) bilateral lambdoid or coronal synostosis, (d) unilateral coronal synostosis, (e) unilateral lamdoid synostosis

2   Materials and Methods

A test group consisted of 129 infants of a regular head structure (Group 1) and 104 patients with various types of craniosynostosis (Group 2). Morphological tests were conducted in order to calculate indices determining the shape of the skull in children under 1 year of age. In anthropometric measurements CT images were used, which were obtained from the Upper Silesian Children's Health Centre in Katowice. CT examinations were performed with a 16-slice scanner (Aquilion S 16, Toshiba, Tokyo, Japan). Standard vendor diagnostic protocols for head CT were modified according to ALARA principle and patients age, with following parameters: spiral mode, 80–120 kV tube voltage, 80–150 mAs tube current, gantry rotation time 0.5 s, FOV 240. Whole head from gonion to vertex, was included into field of view, together with soft tissue of the face. Scanner gantry was not tilted. Reconstructed slice thickness was 0.5 mm, with an increment of 0.5 mm. Children in which 'feed and wrap' technique was not working were examined in general anesthesia. Regional Ethics Board approval was received and all parents gave informed consent for CT scan.

In Group 1 (Table 1) computer tomography was done during the diagnosis of neurological, oncological and other diseases. The patients with a suspected craniosynostosis or other diseases resulting in a possible skull deformation were excluded. The patients with hydrocephalus and after skull injuries were not taken into consideration either. On the day of the CT examination the youngest child was 3 days old, whereas the oldest was 12 months old. The patients were divided into 12 age groups with monthly intervals. Each group consisted of at least six children in order to enable reliable statistical analyses in a further part of the research. A detailed description of sub-groups has been presented in tables below In Group 2 (Table 2) CT images of 104 patients were used. These patients had the examination conducted before the operation. Two patients had also CT done after corrective operations. Designations such as: TRI, SCP, BCP and PCP stand for the name of a condition and mean respectively: TRI - trigonocephaly, SCP - scaphocephaly, BCP - brachycephaly and PCP - plagiocephaly. The age of all patients before the operation was within 0–12 months.

Table 1. Specification of group of children with regular skull shape

Age (months)	1	2	3	4	5	6	7	8	9	10	11	12	Σ
Number	6	12	9	11	9	6	16	13	13	11	14	9	129

Table 2. Specification of group of children with various types of craniosynostosis: SCP - scaphocephaly, TRI - trigonocepfaly, PCP - plagiocephaly, BCP - brachycephaly

Age (months)	SCP	TRI	PCP	BCP	Σ
0–6	14	13	2	0	29
6–12	32	18	8	2	60
12–18	7	4	3	1	15
SUM	**53**	**35**	**13**	**3**	**104**

The CT results made it possible to develop models of skulls which accurately mapped geometrical features of the real structure. Thanks to special engineering

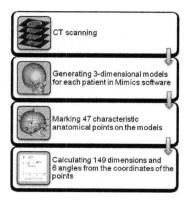

Fig. 2. Procedure of obtaining the database used in statistical analysis

software, the above mentioned models can be modified, improved and used as input data in various types of research and examinations, beginning from the geometrical analysis to advanced numerical simulations.

The research took advantage of Mimics software which enabled finding the location of several dozen characteristic anatomic points of the skull (Fig. 2). These points were selected together with the neurosurgeon, as well as from the literature review. On this basis, some distances were selected and calculated in order to create a database of indices characterizing the shape of the skull and head in children at the first year of age. The analysis of such data made it possible to precisely define characteristic features of the head structure defects and determine the location of deformations on the skull. On the grounds of the determined points, the head perimeter was calculated for all the children; 13 angles and 167 distances. The distances were calculated by joining selected points (Fig. 3) with one another, however, with the consideration of interesting directions of individual dimensions. In this way, a broad database of craniometrical values was created and then subjected to a multidimensional statistical analysis.

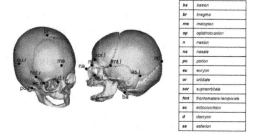

Fig. 3. Exemplary points marked on the models during the morphological analysis

Due to a considerable amount of data, it was necessary to conduct a statistical analysis for the database created. The following software was used for the calculation and visualization of results: StatSoft Statistica v10.0 and MS Excel 2007. On the basis of the analyses performed the graphs of the major dimensions of skulls in children under 12 months were developed. In order to create the description of the database of healthy children the researchers calculated mean values, standard deviations, variances as well as checked regularity of the distribution of the values of individual dimensions. Variance homogeneity was tested in the test group by means of Levene's test in order to apply a proper test of the variance analysis (Welch's test).

3   Results

At first it was performed the multivariety statistical analysis. In order to better understand the variability of such a vast database, a factor analysis was conducted to reduce the variables. Thanks to that, ten factors responsible for variability between subgroups were isolated. Subsequently, post-hoc tests were carried out. With the use of ROC curves the classification of factors was made. They were correlated then with particular types of craniosynostosis.

The analysis of variance conducted revealed that for regular skulls the majority of measurements (89.4 %) was statistically significant, which is connected with a regular growth of the head. While in the case of deformed skulls, at most half of the measurements met the criterion of mean variabilities. On the basis of the variance analysis results, the diversity of patterns of the dimensions of the heads in healthy and sick children was found, which is particularly significant for the prediction of further deformity of the head.

Having conducted a principal component analysis in the factor analysis, it was stated that all angles and distances measured may be reduced to 10 factors which describe almost 80 % (79.46 %) of variances of the skulls variability between both groups of patients. For all these variables the distribution of the factor loading was determined in subsequent classifiers. The list of a precise number of variables in individual classifiers has been presented in Table 3.

The analysis adopted the cutoff point equal 0.7 for loading. Analyzing the results of the factor analysis it should be noted that in the case of a given distance being located both on the right and left side of the skull the table shows only one of them as they are equivalent. The first factor, including 36.619 % of variability variances, consists of 67 variables of the factor loading above 0.70. All of them are highly correlated with the skull perimeter calculated by means of the equation for the ellipsis perimeter, where the maximum length and width of the skull are the diameters. The correlation coefficient equaled to 0.89. It can be thus concluded that these 67 parameters are responsible for the variability related to age. The second classifier includes 14 essential distances from point 'ba' (basion) located on the perimeter of the large opening (foramen magnum) of the occipital bone. It should be noted that for this factor the correlation coefficient with the skull perimeter (and thus with the child's age) was very low and amounted to 0.046.

Table 3. The variable distribution of factors selected in factor analysis

Factor number	Number of variables	Number of variables with the factor loading >0.70	% of variability variances	Exemplary dimensions included in factors
1	87	67	36.619	Euryon left-right (skull width) metopion-opisthocranion (skull length)
2	15	14	8.344	Euryon-porion
3	13	6	6.906	Lambda-bregma nasion-bregma (skull vault height)
4	9	4	6.470	Nasion–basion lambda-basion (skull base height)
5	9	3	6.256	Orbitale-basion
6	7	5	3.614	Lateral orbitale left - right
7	8	1	3.472	Nasion-nasale
8	5	2	2.968	Nasale-porion, nasale-lateral orbitale
9	4	2	2.429	Opisthocranion-basion
10	2	1	2.384	Angle spc.r-n-spc.l (Fig. 9)

Factors 3–10 also include variables which distinguish between a group of children with a regular skull shape and patients with craniosynostosis. These variables are particularly significant as they are not directly connected with growth. It can be stated thus that they constitute the database of the determinants of the abnormal shape of the head. Additionally, it is noteworthy that factors 7 and 10, being variables of the highest factor loading, include the skull angles responsible for 3.47 and 2.38 % of the variability of variances.

In the next phase, the analysis of ROC curves was conducted in order to evaluate the predictive value and classifying value of the previously determined factors.

The surface area under the diagram of ROC-AUC curve, which has values in the range from 0 to 1, defines the ability of the test to distinguish between correct and incorrect results. The higher AUC (and in the same way the more concave ROC function), the bigger diagnostic force of the test.

First of all, the researchers analyzed a classifier between children with a regular head shape and all patients with various types of craniosynostosis. It was found that factors 2, 4 and 10 distinguish irregular skulls from regular ones (Fig. 4). Further on, a classifier between regular skulls and skulls with scaphocephaly was analyzed. The surface area under the curve was the biggest for factors 5 and 10. A subsequent analysis was concerned with a classifier between regular skulls and trigonocephaly. This defect was best distinguished from regular skulls by means of factors 8, 9 and 10. It was found that the best classifiers

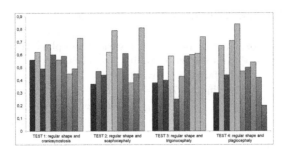

Fig. 4. Results of AUC analysis in four tests. Each column represents factors from first to tenth respectively. Yellow columns represent the factors with the biggest value, that were selected to subsequent analysis (Color figure online)

for the group of children with plagiocephaly were factors 2, 4 and 5. It should be emphasized that the predictive value for factor 10 was exceptionally low for this subgroup.

Within the scope of this work, nine indices and cranial angles were determined for scaphocephaly and trigonocephaly. They were selected on the basis of the results obtained from a prior statistical analysis and consultations with a neurosurgeon. Standard values of indices were examined in age groups of children with a regular skull shape and a comparative analysis was conducted among patients.

Indices for the Assessment of the Skull Shape in Scaphocephaly. In the case of scaphocephaly, it is characteristic that the growth disorder of the skull occurs in the anterior and posterior directions. The length of the skull is thus one of the most important dimensions that should be watched. On the basis of the characteristic anatomical points, the following items were determined: the cephalic index, the index of lateral anterior and posterior length of the cranial vault, the index of anterior and posterior height of the cranial vault, the index of anterior and posterior height of the cranial base and additionally, predicting the changes within eye sockets (on the basis of prior ROC curves analysis) - the nasal-orbital angle.

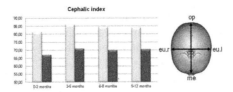

Fig. 5. Obtained values of cephalic index values for healthy children (light grey) and patients with sagittal synostosis (dark grey) in groups of age

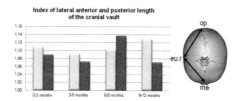

Fig. 6. Obtained values of index of lateral anterior and posterior length of the cranial vault for healthy children (light grey) and patient with scaphocephaly (dark grey) in groups of age.

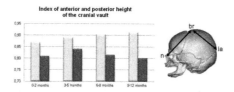

Fig. 7. Obtained values of index of anterior and posterior height of the cranial vault for healthy children (light grey) and patient with scaphocephaly (dark grey) in groups of age.

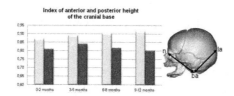

Fig. 8. Obtained values of index of anterior and posterior height of the cranial base for healthy children (light grey) and patient with scaphocephaly (dark grey) in groups of age.

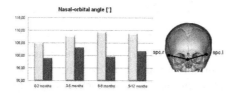

Fig. 9. Obtained values of nasal-orbital angle for healthy children (light grey) and patients with scaphocephaly (dark grey) in groups of age

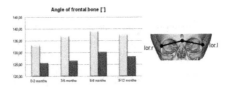

Fig. 10. Obtained values of angle of frontal bone for healthy children (light grey) and patients with trigonocephaly (dark grey) in groups of age

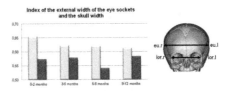

Fig. 11. Obtained values of index of the external width of the eye sockets and the skull width for healthy children (light grey) and patient with trigonocephaly (dark grey) in groups of age.

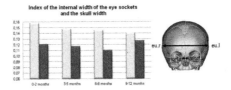

Fig. 12. Obtained values of index of the internal width of the eye sockets and the skull width for healthy children (light grey) and patient with trigonocephaly (dark grey) in groups of age.

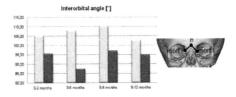

Fig. 13. Obtained values of interorbital angle for healthy children (light grey) and patients with trigonocephaly (dark grey) in groups of age

Indices for the Assessment of the Skull Shape in Trigonocephaly. In patients with trigonocephaly a visible deformation occurs first of all in the frontal and orbital area. It is therefore advisable to examine the dimensions of the angles in the eyes area as well as the distance between the eyes in relation to the skull width - in order to discover hypotelorism (abnormally close eyes). Taking into account the above, the following items were determined: angle of frontal bone, index of the external width of the eye sockets and the skull width, index of the internal width of the eye sockets and the skull width and interorbital angle.

4   Discussion

On the basis of the tests conducted, it was discovered that during the growth of the head with obliterated cranial suture some cranial angles and measurements become subject to alteration which does not occur in a regular growth. In previous studies mostly focused on the analysis of the cephalic index [4,9,11]. The analysis showed that in the case of each defect, except for characteristic deformations of the head (e.g. a triangular forehead in trigonocephaly or elongated skull in scaphocephaly) one can distinguish the dimensions which disturb the growth of other parts of the skull - the parts which are not directly connected to the obliterated cranial suture. This constitutes significant evidence that it is essential to apply complex treatment as soon as possible due to the fact that irreversible deformations of the skull shape may appear with its growth. It refers not only to the cranial vault, which can be relatively easily reconstructed, but to the facial skeleton, cranial base and vertebral column. To sum up the statistical analysis of morphometric tests of the skulls in healthy children and in children with craniosynostosis made it possible to determine a set of dimensions classifying and distinguishing irregular skulls from regular ones.

The results obtained enable better understanding of the skull deformation mechanisms. The results may also constitute the basis for a quantitative evaluation of the effectiveness of craniosynostosis treatment in infants.

In healthy infants under 12 months, the relation of maximum width to length of the skull oscillates between 83.8 ± 6.9 (Fig. 5). For sick children, the value of the index is considerably lower, about 70.0, which is obviously caused by the elongated posterior part of the head in the case of scaphocephaly.

In patients with scaphocephaly the value of the index of anterior and posterior length of the skull calculated from the left and right side in the first months of life is almost identical to the one in healthy children and oscillates between 1.1 ± 0.05 (Fig. 6). However, an interesting phenomenon was observed in children at the age of 6–8 months old. In these children this index is higher than in healthy children, whereas in children above the age of 9 months this index significantly decreases. It may be thus concluded that the occurrence of some deformations in the proportions of the posterior and anterior parts of the head is connected with the children's age.

The index values of the anterior and posterior height of the cranial vault and cranial base are lower in children with scaphocephaly (Figs. 7 and 8). With age the difference between the index values in sick and healthy children increases. It may be thus concluded that these indices can constitute markers for the assessment of the phase and degree of scaphocephaly.

In healthy children under 12 months, the nasal-orbital angle oscillates between $108° \pm 6°$ (Fig. 9), whereas in children with scaphocephaly this angle is lower ($99° \pm 5°$) due to a smaller width of the skull caused by blocking the head growth in lateral directions. The biggest difference in the values of the angle can be noticed in children above 6 months of age.

On the grounds of the diagrams presented in the Figs. 10 and 11, it can be stated that in patients with trigonocephaly the angle of the frontal bone and the interorbital angle may constitute the marker of this defect. During the planning of a surgical procedure, it is essential to take into consideration the increase of these angles in order to obtain a rounder shape of the head. Figures 12 and 13 present the dependence of linear dimensions of the skull, which enables the evaluation of hypotelorism in patients. The values of both indices in patients are lowered in comparison with the children having a regular head shape.

To sum up the analysis of the values of skull indices, it can be stated that it is possible to assess the degree of the skull deformation on the basis of the distances between ten and twenty anatomical points in a proper configuration determined for a particular defect. In addition to that, it should be emphasised that the points constituting the basis for the distances may be relatively easily found on the childs head. The development of standard indices for the group of healthy children enables a quick comparison of the index values in the case of patients, both during the initial diagnosis and during check-ups before the operation (it should be noted that usually the time between a diagnostic CT examination and an operation takes around three months). There is also one more significant observation that the values of the majority of the presented coefficients differ from standard values, especially in patients above 6 months of age. In this period a dynamic irregular growth of the head can be noticed, therefore early diagnosis and treatment of the malformation are necessary to avoid further complications.

The statistical analysis of morphometric tests of the skulls of healthy children and those with craniosynostosis enabled the determination of a set of dimensions distinguishing regular skulls from pathological ones. The results obtained make it possible to better understand the mechanisms which deform the skull. The research results also constitute the basis for a quantitative assessment of effectiveness of the treatment of craniosynostosis in infants. On the grounds of the distances between selected anatomical points, the indices were determined in a proper configuration corresponding to a particular defect. The standard values calculated for the group of healthy children enable a quick comparison of the patient's indices obtained during the initial diagnosis as well as the evaluation of the degree of the skull deformation. The development of standard indices allows also an objective assessment of the treatment progress and effects of the operation during medical check-ups. The examinations of the skulls morphology made it possible to select morphometric features typical of particular types of skull shape defects. They constitute a set of qualifiers which enable the differentiation of the shape defects of not only the cranial vault but also the facial skeleton and the cranial base. In the case of scaphocephaly, it is characteristic that the growth disorder of the skull occurs in the anterior and posterior directions. It is thus the length of the skull which is the most important dimension to watch. Apart from the cephalic index, there are also other important indices for this defect such as the index of the anterior and posterior length of the cranial vault as well as the index of the anterior and posterior height of the cranial vault. In patients with trigonocephaly the deformation occurs first of all in the frontal and orbital area. It is therefore advisable to test the dimensions which characterize the angles in the area of eyes and the distances between eyes as they determine hypotelorism. Moreover, there are further indices typical of children with trigonocephaly. Such indices relate to anthropometric points located within nasal bones. The indices characteristic of trigonocephaly determine the symmetry of the skull. They are based first of all on the distances between points located in the area of the facial skeleton and cranium. The index of the anterior and posterior length of the skull as well as the index of the anterior and posterior height of the cranial base are typical of this kind of defect. In the case of brachycephaly, this malformation is characterized by the index of the anterior and posterior length of the skull as well as the index of the anterior and posterior height of the cranial vault. Assigning individual indices to typical defects of the skull shape may result in the practical application in the decision-making process during diagnosing and selection of treatment suitable for a particular type of craniosynostosis.

References

1. Agrawal, D., Steinbok, P., Douglas, C.: Long-term anthropometric outcomes following surgery for isolated sagittal craniosynostosis. J. Neurosurg. Pediatr. **105**(5), 357–360 (2006)
2. Aviv, R., Rodger, E., Hall, C.: Craniosynostosis. Clin. Radiol. **57**(2), 93–102 (2002)
3. Cotton, F., Rozzi, F., Vallee, B., Pachai, C., Hermier, M., Guihard-Costa, A., Froment, J.: Cranial sutures and craniometric points detected on MRI. Surg. Radiol. Anat. **27**(1), 64–70 (2005)
4. Dvoracek, L., Skolnick, G., Nguyen, D.C., Naidoo, S.D., Smyth, M.D., Woo, A.S., Patel, K.B.: Comparison of traditional versus normative cephalic index in patients with sagittal synostosis: measure of scaphocephaly and postoperative outcome. Plastic Reconstr. Surg. **136**(3), 541–548 (2015)
5. Gzik-Zroska, B., Wolański, W., Gzik, M.: Engineering-aided treatment of chest deformities to improve the process of breathing. Int. J. Numer. Methods Biomed. Eng. **29**(9), 926–937 (2013)
6. Heller, J.B., Heller, M.M., Knoll, B., Gabbay, J.S., Duncan, C., Persing, J.A.: Intracranial volume and cephalic index outcomes for total calvarial reconstruction among nonsyndromic sagittal synostosis patients. Plastic Reconstr. Surg. **121**(1), 187–195 (2008)
7. Larysz, D., Larysz, P., Filipek, J., Wolański, W., Gzik, M., Kawlewska, E.: Morphometric analysis of the skull shape in children with hydrocephalus. Computational vision and medical image processing IV. Proceedings of VIPIMAGE 2013-IV ECCOMAS, Funchal pp. 337–340 (2013)
8. Larysz, D., Wolański, W., Kawlewska, E., Mandera, M., Gzik, M.: Biomechanical aspects of preoperative planning of skull correction in children with craniosynostosis. Acta Bioeng. Biomech. **14**(2), 19–26 (2012)
9. Leikola, J., Koljonen, V., Heliövaara, A., Hukki, J., Koivikko, M.: Cephalic index correlates poorly with intracranial volume in non-syndromic scaphocephalic patients. Child's Nervous Syst. **30**(12), 2097–2102 (2014)

10. Likus, W., Bajor, G., Gruszczyńska, K., Baron, J., Markowski, J.: Nasal region dimensions in children: a CT study and clinical implications. BioMed Res. Int. 2014 (2014)
11. van Lindert, E.J., Siepel, F.J., Delye, H., Ettema, A.M., Bergé, S.J., Maal, T.J., Borstlap, W.A.: Validation of cephalic index measurements in scaphocephaly. Child's Nervous Syst. 29(6), 1007–1014 (2013)
12. Scarr, G.: A model of the cranial vault as a tensegrity structure, and its significance to normal and abnormal cranial development. Int. J. Osteop. Med. 11(3), 80–89 (2008)
13. Sgouros, S., Natarajan, K., Hockley, A., Goldin, J., Wake, M.: Skull base growth in craniosynostosis. Pediatr. Neurosurg. 31(6), 281–293 (2000)
14. Tejszerska, D., Wolański, W., Larysz, D., Gzik, M., Sacha, E.: Morphological analysis of the skull shape in craniosynostosis. Acta Bioeng. Biomech. 13(1), 35–40 (2011)
15. Wolański, W., Gzik, M., Kawlewska, E., Larysz, D., Larysz, P.: The finite element analysis of skull deformation after correction of scaphocephaly. In: Tavares, J., Jorge, R.M.N. (eds.) Computational Vision and Medical Image Processing: Vip-IMAGE 2011, pp. 43–46. Taylor and Francis Group (2012)
16. Wolański, W., Gzik, M., Kawlewska, E., Stachowiak, E., Larysz, D., Rudnik,A., Krawczyk, I., Bazowski, P.: Preoperative planning the lumbar spinestabilization with posterior intervertebral systems. Computational Vision andMedical Image Processing IV: VIPIMAGE 2013, p. 345 (2013)
17. Wolański, W., Larysz, D., Gzik, M., Kawlewska, E.: Modeling and biomechanical analysis of craniosynostosis correction with the use of finite element method. Int. J. Numer. Methods Biomed. Eng. 29(9), 916–925 (2013)

Application of the Ogden Model to the Tensile Stress-Strain Behavior of the Pig's Skin

Sylwia Łagan$^{(\boxtimes)}$ and Aneta Liber-Kneć

Crakow University of Technology, Warszawska 24, 31-155 Crakow, Poland
slagan@mech.pk.edu.pl
http://pk.edu.pl

Abstract. The mechanical properties of a pig's skin which is used as the human skin substitute in the studies carried out *in vitro* are important for a number of applications, including surgery and biomechanics. In this study, uniaxial tensile experiments were performed on porcine skin for the two directions of the samples taken (parallel and perpendicular to the spine) to investigate the tensile stress-strain response. The experimental results show that pig's skin exhibits anisotropic and non-linear behavior. The Ogden model was adopted to describe tensile behavior of the pig's skin. The Ogden model provides a good tensile curve fit for the animal skin tissue in the low range of deformation (first and second stage of elongation curve).

Keywords: Tensile test · Mechanical response · Porcine skin · Ogden model

1 Intoduction

The human skin is a complex tissue which consists of several heterogeneous layers: the epidermis, the dermis, and the hypodermis. Each layer has a unique structure and function [5,13]. Due to the legal regulations and the ethical issues, obtaining human skin for experimental tests is difficult. A literature analysis shows that substitute of human skin like animals' skin is used in the majority of *in vitro* skin examinations. The similarity of anatomical features and mechanical properties makes the pig's skin most commonly used human skin substitute [10,16]. The mechanical examinations carried on towards recognizing skin tissue properties show that it is an anisotropic, viscoelastic and non-linear material [13]. The exact determination of skin's mechanical properties is still an open question, and there is no one and only standard that has been established in determining skin's behavior. Additionally, tests results are influenced by the conditions of samples taken (e.g. a direction of sample taken, a type of animal, parameters of samples storage: medium, temperature, time, humidity). There are several methods of samples storage, e.g. cooling, freezing [5].

The determination of mechanical properties of skin is essential both in engineering and medicine, in such fields like surgery and dermatology to predicting

© Springer International Publishing AG 2017
M. Gzik et al. (eds.), *Innovations in Biomedical Engineering*, Advances in Intelligent Systems and Computing 526, DOI 10.1007/978-3-319-47154-9_17

the effect of surgical treatment. The knowledge acquired in experimental tests *in vivo* and *in vitro* is used for designing surgical tools, medical robots and in criminology to estimation the history of damage formation and the nature of skin lesions due to mechanical injuries or traffic accidents [13].

Constitutive modeling of biological tissues is important in many fields such as biomechanics of collisions [4,7,12], rehabilitation, tissue engineering, surgical simulations [3,9], drug delivery systems. For skin, existing hyperelastic models such as Neo-Hookean [1], Mooney-Rivlin [15], Ogden [2,15] have been employed.

In this study, *in vitro*, tensile uniaxial stress versus strain response for pig's skin tissue and the approximation of experimental results with the use of the Ogden model were presented.

2   Material and Methodology

The pieces of skin for examinations were taken from the back of a 9-month domestic pig (the weigh of animal was 135 kg). Hairs and the fat were removed from the skin using a sharp scalpel blade and then skin samples were cut in two directions: parallel and perpendicular in the reference to the spine. All samples had the same dimensions: the length 100.0 ± 0.2 mm, the measurement base for all samples was 50 ± 0.2 mm, the width 10.0 ± 0.2 mm and the average thickness was 2.2 ± 0.2 mm. The samples were stored at the temperature of $-18\,°C$ wrapped in polypropylene foil. The tests were carried out after 1 hour from defrosting in the temperature of $22 \pm 2\,°C$. The uniaxial tensile tests were carried out with the use of the MTS Insight 50 testing machine, the range of measuring head was 1 kN. The samples were mounted using flat clamps and they were elongated at the constant rate of 5 mm/min (the strain rate of 0.0017 1/s), which is commonly used for soft tissues [17]. Each set of samples for tension testing (the samples divided according to the direction of their taking) contained minimum 5 samples. In the results the average stress-strain curves were presented. Next, the Ogden model with two material constants was used to describe the tensile behavior of the pig's skin.

3   Results of Tensile Test

The characteristic tensile curves for the parallel and the perpendicular directions of sample taking were presented in Figs. 1, 2 and 3. The elongation curves for the skin present non-linear characteristic with two quasi-linear segments. The shape of the curves allows to distinguish three phases, what is specific for soft tissues. The first phase (I) showed in Figs. 1 and 2, is known as "toe region", in which the elastin fibres are mainly responsible for stretching mechanism, while the contribution of the collagen fibres is negligible. In the second phase (II) of stretching, the collagen fibres align themselves in the direction of applied load and become straighter, the force-extension relation becomes approximately linear. In the third phase (III), the ultimate tensile strength is reached [5,6]. In dependence of sample direction taking, the curves had different slope and the

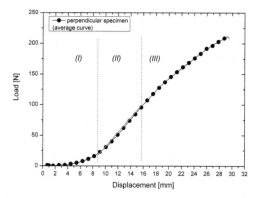

Fig. 1. The average tension curve for perpendicular samples pig's skin tissue with specific phases *(I)*, *(II)* and *(III)*.

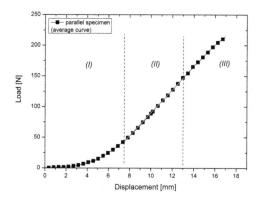

Fig. 2. The average tension curve for parallel samples pig's skin tissue with specific phases *(I)*, *(II)* and *(III)*.

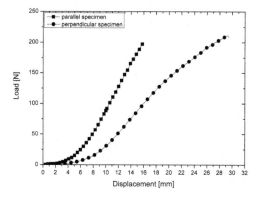

Fig. 3. The comparison of elongation curves for parallel and perpendicular samples.

range of maximal extension. The tensile test of skin samples was carried out to characterize the mechanical parameters of skin material, the tensile strength for the perpendicular samples was $11.87 \pm 1.69\,\mathrm{MPa}$, $10.65 \pm 1.75\,\mathrm{MPa}$ for parallel samples and the strain was respectively 0.66 ± 0.05 and 0.34 ± 0.02.

4   Constitutive Model

To describe the measured constitutive response of skin tissue, the Ogden model is commonly employed [15]. The Ogden model is used to describe non-linear behavior of hyperelastic material, such as polymers, rubber and soft tissue. The model assumes that materials behavior may be characterized by a strain energy density function. On the base on this function stress-strain relationship is obtained. A strain energy density function W is given as (1):

$$W(\lambda_1, \lambda_2, \lambda_3) = \frac{2\mu}{\alpha^2}(\lambda_1^\alpha + \lambda_2^\alpha + \lambda_3^\alpha - 3) \qquad (1)$$

where α and μ are material constants - shear modulus and strain hardening exponent. For incompressible material, the principal stretch ratios are described by the formula (2):

$$\lambda_1 \lambda_2 \lambda_3 = 1 \qquad (2)$$

A strain energy function can be given as the function of two independent stretches with the use of formulas (1) and (2):

$$\hat{W}(\lambda_1, \lambda_2) = W(\lambda_1, \lambda_2, \lambda_1^{-1}\lambda_2^{-1}) = \frac{2\mu}{\alpha^2}(\lambda_1^\alpha + \lambda_2^\alpha + \lambda_1^{-\alpha}\lambda_2^{-\alpha} - 3) \qquad (3)$$

Under plane stress condition it is assumed $\sigma_3 = 0$, nominal stress σ_i is described by dependence [14]:

$$\sigma_1 = \frac{\partial \hat{W}}{\partial \lambda_1}, \quad \sigma_2 = \frac{\partial \hat{W}}{\partial \lambda_2} \qquad (4)$$

For uniaxial elongation carried out by the load in the direction of the long axis, the nominal stress can be given as (5):

$$\sigma_1 = \frac{2\mu}{\alpha}[\lambda^{\alpha-1} - \lambda^{-1-(\frac{\alpha}{2})}], \quad \sigma_2 = 0 \qquad (5)$$

The materials constants for the Ogden model (α i μ) can be obtained experimentally. During the calculation of the Ogden model, the values of shear modulus and strain hardening exponent were set up as variables larger than zero. The procedure of calculation was carried out until the value of R^2 (coefficient of determination) was higher than 0.99.

4.1   Results and Discussion

In Fig. 4, the tensile stress-strain curves fitted with the Ogden model at 0.0017/s strain rate were shown. The Ogden model provided a good approximation of the experimental data obtained in the tensile test for pig's skin but only for low stretching ratio value, first and second stage of stress-stain curves (Fig. 5). This corresponds to a range of elastic deformation of elastin and collagen fibers, where initially the non-linear shape of the stress-strain curve changes the character on the similar to a straight line. For the third stage of elongation, the stress-stain curves didn't fit with the Ogden model (for stretching ratio above 1,15 for perpendicular samples and 1,3 for parallel samples). The Ogden constants determined experimentally for two directions of samples taken were summarized in Table 1.

In our research, one value of the strain rate and variable values of shear modulus and strain hardening exponent were used. However in the literature,

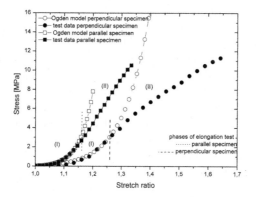

Fig. 4. The engineering stress versus stretch ratio response of pig's skin, experimental data and the Ogden fit for the first and second phase of elongation test.

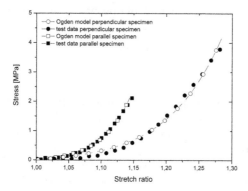

Fig. 5. The comparison of theoretical Ogden model curves and stress-stretch ratio curves for parallel and perpendicular samples in the total range of elongation.

Table 1. Ogden constants (α and μ) evaluated from uniaxial tensile stress versus strain response of pig's skin.

Direct of sample	Shear modulus μ (MPa)	Strain hardening exponent α
Parallel	0.78387 ± 0.01388	28.10237 ± 0.2113
Perpendicular	0.64764 ± 0.01862	17.02676 ± 0.1708

the noticeable influence of the strain rate on changing the value of the Ogden coefficient μ and its negligible influence on the Ogden exponent α was observed [14]. The data used by Manan et al. [11] for numerical investigation of influence of the Ogden coefficients (μ and α) on stress-stretch ratio curves showed its quasi-linear dispersion. According to [11] the low value of shear modulus will influence the stress-stretch ratio curve linearly, where by increasing the values will cause the curve to behave highly non-linear.

In the literature, elongation curves fitting by the Ogden model are shown for the elastic behavior of the material. In the research carried out by Shergold et al., the Ogden material model was used to detail the mechanical characteristics of pig's skin under uniaxial tension [15]. The results showed that the Ogden model provides a good curve fit for the pig's skin. A good elongation curve fit was obtained by Lim et al. for the stretch ratio of about 2,3 for specimen perpendicular to spine and 1,4 for the specimen parallel to spine [8]. The value of shear modulus for perpendicular and parallel pig's skin samples agrees with the shear modulus reported by Shergold et al. (0,4–7,5 MPa in dependence on strain rate and constant $\alpha = 12$). In our research, the parallel specimens have higher values of strain hardening exponent (about 40 %) and shear modulus (about 17 %) than perpendicular samples. The low strain rate shear modulus of human skin $\mu = 0.11$ MPa and $\alpha = 9$ are close to our values. The study conducted by Ni Annaidh et al., shows the value of mechanical properties for human skin: ultimate tensile stress 21,6 $\pm$ 8,4 MPa, but in the literature 1–32 MPa, failure strain 0,54 $\pm$ 0,17, but in the literature 0,17–2,07 [13]. Wide range of values depends on age, orientation/location of specimens, conditions of *in vivo* or *in vitro* tests.

5   Conclusions

An analysis of the stress versus strain response for pig's skin tissue under quasi-static uniaxial tensile test of samples taken in two directions, parallel and perpendicular with respect to the long axis of the animal (identified by the axis of the spine) was performed. The experimental results indicate the non-linear nature of the behavior and the effect of anisotropy of skin tissue on the stress-strain characteristics. Presented results demonstrate that the Ogden model can provide a good approximation to experimental data, particularly in the range of low stretch ratio. For the good approximation of constitutive model, it is essential to obtain the values of material constants for different strain rates, particularly shear modulus which is dependent on strain rate [8,15]. The understanding of skin behaviour under applied load is important for the production of skin substitutes, temporary and permanent. The anisotropic tensile properties are significant for surgery simulation and skin graft. Mechanical properties of pig's skin should be investigated and compared with human data.

Acknowledgements. The work was realized due to statutory activities M-1/6/2015/DS.

References

1. Delalleau, A., Josse, G., Lagarde, J.M., Zahouani, H., Bergheau, J.M.: A nonlinear elastic behavior to identify the mechanical parameters of human skin in vivo. Skin Res. Technol. **14**(2), 152–164 (2008)
2. Evans, S.L.: On the implementation of a wrinkling, hyperelastic membrane model for the skin and other materials. Comput. Methods Biomech. Biomed. Eng. **12**(3), 319–332 (2009)
3. Famaey, N., Vander Sloten, J.: Soft tissue modelling for applications in virtual surgery and surgical robotics. Comput. Methods Biomech. Biomed. Eng. **11**(4), 351–366 (2008)
4. Forbes, P.D., Cronin, D.S., Deng, Y.C., Boismenu, M.: Numerical human model to predict side impact thoracic trauma. In: IUTAM Symposium on Impact Biomechanics: From Fundamental Insights to Applications, Dublin (2005)
5. Geerligs, M.: Skin layer mechanics. Ph.D. thesis, Technische Universiteit Eidhoven (2010)
6. Hendriks, F.M.: Mechanical behavior of human skin in vivo: a literature review. Nat. Lab. Unclassified report 820, Philips Research Laboratories (2001)
7. Ivancic, P.C., Pearson, A.M., Tominaga, Y., Simpson, A.K., Yue, J.J., Panjabi, M.M.: Mechanism of cervical spinal cord injury during bilateral facet dislocation. Spine **32**(22), 2467–2473 (2007)
8. Lim, J., Hong, J., Chen, W.W., Weerasooriya, T.: Mechanical response of pig skin under dynamic tensile loading. Int. J. Impact Eng. **38**, 130–135 (2011)
9. Lim, Y., Kim, K., Park, K.: ECG recording on a Bed Turing Steep without direct skin-contact. IEEE Trans. Biomed. Eng. **54**(4), 718–725 (2007)
10. Liu, Z., Yeung, K.: The preconditioning and stress relaxation of skin tissue. J. Biomed. Pharmaceut. Eng. **2**(1), 22–28 (2008)
11. Manan, N.F.A., Noor, S.N.A.M., Azmi, N.N., Mahmud, J.: Numerical investigation of Ogden and Mooney-Rivlin material parameters. ARPN J. Eng. Appl. Sci. **10**(15), 6329–6335 (2015)
12. Muggenthaler, H., Merten, K., Peldschus, S., Holley, S., Adamec, J., Praxl, N., Graw, M.: Experimental tests for the validation of active numerical human models. Forensic Sci. Int. **177**(2–3), 184–191 (2008)
13. Annaidh, A.N., Bruyere, K., Destrade, M., Gilchrist, M.D., Ottenio, M.: Characterizing the anisotropic mechanical properties of excised human skin. J. Mech. Behav. Biomed. Mater. **5**(1), 139–148 (2012)
14. Ogden, R.W., Saccomandi, G., Sgura, I.: Fitting hyperelastic models to experimental data. Comput. Mech. **4**(6), 11 (2004)
15. Shergold, O.A., Fleck, N.A., Radford, D.: The uniaxial stress versus strain response of pig skin and silicone rubber at low and high strain rates. Int. J. Impact Eng. **32**, 1384–1402 (2006)

16. Swindle, M.M., Makin, A., Herron, A.J., Clubb, F.J., Frazier, K.S.: Swine as models in biomedical research and toxicology testing. Vet. Pathol. **49**(21), 344–356 (2012)

17. Żak, M., Kuropka, P., Kobielarz, M., Dudek, A., Kaleta-Kuratewicz, K., Szotek, S.: Determination of the mechanical properties of the skin of pig fetuses with respect to its structure. Acta Bioeng. Biomech. **13**(2), 37–43 (2011)

Virtual Therapy Simulation for Patient with Coarctation of Aorta Using CFD Blood Flow Modelling

Bartłomiej Melka[1]([⊠]), Wojciech Adamczyk[1], Marek Rojczyk[1],
Andrzej J. Nowak[1], Adam Golda[2], and Ziemowit Ostrowski[1]

[1] Institute of Thermal Technology, Biomedical Engineering Lab,
Silesian University of Technology, Konarskiego 22, 44-100 Gliwice, Poland
{bartlomiej.melka,ziemowit.ostrowski}@polsl.pl
[2] Department of Cardiology, Gliwice Medical Centre, Kosciuszki 29,
44-100 Gliwice, Poland
http://www.itc.polsl.pl/ostrowski

Abstract. The paper presents a numerical method of blood flow simulation in two geometries. The first geometry covered the ascending and descending parts of aorta and its main branches in patient with a congenital heart disease - coarctation of aorta (inborn narrowing of the descendent aorta). The second geometry used in the flow field analysis mimicked the state of the vessel after a successful percutaneous intervention and thus without pathological narrowing (virtual therapy). The blood was treated as a non-Newtonian fluid. The pulsating flow was set at the inlet to ascending aorta. The lumped model based on electrical analogy using three-element-Windkessel model was created to calculate pressure at the outlets. In the publication the fields of velocity and pressure were presented. The obtained outflow streams were modified after virtual therapy.

Keywords: CFD · Blood flow · Coarctation of the aorta · Lumped model · non-Newtonian flow

1 Introduction

In the last years the Computational Fluid Dynamics (CFD) was gaining a wider application in bio-engineering. Combining a numerical flow simulation with images obtained from a computed tomography or magnetic resonance may give a novel quality for a non-invasive blood flow analysis in the medicine and thus help to better identify the pathological changes within the circulatory system or set more accurate diagnoses [1]. The CFD implementation could model and visualize the blood flow before intended endovascular therapy or surgical intervention and show the consequences for the patient prior the invasive procedure [2].

Nowadays the multiphase approach of blood flow CFD modeling is the state of art [3–5]. It is proved to be essential especially in the simulations of the blood

M. Gzik et al. (eds.), *Innovations in Biomedical Engineering*, Advances in Intelligent Systems and Computing 526, DOI 10.1007/978-3-319-47154-9_18

flow in the coronary arteries [3]. To obtain more precise results a coupled model with mechanic solver has to be implemented in order to take in account the influence of elasticity of vessel walls and their deformation caused by the blood flow [6]. This coupled approach is used as Fluid Structure Interaction (FSI). In the current publication the authors intended to present a single-phase blood flow model with rigid walls.

There are many congenital heart diseases described in the literature where the cardiovascular abnormalities cause the alternations of the blood flow within the circulatory system. Coarctation of aorta (CoA) is one of the most frequent inborn cardiovascular defects. This defect is a pathological narrowing of the descending aorta causing a pressure drop in the descending aorta and consequently hypoperfusion of the lower parts of the human body. The upper parts of the body in this disease are exposed to arterial hypertension with all consequences like coronary artery disease or stroke. The curative therapy for CoA includes a surgical or percutaneous intervention intending to remove or dilate the narrowed site.

Up till now the application of the CFD methods is not a validated approach for clinical use. The main barriers for the implementation of numerical blood flow simulation in the clinical practice are time demanding pre-processing of the scan images and long calculation times caused by the unsteady flow phenomena. Usually for the blood flow simulation of the selected part of vascular system using CFD a lumped model is added to create a boundary conditions which simulates the remaining part of the circulatory system [7–10]. In this study a three-element-Windessel model was implemented for this purpose.

In the current work the authors present a blood flow distributions in the coarcted aorta before and after the virtual therapy. This virtual therapy could help to estimate the alternations of the blood flow within aorta and its main branches as a consequence of a real surgical therapy.

2   Numerical Model

In the research, models were built on the base of two geometries. The first one was converted from the surface format collected from a real 8-year old female patient by MRA imaging (Gadolinium – enhanced Magnetic Resonance Angiography). The original geometry is presented in Fig. 1. The second geometry was rebuilt from the first one in the region of CoA. In order to implement the reconstruction, the lumen before and behind the coarctation was smoothed and in consequence the narrowing was removed.

The mesh in both cases exceeded about 1.2 million of elements. The meshes were of a hybrid-type. In the first part of the inlet and main part of descending aorta hexahedral elements were used. In the bifurcation region mostly the tetrahedral elements were applied. The tetrahedral cells were chosen since this domain part was geometrically complex. The first layer of the boundary layer mesh was about 0.1 mm. Moreover, the boundary layer mesh was built from five layers and the growth ratio was at the level of 1.1. The sensitivity analysis of

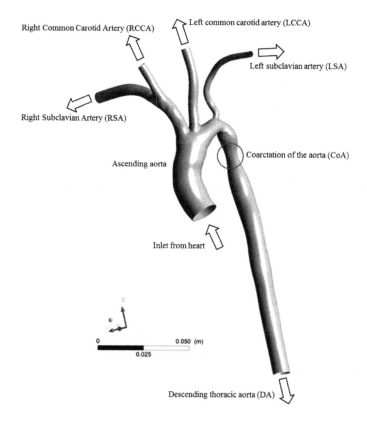

Fig. 1. The geometry with outlets description

the meshes leaded to a conclusion, that the mesh density did not influence the solution.

Seven main boundary conditions were assigned to the numerical domain. At the inlet, the pulsating velocity function was imitating the work of heart. This function is presented in Fig. 2. The vessel walls were treated in the model as rigid and in this boundary the no slip wall condition was used. The rest of boundary conditions were used as the pressure outlets, which were calculated separately for each one on the base of the Windkessel model.

The modeled fluid was treated as single phase and non-Newtonian. The non-Newtonian properties of the flow were implemented using Carreau model for the local viscosity calculation by (1), in accordance with [11]. The value of density used in calculations was $1055 \, \mathrm{kg \, m^{-3}}$.

$$\eta = \eta_\infty + (\eta_0 - \eta_\infty)\left[1 + (\lambda\dot{\gamma})^2\right]^{\frac{n-1}{2}} \tag{1}$$

where η means the local non-Newtonian viscosity and the local share rate $\dot{\gamma}$ is a scalar and was calculated locally from (2), the rest constants were: infinite shear viscosity $\eta_\infty = 0.0034\,\mathrm{Pa\,s}$, zero share viscosity $\eta_0 = 0.056\,\mathrm{Pa\,s}$, time constant $\lambda = 3.313\,\mathrm{s}$, Power Law index $n = 0.355$.

$$\dot{\gamma} = \sqrt{\frac{1}{2}\bar{\bar{D}} : \bar{\bar{D}}} \tag{2}$$

where $\bar{\bar{D}}$ is the rate of deformation tensor and is defined by (3).

$$\bar{\bar{D}} = \left(\frac{\partial u_j}{\partial x_i} + \frac{\partial u_i}{\partial x_j}\right) \tag{3}$$

where u is the velocity component and x is the Cartesian coordinate.

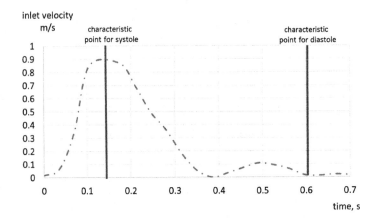

Fig. 2. Pulsatile velocity profile set at the inlet to the domain

The model domain contains five outflows represented by the pressure boundary conditions. The Windkessel model applied as the lumped parameter model was used at the outlets to set the proper overpressure simulating the vascular system response to the flow. The three-element Windkessel model [12] can be expressed by (4).

$$\left(1 + \frac{R_p}{R_d}\right) I(t) + C R_p \frac{dI(t)}{dt} = \frac{P(t)}{R_d} + C\frac{dP(t)}{dt} \tag{4}$$

where $I(t)$ is the blood flow out of the pump (heart) as a function of time, R_p is the resistance encountered by blood as it enters the aortic or pulmonary valve, while R_d is the resistance of blood as it passes from the aorta to the narrower arterioles, C is the constant ratio of air pressure to air volume (capacitance of the capacitor), $P(t)$ is blood pressure as a function of time.

R_p and R_d were constants and were adopted according to the values from Table 1. They were implemented from [13]. Created lumped model was applied in the similar way in [14].

Table 1. LPM model parameters

Artery name	Abbrev	R_p (kg m^{-4} s^{-1})	C (m^4 s^2 kg^{-1})	R_d (kg m^{-4} s^{-1})
Right subclavian	RSA	0.885×10^8	7.13×10^{-10}	1.3858×10^9
Right common carotid	RCCA	1.122×10^8	5.62×10^{-10}	1.7571×10^9
Left common carotid	LCCA	1.124×10^8	5.62×10^{-10}	1.7611×10^9
Left subclavian	LSA	2.895×10^8	2.12×10^{-10}	4.5361×10^9
Descending thoracic aorta	DA	0.271×10^8	2.92×10^{-9}	0.3122×10^9

The solver used to create and calculate solution was ANSYS® Fluent in the pressure based approach. The solver contained governing equations based on the mass and momentum conservation principles and they can be expressed by (5) and (6) as follows:

$$\frac{\partial \rho}{\partial t} + \nabla \cdot (\rho \mathbf{v}) = 0 \tag{5}$$

where ρ is the density, t is the time and $\mathbf{v}$ is the velocity.

$$\frac{\partial \rho}{\partial t} (\rho \mathbf{v}) + \nabla \cdot (\rho \mathbf{v} \mathbf{v}) = -\nabla p + \nabla \cdot \bar{\bar{\tau}} \tag{6}$$

where p is a static pressure and $\bar{\bar{\tau}}$ is the stress tensor, which can be calculated for the non-Newtonian fluid from (7).

$$\bar{\bar{\tau}} = \eta \left(\nabla \mathbf{v} + \nabla \mathbf{v}^T \right) \tag{7}$$

3 Results

All results presented in this section are referred to the maximum flow corresponding to the characteristic point of the systole (marked in Fig. 2). The results are presented as the instantaneous values.

The velocity field in the model with CoA is presented in Fig. 3 for the maximum flow during the systole (point marked in Fig. 2). The maximum velocity occurs in the region of the coarctation and reaches about 3.2 m/s.

After applying virtual therapy (narrowing removal), the maximum speed decreased to 2.7 m/s. The velocity profile in the reconstructed region with main aorta bifurcations is presented in Fig. 4. In Figs. 3 and 4, it is visible that the velocity profile did not change significantly after the coarctation reconstruction in the region of the main aorta bifurcations. The main change after virtual

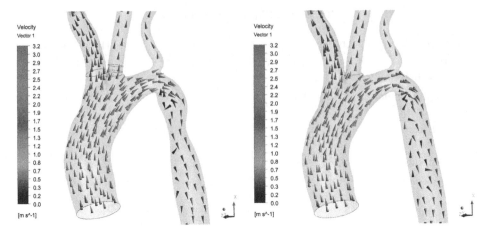

Fig. 3. Velocity field in m/s in model with CoA

Fig. 4. Velocity field in m/s in model after virtual therapy

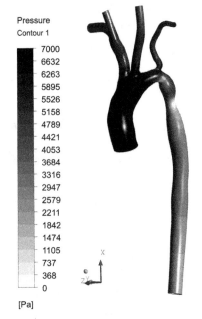

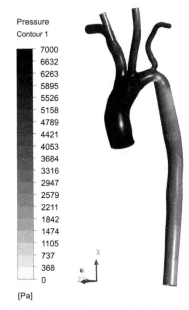

Fig. 5. Pressure field in Pa in model with coarctation

Fig. 6. Pressure field in Pa in model after virtual therapy

therapy can be noticed in the velocity field in the region of narrowing. The velocity decreased in this region.

The static pressure profile on the walls region for the original geometry with coarctation is presented in Fig. 5. While, in Fig. 6 the same profile is shown for the reconstructed geometry. From presented pressure fields, one can notice that the local static pressure minimum in the region of CoA vanished after

Table 2. Mass flows and pressures at the outlets.

Artery	Mass flow (kg/s)		Overpressure with CoA (Pa)	
	With CoA	After Virt. therapy	With CoA	After Virt. therapy
Inlet	0.212	0.212	6979	6722
RSA	0.044	0.040	4253	3734
RCCA	0.032	0.030	3997	3565
LCCA	0.035	0.033	4354	3897
LSA	0.010	0.009	3281	2799
DA	0.091	0.099	2617	2769

geometry changing. Additionally, the pressure values at the outlets are presented in Table 2. The pressure fields indicate decrease of the static pressure on the vessel walls after virtual therapy. The maximum pressure differences between inlet and outlets reached 4362 Pa before coarctation removal and after that was 3953 Pa. Moreover, the flow after the CoA removal increased by 9 % in the descending aorta.

4   Conclusions

In this paper a numerical models of blood flow through aorta with congenital coarctation and after a virtual therapy were presented. The first model covered the geometry converted magnetic resonance angiography of an 8-year old patient with the CoA (with an approximately 65 % lumen reduction of the proximal part of descending aorta). The virtual therapy included the reconstruction of the abnormal narrowing to average diameter corresponding to the next section of descending aorta. The models presented the pulsating blood flow as a non-Newtonian single phase fluid coupled with lumped model setting the pressure at the outlets. The lumped model was built on the base of three-element-Windkessel model.

The stream flowing through descending aorta increased by 9 % after elimination of the coarctation in comparison to flow before virtual therapy. Moreover, the removal of CoA caused the velocity decrease in the modified region. Also the pressure difference between main inlet and descending aorta outlet has been reduced after virtual therapy.

Acknowledgements. This research is supported by National Science Centre (Poland) within Project Nos. 2014/13/B/ST8/04225 and 2014/15/D/ST8/ 02620 (Thanks for making GeoMagic Design X software available to the research team). This help is gratefully acknowledged herewith.

References

1. DeCampli, W., Argueta-Morales, R., Divo, E., Kassab, A.: Computational fluid dynamics in congenital heart disease. Cardiol. Young **22**(6), 800–808 (2012)
2. Morris, P.D., Narracott, A., Von Tengg-Kobligk, H., Soto, D.A.S., Hsiao, S., Lungu, A., Evans, P., Bressloff, N.W., Lawford, P.V., Rodney Hose, D., Gunn, J.P.: Computational fluid dynamics modelling in cardiovascular medicine. Heart **102**(1), 18–28 (2016)
3. Huang, J., Lyczkowski, R.W., Gidaspow, D.: Pulsatile flow in a coronary artery using multiphase kinetic theory. J. Biomech. **42**(6), 743–754 (2009)
4. Ostrowski, Z., Melka, B., Adamczyk, W., Rojczyk, M., Golda, A., Nowak, A.J.: CFD analysis of multiphase blood flow within aorta and its thoracic branches of patient with coarctation of aorta using multiphase Euler–Euler approach. J. Phys. Conf. Ser. (2016, accepted for publication, in press)
5. Gidaspow, D., Huang, J.: Kinetic theory based model for blood flow and its viscosity. Ann. Biomed. Eng. **37**(8), 1534–1545 (2009)
6. Reymond, P., Crosetto, P., Deparis, S., Quarteroni, A., Stergiopulos, N.: Physiological simulation of blood flow in the aorta: comparison of hemodynamic indices as predicted by 3-D FSI, 3-D rigid wall and 1-D models. Med. Eng. Phys. **35**(6), 784–791 (2013)
7. De Pater, L., Van den Berg, J.W.: An electrical analogue of the entire human circulatory system. Med. Electron. Biol. Eng. **42**, 161–166 (1964)
8. Westerhof, N., Bosman, F., Cornelis, J., Noordergraaf, A.: Analog studies of the human systemic arterial tree. J. Biomech. **2**, 121–143 (1969)
9. Westerhof, N., Elzinga, G., Sipkema, P.: An artificial arterial system for pumping hearts. J. Appl. Physiol. **31**, 776–781 (1971)
10. Yoshigi, M., Keller, B.B.: Characterisation of embryonic aortic impedance with lumped parameter models. Am. J. Physiol. **273**, 19–27 (1997)
11. Cho, Y., Kensey, K.R.: Effects of the non-Newtonian viscosity of blood on flows in a diseased arterial vessel. Biorheology **28**(3), 241–262 (1991)
12. Broemser, P., Ranke, O.: Ueber die Messung des Schlagvolumens des Herzens auf unblutigem Weg. Zeitung fur Biologie **90**, 467–507 (1930)
13. http://www.vascularmodel.com. Accessed 30 Apr. 2016
14. Rojczyk, M., Ostrowski, Z., Adamczyk, W., Melka, B., Bandoła, D., Gracka, M., Knopek, A., Golda, A., Nowak, A.J., Golda, A.: CFD analysis of blood flow within aorta of patient with coarctation of aorta. Stud. Inf. (2016, in review)

Evaluation of Locomotor Function in Patients with CP Based on Muscle Length Changes

Katarzyna Nowakowska[1]([✉]), Robert Michnik[1],
Katarzyna Jochymczyk-Woźniak[1], Jacek Jurkojć[1], and Ilona Kopyta[2]

[1] Department of Biomechatronics, Faculty of Biomedical Engineering, Silesian
University of Technology, F. D. Roosevelta 40, 41-800 Zabrze, Poland
{katarzyna.nowakowska,robert.michnik,katarzyna.jochymczyk-wozniak,
jacek.jurkojc}@polsl.pl
[2] Department of Paediatrics and Developmental Age Neurology, Chair of Paediatrics,
Medical University of Silesia, Medyków 16, 40-752 Katowice, Poland
ilonakopyta@autograf.pl
https://www.polsl.pl/Wydzialy/RIB
http://www.sum.edu.pl/

Abstract. The aim of this study was to analyze locomotor function of children with cerebral palsy based on changes in muscle length and to evaluate if the muscle length changes may be used as a diagnostic indicator. The study group consisted of 23 people with normal gait and 3 patients with cerebral palsy. Locomotor function tests were performed using the BTS Smart system, while the length of the muscles were determined using mathematical modeling methods with the help of Anybody Modeling System software. In this study the muscle group functioning in connection with the knee joint were analyzed. The results of muscle length changes for children with CP were compared to those of people with no evidence of impaired locomotor function, as well as to the values of GGI and GDI indicators and to kinematic parameters.

Keywords: Muscle length · Gait analysis · Musculo-skeletal model · Anybody modeling system

1 Introduction

Biomechanical studies are being used in the analysis of locomotor function more and more commonly. They allow the assessment of the gait through a series of kinematic and kinetic gait parameters i.e. joint angle changes, ground reaction, torque and force in the individual joints. Frequently patient diagnostics requires obtaining information concerning the function of individual muscles. EMG tests used for this purpose allow for assessment of muscle activity, but only of those directly beneath the skin. Meanwhile somewhat more problematic is the appointment of forces generated by muscle groups, because there is no possibility of direct measurements [12]. Muscle strength is dependent on: the muscle fiber length change rate (the speed of muscle shortening), the cross section of

© Springer International Publishing AG 2017
M. Gzik et al. (eds.), *Innovations in Biomedical Engineering*, Advances in Intelligent
Systems and Computing 526, DOI 10.1007/978-3-319-47154-9_19

the muscle, energy production efficiency in muscle cells, intramuscular temperature or fatigue. For a detailed description of muscle function during walking it is necessary to characterize the muscle fiber length changes, which is also very difficult to perform. So far to directly measure the length of sarcomeres either laser diffraction [6] or microendoskopy [9,10] methods were used. Attempts were also made to assess muscle length using imaging techniques and mathematical modeling [2–5,11,13,14]. However, none of the existing methods allows for the direct measurement of changes in muscle length during movement [1]. Without evaluating muscle length changes it is not possible to determine the operating characteristics of the muscle, i.e. determining whether the muscle during activity works concentrically or eccentrically. In addition, in patients with impaired muscle functions caused by, for example, spasticity, knowledge of the course of the changes in their length may allow for easier evaluation of abnormalities [14].

The aim of this study was to determine the course of length change in selected muscles during gait for a group of healthy children and patients with cerebral palsy. Gait kinematics studies and musculo-skeletal system modeling methods were used to achieve this. The paper presents an initial evaluation of the possibilities of using designated changes in muscle length as a diagnostic indicator.

2   Materials and Methods

Locomotor function tests were carried out in the Upper Silesian Child Health Care Center in Katowice using the optical system BTS SMART. The system for gait analysis consists of: a set of markers placed in specific anatomical points on the body of the tested person, a set of eight cameras registering the markers' position change (with a sampling frequency of 250 Hz), two video cameras and two dynamometric platforms manufactured by Kistler. Before examining gait necessary anthropometric measurements were taken. During the study, each patient performed a static test requiring standing still and then walked through the measuring path with his own natural speed. Kinematic and dynamic gait parameters registered during the experiment allowed for numerical simulation in the Anybody Modeling System program. The calculations used a modified Gait Full Body model allowing for simulation of the muscular system function during gait. The musculo-skeletal models were scaled off of the person's anthropometric parameters and registered marker location. The use of mathematical modeling in Anybody software allowed us to determine the trajectory of length changes in selected muscles during walking. For the studied group of patients, using self-developed applications written in Matlab, gait indicators: Gillette Gait Index (GGI) and Gait Deviation Index (GDI) were calculated.

The control group (standard) consisted of 23 people (13 boys and 10 girls) ranging in age from 7 to 16 years with no locomotor function impairment. In addition three patients with spastic forms of cerebral palsy, who have been qualified for treatment using botulinum toxin had their gait analyzed. The P2 patient was diagnosed with bilateral spastic paralysis of the lower limbs (diplegia), while patients P1 and P3 were diagnosed with right hemiplegia. The characteristics of the group studied have been presented in Table 1.

Table 1. Characteristics of control group and patients with CP

	Control group	P1	P2	P3
Number (males/females)	23 (13/10)	F	F	M
Age [years]	12 ± 4	12	3	3
Height [m]	1.57 ± 0.19	1.4	1.0	1.0
Body weight [kg]	47.28 ± 13.68	26	16	15
BMI [kg/m^2]	18.7 ± 2.4	13	16	15

3 Results

The determined values of gait parameters: Gillette Gait Index and Gait Deviation Index, together with the values of selected parameters GGI consists of for the group of patients with normal gait and patients with cerebral palsy are presented in Fig. 1. Based on medical diagnosis and set parameters of GGI all patients with cerebral palsy were evaluated as having problems with knee joint function, which is for most part the result of muscle malfunction. As part of this study length change of muscles associated with the joint were therefore analyzed. The knee angle in flexion during the gait cycle for the group of patients with normal gait and patients with cerebral palsy are presented in Fig. 2.

		Control group	P1		P2		P3	
			right	left	right	left	right	left
GDI		100±10	73.3	63.14	76.11	65.75	47.63	70.73
GGI		15.71±5.68	84.92	78.67	220.51	251.66	383.49	120.02
P11	Angle in knee at initial contact [°]	11.51 ±4.41	25.17	23.35	33.37	45.95	38.15	16.3
P12	Time to peak knee flexion [% of gait cycle]	70.46±1.16	70.08	66.9	78.05	71.31	74.62	71
P13	Range knee flexion-extension [°]	58.88 ±3.74	53.3	48.7	40.2	28.82	55.8	63.8

■ avg ± σ   ■ avg ± 2σ   ■ avg ± 3σ   ■ avg ≥ 3σ

Fig. 1. Values of gait parameters: Gillette Gait Index and Gait Deviation Index for the group of children with normal gait and patients with cerebral palsy

The results acquired for the group of healthy children formed a standard courses of selected muscles' length changes, where results obtained by patients with cerebral palsy (Figs. 3 and 4) were then applied for comparison. Changes in the value of muscle length (L_M) have been normalized to their length during the static test (while standing still; L_{MO}) and related to the gait cycle.

Figure 5 shows the parameters characterizing the length change of selected muscles during walking for healthy children and for patients with CP, i.e. the average length of the muscle ($L_{M_{avg}}$) and range of length variation (ΔL_M) in a single gait cycle.

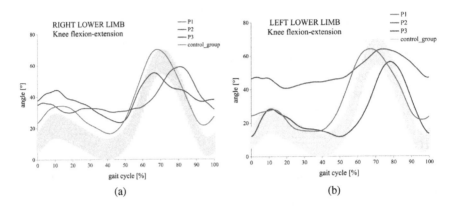

Fig. 2. The knee angle in flexion during the gait cycle for (a) right lower limb, (b) left lower limb

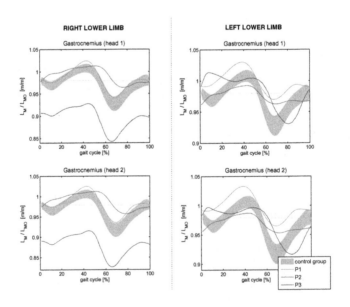

Fig. 3. Waveforms length change courses of selected muscles (Gastrocnemius head 1 and 2) during gait for children with normal gait and patients with cerebral palsy

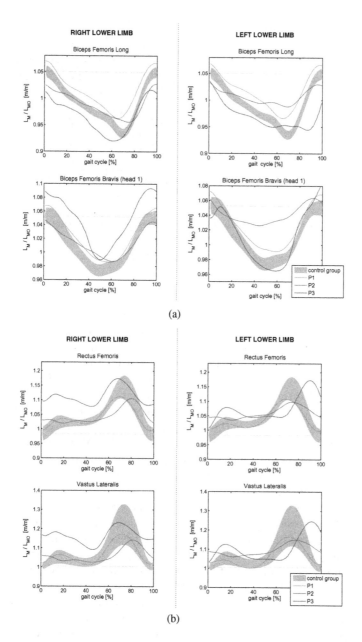

Fig. 4. Waveforms length change courses of selected muscles (a) Biceps Femoris Long and Biceps Femoris Bravis, (b) Rectus Femoris and Vastus Lateralis during gait for children with normal gait and patients with cerebral palsy

muscle		Control group		P1		P2		P3	
		$L_{M/L_{MO}}$ [m/m]							
		$L_{M\ śr}$	ΔL_M	$L_{M_{avg}}$	ΔL_M	$L_{M_{avg}}$	ΔL_M	$L_{M_{avg}}$	ΔL_M
Gastrocnemius (head 1)	R	0.974±0.023	0.081±0.013	0.983	0.084	0.991	0.049	0.897	0.085
	L			0.999	0.06	0.976	0.031	0.983	0.083
Gastrocnemius (head 2)	R	0.969±0.026	0.09±0.013	0.982	0.089	0.989	0.055	0.881	0.089
	L			0.999	0.068	0.969	0.034	0.97	0.081
Rectus Femoris	R	1.048±0.048	0.161±0.027	1.043	0.117	1.046	0.086	1.113	0.096
	L			1.04	0.109	1.06	0.064	1.076	0.166
Biceps Femoris Long	R	0.992±0.036	0.116±0.016	1.014	0.107	0.989	0.071	0.967	0.095
	L			1.016	0.102	1.006	0.045	0.969	0.09
Biceps Femoris Bravis (head 1)	R	1.011±0.029	0.079±0.014	1.023	0.082	1.014	0.059	1.048	0.104
	L			1.025	0.082	1.041	0.037	1.012	0.12
Vastus Lateralis	R	1.08±0.07	0.219±0.108	1.07	0.162	1.062	0.117	1.163	0.141
	L			1.064	0.164	1.096	0.09	1.106	0.213

avg ± σ   avg ± 2σ   avg ± 3σ   avg ≥ 3σ

Fig. 5. Characteristics of length changes of selected muscles during gait for children with normal gait and patients with cerebral palsy

4   Discussion

In the case of many diseases accurate diagnostics needs information concerning the functioning of muscles. A comprehensive assessment of muscle function is not possible without specifying its length changes during motion. Acquired in this study courses of muscle length changes during gait for the normative group (the templates) overlap with the results of other authors [1,7,8,14]. There is however few papers in which the same problem was evaluated for children with cerebral palsy [14]. Determining muscle lengths change courses during gait for this disease is extremely valuable because of the occurring muscle spasticity, contractures and lack of synergy between agonist and antagonist muscles. Moreover, in the case of pathological gait of patients with cerebral palsy compensatory mechanisms can be observed. Inactive or insufficiently active muscles are replaced by excessive activity of other muscle groups.

Therefore, in this study, the muscle length changes during walking in patients with cerebral palsy were calculated. For all the studied patients the greatest disturbances were noted in the knee joint function. Flexion of the knee at the initial contact for all patients is measured as outside the norm both for the right and left lower limb (gait of all patients is characterized by increased flexion). Moreover, deviations from the standard values were observed for time to maximum knee flexion and range of flexion-extension in the knee joint. The greatest length change disorders of selected muscles during walking with respect to the standard charts were recorded for the patient P3, and lowest for patient P1, which is in line with the general evaluation of patients' gait described by Gait Deviation Index and Gillette Gait Index (Fig. 1). Analyzing the parameters characterizing the muscle length change during gait, i.e. the average length of the muscle ($L_{M_{avg}}$), the range of length variation (ΔL_M) in a single gait cycle (Fig. 5) and the muscle length change courses (Figs. 3 and 4) in patients with CP, an asymmetry between the left and right lower limb muscle function was observed.

The lowest deviation from the normal value, both for the obtained gait index values and individual performance indicators, as well as the muscle length change courses was observed in patient P1. For patient P2 a reduced range of flexion-extension of the knee joints in both lower limbs was observed. For the left lower limb it is nearly two times lower than the standard range. Reduced range of flexion-extension of the knee joints is associated with a reduced range of length change in most analyzed muscles during gait. Whereas the P3 patient's results of knee flexion at initial contact and the time to the maximum knee flexion significantly differ from normative data for the right lower limb. Based on the obtained muscle length change courses we can assume that the increased flexion of the knee joint in the right leg could be the result of improper function of the gastrocnemius muscle, which in relation to the standard is excessively shortened throughout the gait cycle. Excessive contracture of the gastrocnemius muscle, which is the main flexor of the knee interferes with the function of other skeletal muscles.

5   Conclusion

1. The paper presents the possibility of using mathematical modeling methods to determine the change in length of muscle fibers.
2. The results for the group of healthy people have been used to form standard normalized muscle length change courses during walking.
3. The obtained courses of muscle length change, supported by other parameters of gait and the knowledge and experience of the doctor can help determine which muscles work improperly.
4. Thanks to the research methodology the symmetry of muscle function between the right and left lower limb can be assessed.

Acknowledgements. The study was supported by the research grant DEC-2011/01/B/NZ7/02695 of the National Science Center.

References

1. Arnold, E.M., Delp, S.L.: Fibre operating lengths of human lower limb muscles during walking. Philos. Trans. R. Soc. B Biol. Sci. **366**, 1530–1539 (2011)
2. Arnold, E.M., Ward, S.R., Lieber, R.L., Delp, S.L.: A model of the lower limb for analysis of human movement. Ann. Biomed. Eng. **38**, 269–279 (2010)
3. Chleboun, G.S., France, A.R., Crill, M.T., Braddock, H.K., Howell, J.N.: In vivo measurement of fascicle length and pennation angle of the human biceps femoris muscle. Cells Tissues Organs **169**, 401–409 (2001)
4. Cutts, A.: The range of sarcomere lengths in the muscles of the human lower limb. J. Anat. **160**, 79–88 (1988)
5. Cutts, A.: Sarcomere length changes in muscles of the human thigh during walking. J. Anat. **166**, 77–84 (1989)

6. Fleeter, T.B., Adams, J.P., Brenner, B., Podolsky, R.J.: A laser diffraction method for measuring muscle sarcomere length in vivo for application to tendon transfers. J. Hand Surg. **10**, 542–546 (1985)

7. Krogt, M.M., Doorenbosch, C.A.M., Harlaar, J.: Muscle length and lengthening velocity in voluntary crouch gait. Gait Posture **26**, 532–538 (2007)

8. Lieber, R.L., Friden, J.: Musculoskeletal balance of the human wrist elucidated using intraoperative laser diffraction. J. Electromyogr. Kinesiol. **8**, 93–100 (1998)

9. Llewellyn, M.E., Barretto, R.P., Delp, S.L., Schnitzer, M.J.: Minimally invasive high-speed imaging of sarcomere contractile dynamics in mice and humans. Nature **454**, 784–788 (2008)

10. Maganaris, C.N.: Force-length characteristics of in vivo human skeletal muscle. Acta Physiol. Scand. **172**, 279–285 (2001)

11. Michnik, R., Nowakowska, K., Jurkojć, J., Kopyta, Jochymczyk-Woźniak, K.I., Mandera M.: Wykorzystanie metod modelowania obciążeń układu szkieletowo-mięśniowego u pacjenta z mózgowym porażeniem dziecięcym (The use of musculosceletal system load modling methods in patients with cerebral palsy). Modelowanie Inżynierskie, Tom 24, Zeszyt 55, 2015, s. 74–80 (in Polish)

12. Orendurff, M.S., et al.: Length and force of the gastrocnemius and soleus during gait following tendo Achilles lengthenings in children with equinus. Gait Posture **15**, 130–135 (2002)

13. Ward, S.R., Eng, C.M., Smallwood, L.H., Lieber, R.L.: Are current measurements of lower extremity muscle architecture accurate? Clin. Orthop. Rel. Res. **467**, 1074–1082 (2009)

14. Wren, T.A., Do, K.P., Kay, R.M.: Gastrocnemius and soleus lengths in cerebral palsy equinus gait: differences between children with and without static contracture and effects of gastrocnemius recession. J. Biomech. **37**(9), 1321–1327 (2004)

The Loads Acting on Lumbar Spine During Sitting Down and Standing Up

Katarzyna Nowakowska[1(✉)], Marek Gzik[1], Robert Michnik[1],
Andrzej Myśliwiec[2], Jacek Jurkojć[1], Sławomir Suchoń[1], and Michał Burkacki[1]

[1] Department of Biomechatronics, Faculty of Biomedical Engineering,
Silesian University of Technology, ul. F. D. Roosevelta 40, 41-800 Zabrze, Poland
{katarzyna.nowakowska,marek.gzik,robert.michnik,jacek.jurkojc,
slawomir.suchon,michal.burkacki}@polsl.pl
[2] Department of Kinesitherapy and Special Methods of Physiotherapy,
Academy of Physical Education in Katowice, ul. Mikołowska 72a,
40-065 Katowice, Poland
https://www.polsl.pl/Wydzialy/RIB
http://awf.katowice.pl/uczelnia/wydzial-fizjoterapii

Abstract. The paper presents an analysis of the loads acting on lumbar spine during movement of sitting down and getting up from a chair. The study was conducted on a group of 30 people (parents of disabled children) complaining about chronic low back pain. Basing on kinematics, obtained during experiment from APAS system, simulations were performed in the Anybody Modeling System environment. The use of methods, mathematical modeling and static optimization, allowed to determine the magnitude of the loads acting on musculoskeletal system. The results of reactions in the L5-sacrum joint, the muscular forces of erector spinae and the transversus abdominis are significantly correlated with the kinematics of the movement.

Keywords: Mathematical modeling · Loads · Muscle strength · Anybody Modeling System · Lumbar spine

1 Introduction

Back pain relates to almost half of the adult population. About 6–9 % of people with back pain consults annually with doctor [4]. Among the risk factors it can be calculated: the wrong posture, work in non-ergonomic positions, lifting, obesity, insufficient rest, incorrect positions while sitting or excessively long time in sitting position [17]. Morloc et al., who monitored the frequency and duration of daily activities, report that the most common form of human activity during the day is seating that occupies a total of approximately 44 % of the time [14]. Another interesting issue is the problem of physical activity. On the one hand researches indicate a sedentary lifestyle as a factor increasing the likelihood of becoming ill, on the other hand, according to some authors, above-average physical activity is one of the risk factors [10,19].

© Springer International Publishing AG 2017
M. Gzik et al. (eds.), *Innovations in Biomedical Engineering*, Advances in Intelligent
Systems and Computing 526, DOI 10.1007/978-3-319-47154-9_20

Low back pain causes a number of changes in the body and has impact on social and career field. The emergence of this pain in youth signals probability of occurring in the later years, which should suggest early diagnosis and consequently prevention efforts. For the rise of lumbar spine pain, beyond overloading of the musculoskeletal system, may correspond to the failure of the muscular system, as well as disorders of motor control mechanisms in statics and in the course of the movement. For this control of local short muscles, acting with stabilizing effect, are responsible [7–9]. One of stabilizing muscle is transverse abdominal muscle. Transversus abdominis (TRA) is the deepest located muscle from the abdominal group and belongs to the local stabilizers, thereby directly affecting segmental control in the lumbar region. It has no motor function, and its task is to control the neutral zone and increase the stiffness of the spine segment [15,16]. It also controls rotational and translational movements [9]. TRA and the internal oblique abdominal muscles stabilize the sacroiliac joints, which ensures the stability of the entire lumbo-pelvic-hip complex.

Motor disabled children care induces many factors that can cause the formation of pain. Activities performed by the parent associated with the child care can be compared to the work of the disabled person or assistant nurses [1]. These people are exposed to lift their children which cause repetitive, monotonous motions performed in the awkward positions and also the inclination of the body while performing nursing activities. Relevant information from the biomechanics, medicine and ergonomics point of view, is the knowledge of the mechanism loading the spine and the size of the load acting on musculoskeletal system while performing different tasks. Currently, the loads on musculoskeletal system can be determined by: implants measuring EMG signals and mathematical models [3,18,20]. The only direct method for determining response in the measuring joints are implants (eg. Intradiscal pressure transducer or telemetric prosthesis of vertebral body VBR). Unfortunately, this method involves performing an invasive surgical procedure and the measurements may only be made at the implantation site. Therefore noninvasive mathematical models of the musculoskeletal system are more frequently used [2,6,12,13,20].

The aim of this study was to determine the size of the load acting on musculoskeletal system within the lumbar spine region, occurring during the movement of standing up and sitting down, mainly the influence of the kinematics on the results of the reaction forces in the intervertebral joint L5-sacrum and the values of selected muscle strength.

2   Materials and Methods

The study group consisted of 30 people (parents with motor disabled children) who complained of chronic low back pain. Group characterization is presented in Table 1.

In first stage of our study, kinematic analysis of sitting down and standing up from chair was made using APAS optical system. Obtained kinematics data was used as input data for simulations in AnyBody Modeling System software.

Table 1. Study group characterization

	Age (years)	Body weight (kg)	Height (cm)
Males	37.67 ± 1.15	76.67 ± 1.53	174 ± 5
Females	43.39 ± 9.10	65.30 ± 7.32	161.95 ± 3.92
Whole group	43.05 ± 8.96	66.66 ± 7.83	163.51 ± 5.84

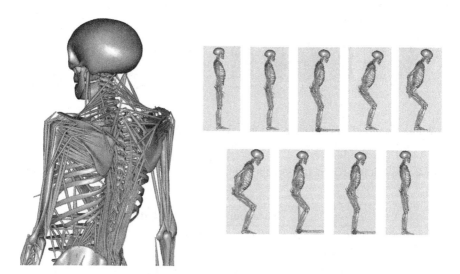

Fig. 1. Lumbar spine model and motion analyzed in Anybody Modeling System software.

The model of whole body (Standing Model) was used. Model parameters were scaled using ScalingLengthMassFat method according to height, body mass and percentage of body fat of a measured person. The analyzed model of lumbar spine contains 5 vertebras, pelvis, thorax, joints, over 180 actons of back and abdomen muscles and model of intra-abdominal pressure (Fig. 1). The used methods of mathematical modelling and static optimization allowed to determine loads acting on muscle-skeletal system around the lumbar spine. The muscle activities were estimated according to a 3rd order polynomial optimization. The muscle activity is defined as the muscle force divided by its strength. This paper presents the results of described studies, investigating impact of kinematics on force reaction in L5-Sacrum joint and activity of abdominal and back muscles.

3   Results

Maximum values of loads in lumbar spine and values of muscle forces are presented in Fig. 2. The values were normalized respectively to the body weight value (BW).

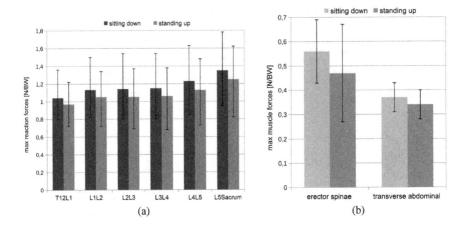

Fig. 2. (a) Range of maximum reaction forces in lumbar spine segments, (b) muscle activity during sitting down and standing up

Table 2. Reaction force in L5-Sacrum joint versus body tilt and knee and hip joints angle

	Knee joint	Hip joint	Body tilt
Pearson's correlation coefficients			
Sitting down	−0.46	0.73	0.82
Standing up	−0.39	0.77	0.84

The analysis of results shows influence of angle in knee and hip joints and body tilt angle on resultant reaction force in L5-Sacrum joint and also force value of erector spinae muscle and transverse abdominal muscles. Determined Pearson's correlation coefficients are shown in Tables 2 and 3. These results are statistically significant. Figure 3 presents scatterplots for selected relationship.

Table 3. Abdominal and back muscles activity versus body tilt and knee and hip joints angle

	Knee joint	Hip joint	Body tilt
Pearson's correlation coefficients			
Erector spinae muscles	−0.41	0.76	0.84
Transverse abdominal muscle	−0.39	0.63	0.83

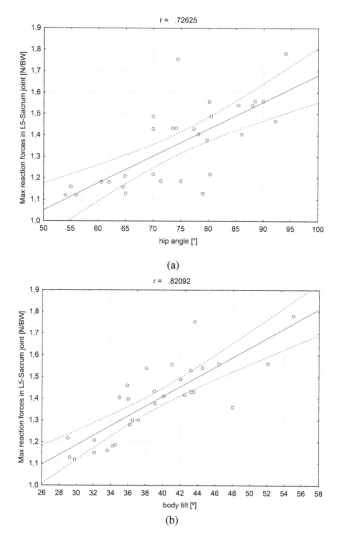

Fig. 3. Maximum reaction forces in L5-Sacrum joint during sitting down versus (a) hip joint angle, (b) body tilt

4 Discussion

The problems of overload among disabled children's parents are very complex issue. The research carried out on attendants of bedridden patients, presented in [20], shows that static and dynamic overloads cannot be omitted as factors causing spine pain. Undesirable position is taken during feeding, hygiene, bedding, dressing or undressing and conversation with disabled person. Nachemson's diagram (1976) illustrating load on third lumbar disc in various positions clearly shows consequences of everyday tasks performed by disabled children attendant. Only 20 degrees body tilt increases compression value in fourth lumbar spine intervertebral disc by 50 %. The same body position with 20 kg in hands increases this value by 220 % [10]. Researchers from Medical University Charite in Berlin have used telemetric implant of vertebral body VBR to measure loads in lumbar spine during 1000 different daily activities. They put sitting down and standing up from chair in first 10 of most overloading activities with value of 1200 N resultant reaction force measured in Th12-L1 joint [17].

The results show that most significant loads occur in at the moment of separation of the body from the chair (standing up) and also at the moment before the first contact with a chair (sitting down). Load values are different in sections of lumbar spine. Greater resultant reaction force is present in lower sections of lumbar spine. Resultant reaction forces in T12-L1 segment, acquired in simulations, are consistent with in vivo measurements by Rohlmann et al. [17] with VBR implants. Average value of maximum reaction during sitting down and standing up for 4 patients oscilates between 0.85 and 1.33 [N/BW] [17], while average reaction value in numerical studies was between 0.80 and 1.36 [N/BW]. However, in case of results obtained with VBR method, acquired values are lower because some portion of load is transferred through implant itself, stabilization device and bones.

The forces generated by the muscles around the lumbar spine were analyzed. The most activated muscles during sitting down and standing up were erector spinae muscle and transverse abdominal muscle. Average value of maximum muscle forces of erector spinae muscle were 56 ± 13 %BW during sitting down and 47 ± 20 %BW during standing up. Among abdominal muscle most engaged was transverse abdominal muscle: 37 ± 6 %BW (sitting down), 34 ± 6 %BW (standing up). The action of the transverse abdominal muscle affects the lateral stability of lumbar spine and lumbo-pelvic-hip complex [5]. It is possible due to abdominal pressure, which reduces spine compression during rest and activity [19]. Correct tension control of deep stabilizing muscles including transverse abdominal muscle reduces occurring of neutral zones and sharing forces which may cause overload of lumbar spine.

The influence of kinematics during sitting down and standing up on loads around lumbar spine was also examined. Angle in knee and hip joints and body tilt affects reaction forces in L5-Sacrum joint as well as abdomen and back muscles activity. The following relations were found:

- lower loads in lumbar spine are linked with greater angle in knee joints,
- greater angle in hip joint or body tilt moves body center mass which causes greater forces.

The results shows how kinematics of activity, especially body tilt and hip joint angle affect loads in the lumbar spine. Incorrect performance of simple activities contributes to increased loads which lead to increasing of strains and deformations. With no doubt this has a destructive effect on human musculoskeletal system and increases pain [6].

5   Conclusion

1. Sitting down and standing up may increase loads in L5-Sacrum segment up to 180 % comparing to standing pose.
2. The most activated muscles during sitting down and standing up were erector spinae muscle and transverse abdominal muscle.
3. Reactions forces in L5-Sacrum joint and muscular force of erector spinae and transverse abdominal muscles are significantly correlated with kinematics (hip joint angle and body tilt).
4. The results may become helpful in validation and modification of therapeutic exercises in order of better abdominal muscles activation and better control of pelvis position which may reduce pain of lumbar spine and improves society quality of life.

Acknowledgements. The study was conducted within *3 Year Healthy Community Project* conditioned upon Special Olympics Poland (Olimpiady Specjalne Polska). Grant was approved and financed by Special Olympics Inc. on 25th April 2016.

References

1. Brulin, Ch., Höög, J., Sundelin, G.: Psychosocial predictors for shoulder/neck and low back complaints among home care personnel. Adv. Physiother. **3**, 169–178 (2001)
2. Damsgaard, M., et al.: Analysis of musculoskeletal systems in the AnyBody Modeling System. Simul. Model. Pract. Theory **14**, 1100–1111 (2006)
3. Dreischarf, M., et al.: In vivo implant forces acting on a vertebral body replacement during upper body flexion. J. Biomech. **48**(4), 560–565 (2015)
4. Foster, N.: Barriers and progress in the treatment of low back pain. BMC Med. **9**, 108 (2011)
5. Gnat, R., Saulicz, E., Kokosz, M., Kuszewski, M.: Biomechanical aspects of modem models of pelvis stability. Polish J. Physiother. **6**(4), 280–288 (2006)
6. Gzik, M., Joszko, K., Pieniążek, J.: Badania modelowe w ocenie stanu fizycznego kręgosłupa lędźwiowego po leczeniu kręgozmyku (Analysis of interactions in the human lumbar spine after treatment spondylolisthesis). Modelowanie Inżynierskie, t. 13, nr. 44, 2012, s. 109–116 (in Polish)
7. Hodges, P.W., Richardson, C.A.: Delayed postural contraction of transversus abdominis associated with lower back pain. J. Spinal Disord. **11**, 46–56 (1998)
8. Hodges, P., Kaigle Holm, A., Holm, S., et al.: Intervertebral stiffness of the spine is increased by evoked contraction of transversus abdominis and the diaphragm: in vivo porcine studies. Spine **28**, 2594–2601 (2003)
9. Hoskins, W., et al.: Low back pain in junior Australian rules football: a cross-sectional survey of elite juniors, non-elite juniors and non-football playing controls. BMC Musculoskel. Disord. **11**, 241 (2010)
10. Jensen, G.: Biomechanics of the Lumbar intervertebral disk: a review. Phys. Ther. **60**, 765–773 (1980)
11. Knibbe, J.J., Knibbe, N.E.: Static load in the nursing profession; the silent killer. Work **41**(1), 5637–5638 (2012)

12. Koblauch, H.: Low back load in airport baggage handlers. Ph.D. Thesis, Denmark (2015)
13. Morlock, M., et al.: Duration and frequency of every day activities in total hip patients. J. Biomech. **34**(7), 873–881 (2001)
14. Nelson, A., Baptiste, A.S.: Evidence-based practices for safe patient handling and movement. Online J. Issues in Nurs. **9**(3), 366–379 (2004)
15. Panjabi, M.M.: The stabilizing system of the spine. Part II: Neutral zone and stability hypothesis. J. Spinal Disord. **5**, 390–397 (1992)
16. Plouvier, S., et al.: Low back pain around retirement age and physical occupational exposure during working life. BMC Public Health **28**(11), 268 (2011)
17. Rohlmann, A., Pohl, D., Bender, A., Graichen, F., Dymke, J.: Activities of everyday life with high spinal loads. PloS ONE **9**(5), e98510 (2014)
18. Sato, T., et al.: Low back pain in childhood and adolescence: assessment of sports activities. Eur. Spine J. **20**(1), 94–99 (2011)
19. Stambolin, D., Eltoukhy, M., Asfaur, S.: Development and validation of a three dimensional dynamic biomechanical lifting model for lower back evaluation for careful box placement. Int. J. Ind. Ergon. **54**, 10–18 (2016)
20. Wilke, H., et al.: New in vivo measurements of pressures in the intervertebral disc in daily life. Spine **24**(8), 755–762 (1999)

Quantitative Assessment of the Parameters Determining Habitual Patella Dislocation

Ewa Stachowiak[1]([✉]), Zbigniew Pilecki[2], and Alicja Balin[1]

[1] Biomechatronics Department, Silesian University of Technology, Zabrze, Poland
ewa.stachowiak@polsl.pl
[2] Chorzów Pediatrics and Oncology Center, Chorzów, Poland
http://www.polsl.pl/Wydzialy/RIB/RIB3/Strony/witamy.aspx

Abstract. In this paper a mathematical way of calculating the existing parameters on the basis of magnetic resonance images is introduced together with assessment of statistical significance in the analysis of patellar instability. 11 anthropometrical parameters were calculated, in various variants, using own methodology. Next, a statistical analysis was performed in order to evaluate their significance in patellar instability assessment. The most significant were Insal-Salvati ratio, trochlear depth, lateral tilt of the patella, lateralisation of tibial tuberosity, patellofemoral angle and sculus angle. The relation between patellar stability and the parameters selected as the most significant was studied with a computer simulation in the multi-body dynamics model.

1 Introduction

The patellar instability is one of the most common knee disorders among the young, it covers 2–3 % of all the knee injuries. Among the elements influencing the stability of the patellofemoral joint both passive and active stabilizers are identified. The passive ones contain: geometry of the patellofemoral joint, as well as ligaments of the knee. The active stabilizing is performed by the muscles, especially thigh quadriceps.

In the Chorzow Pediatrics and Oncology Center (ChPiOC) large numbers of patellar instability are diagnosed among patients below 18 years old. Among these about 50 pro year are qualified for surgery for restoring the stability of the patella.

Currently used methods of patellofemoral joint stability evaluation are based on clinical assessment and anthropometrical parameters determined on X-ray images, which, however, are two-dimensional and do not provide full information about the joint morphology.

Attempts at assessment of the patellofemoral joint based on quantitative anthropometrical parameters have been performed since 1840s [2] and are still conducted. Numerous methods of knee joint parameters assessment based on X-ray images can be found in the literature [2,15] Thanks to the progress in technology, the three-dimensional medical imaging, e.g. MR or CT, is getting more and more accessible. In the papers published during last years definitions

© Springer International Publishing AG 2017
M. Gzik et al. (eds.), *Innovations in Biomedical Engineering*, Advances in Intelligent
Systems and Computing 526, DOI 10.1007/978-3-319-47154-9_21

of parameters for patellar instability based on 3D imaging can be found. It is worth mentioning that most authors support the claim that MR imaging gives best results thanks to the fact that it includes soft tissues [1,13,14].

The aim of this work is to define the parameters which are statistically most significant for patellar stability assessment based on MR images as well as to conduct a simulation of the kinematics of the joint, which allows for model studies of their influence of the patellofemoral joint motion.

2   Materials and Methods

2.1   Patients

MRI scans performed in diagnostic purposes for patients of Chorzow Pediatrics and Oncology Center (ChPiOC) were used for anthropometrical analysis. Studies were acquired with magnetic resonance 1.5 T, distance between slices 1.5 mm, pixel size 0.39 mm, resolution of each slice 384×384 px. Study group contained 16 patients aged 14–18, who had habitual patella dislocation diagnosed during clinical studies. Control group consisted of 23 patients aged 13–18, treated for reasons other than patella instability. In this group, MRI scans did not show pathologies for patellofemoral structures. On the whole, anthropometrical analysis of 39 patients was done, who had MRI scans of knee joint for diagnostic purposes performed in 2014–2015.

2.2   Anthropometrical Analysis

In order to calculate the anthropometrical parameters, the list of 34 landmarks for further calculations of anthropometrical indexes was proposed. A library which allows to quickly input 34 landmarks was created in Mimics Innovation Suite software. These points were crucial. The list of these points with the description of their localisation is given in the Table 1. Based on Cartesian coordinates of points presented above, anthropometrical indexes for quantitative assessment of patellar instability were calculated. The first set of the analysed parameters were the ones used for assessment of the height of the patella location: Insal-Salvati ratio [9,11,15], Blackburn-Peel ratio [2,15], Caton-Deschamps ratio [3,6]. It should be pointed out that all of these parameters were assessed during knee extension, while in case of RTG assessment usually the knee is flexed by angle about 30 °C.

The next studied parameter was the lateralization of the tibial tuberosity, which has incorrect value for 56–93 % of patients with patella instability [14]. Next, the parameters which describe the morphology of condyles joint surface and patella joint surface were evaluated. Among these parameters trochlear depth (3 variants) [1,5], asymmetry of the femur condyles, sculus angle [1,13], and patella angle 16 were assessed. In the end, the parameters which describe the patella position relative to the distal humerus of the femur-lateral patella dislocation, patellofemoral angle, lateral tilt of the patella (which can be calculated in two ways [4], were analyzed.

Table 1. The list of anthropometrical landmarks, which are applied in order to calculate parameters for assessment stability of the patella

No	Localisation	No	Localisation
1	Top point of the patella	18	Vertex of the patella auricular surface (c)
2	Bottom point of the patella	19	Lateral point of the patella
3	Central point of the patellar tendom attachment	20	Medial point of the patella
4	Posterior point of the patellar tendom attachment	21	Posterior point of the lateral condyle of the femur (b)
5	Bottom point of the joint surface of the patella (b)	22	Posterior point of the lateral condyle of the femur (c)
6	Bottom point of the joint surface of the patella (c)	23	Posterior point of the medial condyle of the femur (b)
7	Top superior point of the tibial plateu (b)	24	Posterior point of the medial condyle of the femur (c)
8	Top anterior point of the tibial plateu (c)	25	External point of articular surface of the lateral condyle (b)
9	Top anterior point of the tibial plateu (b)	26	External point of articular surface of the lateral condyle(c)
10	Top anterior point of the tibial plateu (c)	27	External point of articular surface of the medial condyle(b)
11	Anterior point of the lateral condyle of the femur (b)	28	External point of articular surface of the lediall condyle(c)
12	Anterior point of the lateral condyle of the femur (c)	29	External point of articular surface of the patella (b)
13	Anterior point of the medial condyle of the femur (b)	30	External point of articular surface of the patella (c)
14	Anterior point of the medial condyle of the femur (c)	31	External point of articular surface of the patella (b)
15	Condyle intercondylar fossa (b)	32	External point of articular surface of patella (c)
16	Condyle intercondylar fossa (c)	33	Lateral point of patellar tendom attachment
17	Vertex of the patella articular surface (b)	34	Lateral point of patellar tendom attachment

b point marked on bone, *c* point marked on cartilage

2.3   Statistical Analysis

The calculated parameters were analyzed statistically using STATISTICA 12 software. First, a test of the normality of the distribution was performed using Kolmogorov-Smirnov test (K-S test). For all of the studied parameters, on the assumption of 10 intervals, p parameter (the value of the probability of error) was higher than 0.05, which indicates the normality of the distribution.

Next, the statistical significance for all of the parameters was studied using a t-test. Parameters which had p value lower than 0.05 were assumed significant for the differentiation between groups, these values are marked in Table 2.

2.4   Model of the Kinematics of the Knee Joint

Based on the MR images of a 17-year-old woman, using Mimics Innovation Suite 3D, a three-dimensional model of the knee joint has been created. The model includes: femur, fibula, tibia, patella, femoral cartilage, tibial cartilage and patellar cartilage. Based on the resultant 3D geometry other variants simulating pathologies were created, i.e. patella alta, lateralisation of tibial tuberosity, lateral tilt of the patella, decreased patellofemoral angle, reduction of the trochlear depth and lateralization of the patella.

To perform the simulation, the models were imported to Madymo software. For all bodies kinematic properties (center of gravity mass, inertia) were implemented. Femur was fixed, for another bodies all degrees of freedom were free. Motion of these elements was limited and stabilized by implemented ligaments and shapes of joint surfaces. Ligaments are implemented as elements working on extension, with mechanical properties taken from literature [12]. Patella was loaded by the resultant force of quadriceps from gait cycle. This force was examined during experimental research using motion capture, Xsens. The same value of this force was applied in all variants of the model.

3   Results

This chapter presents the results of anthropometrical parameters related to the morphology of the patellofemoral joint, together with their statistical significance presented in the form of the p-parameter (Table 2).

Among the parameters for the patella height assessment, the most significant differences were observed between the study group and the control group for the Insal Salvati ratio ($p < 0.02$). Another parameter which highly correlates with patellar instability is the trochlear depth ($p < 0.01$). Anthropometric analysis also showed a strong dependence between the patellar stability and the lateral patella position ($p < 0.01$) and between the patellar instability and the value of the sculus angle ($p < 0.005$). A relationship between patellar instability and the value of the patellofemoral angle was also observed, which resulted from the patella tilt in correlation to the femur imaged on transverse plane.

By a method of computer simulation, the influence of knee joint geometry modification on patella trajectory during the knee extension motion was analysed. The resultant patella dislocation and patella dislocation in transverse axis of the body, which shows increased values in clinical studies, were presented on the figures below (accordingly Figs. 1 and 2).

Table 2. Comparison of the results of the anthropometrical analysis with assessment of the statistical significance, described by p (p value, probability value)

		Study group		Control group		p
		Mean	STD	Mean	STD	
Insal-Salvati ratio	Midpoint of PT att.	1.512	0.26393	1.252	0.2559	0.002959
	Postr point PT	1.4218	0.27525	1.2146	0.23677	0.016372
Blackburn-Peel ratio	Midpoint of PT att.	0.9506	0.21275	0.9548	0.18933	0.948876
	Post. point PT att.	0.8367	0.23909	0.8503	0.22295	0.856917
Caton-Deschampes ratio	Midpoint of PT att.	1.354	0.23109	1.2252	0.17895	0.057482
	Posterior point PT att.	1.1205	0.23578	1.0471	0.20946	0.312876
Trochlear depth v.1	b	6.2772	1.79771	8.096	1.88266	0.004537
	c	4.4175	3.03063	6.0072	2.46223	0.079405
Trochlear depth v.2	b	6.4755	1.79542	8.2107	1.89109	0.006632
	c	5.2754	1.79859	6.7815	1.57668	0.008713
Trochlear depth v.3	b	7.9492	2.26813	9.599	2.50176	0.042316
	c	6.3283	1.85293	8.2405	1.92904	0.003751
Lateralisation of the patella	b	8.1624	9.99836	−1.4683	9.71842	0.004702
	c	8.6726	8.35128	0.2775	9.6383	0.007635
Lateralisation of the tibial tuberosity	b	14.6997	8.36828	7.1371	4.64944	0.001062
	c	14.5564	7.73928	6.9778	4.76556	0.000654
Condyles asymmetry	b	0.6021	0.15724	0.7275	0.24889	0.083459
	c	0.6051	0.15788	0.7348	0.22619	0.055221
Sculus angle	b	133.3985	10.36325	126.6641	9.70372	0.045135
	c	110.7017	16.02788	113.4393	9.89529	0.513365
Patello-femoral angle	b	−8.3618	20.01415	11.4976	9.67333	0.000198
	c	−5.9133	21.13361	10.1353	10.26511	0.003703
Patella tilt angle	External points of the patella	−2.0099	20.62972	−7.6808	4.62605	0.208566
	b articular surface	5.8892	21.0248	12.9002	11.06144	0.18307
	c articular surface	6.6571	21.58547	13.0886	10.7299	0.225894
Patella angle	b	122.9699	12.69385	126.6606	8.99618	0.294044
	c	119.6219	12.27239	125.032	8.75381	0.116017

b indexes for points marked on bone, c indexes for points marked on cartilages

In case of slight lateralisation of the tibial tuberosity (around 5 mm in comparison to a healthy joint), and patella alta (patella placed around 7 mm higher than in a healthy joint), there were no significant differences observed for the

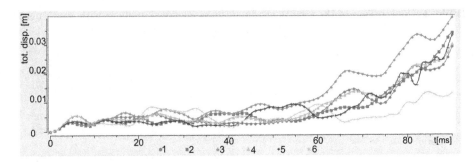

Fig. 1. Values of the patella displacement obtained during simulations: *1* normal joint, *2* patela alta, lateralisation of tibial tuberosity, *4* lateral tilt of the patella, *5* reduction of the trochlear depth, *6* lateralization of the patella

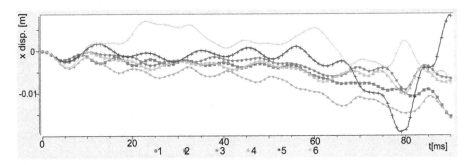

Fig. 2. Values of the lateral displacement of the patella obtained during simulations: *1* normal joint, *2* patela alta, lateralisation of tibial tuberosity, *4* lateral tilt of the patella, *5* reduction of the trochlear depth, *6* lateralization of the patella

patella trajectory. In case of patella lateralisation, the increase of the value of patella lateral movement in was observed for the initial phase of movement (for knee flexion around 40 °C).

A significant increase of total patella displacement, together with displacement in the transverse axis was observed in the case of a decrease of the trochlear depth and a decrease of the patellofemoral angle.

4   Conclusions

In this study analysis of an impact of particular antropometrical parameters on patellar stability was presented. In this study analysis of patellar stability effect of antropometrical parameters was presented. The analysis was done using statistical tests and computer simulations. Firstly, statistical studies made it possible to choose indices that were studied during computer simulations.

Performed studies have confirmed that reduction of trochlear depth affects the stability of the patella. In cases of patella lateralisation and the change of the patello-femoral angle significant changes were observed. It should be taken into consideration that during statistical tests there was no remarkable correlation between the angle of the patella and its stability.

During further research other simulations will be performed. They will include assessment of stability of the patella related to the value of the anthropometrical parameters. The values of these parameters may change in specific ranges suitable for either normal or pathological knee. simulations to assessment the stability of the patella according to values of anthropometrical parameters will be performed. Ranges of the parameters will be adequate to as well results for normal knee as for pathological.

The results may appear useful help for surgical techniques used when restoring stability of patella which could reduce the proportion of postoperative complications.

Dynamic simulations were created and were based on medical images. They may be a useful tool to the patient-oriented planning of a surgery. Creation of the individual model can help with prediction of post-operative clinical results and it may also help to choose the better surgical technique.

References

1. Balcarek, P., Walde, T.A., Frosch, S., et al.: Patellar dislocations in children, adolescents and adults: a comparative MRI study of medial patellofemoral ligament injury patterns and trochlear groove anatomy. Eur. J. Radiol. 415–420 (2011)
2. Blackburne, J.S., Peel, T.E.: A new method of measuring patellar height. J. Bone Joint Surg. **59**, 241–242 (1977)
3. Caton, J., Deschamps, G., Chambat, P., Lerat, J.L., Dejour, H.: Les rotules basses. A propos de 128 observations. Revue de Chirurgie Orthopédique et Traumatologique 317–325 (1982)
4. Dejour, H., Walch, G., Nove-Josserand, L., Guier, C.: Factors of patellar instability: an anatomic radiographic study. Knee Surg. Sports Traumatol. Arthrosc. **2**, 19–26 (1994)
5. del Mar, M., Martín, C., Santiago, F.L., Calvo, R.P., Álvarez, L.G.: Patellofemoral morphometry in patients with idiopathic patellofemoral pain syndrome. Eur. J. Radiol. 64–67 (2010)
6. Fabricant, P.D., Ladenhauf, H.N., Salvati, E.A., Green, W.D.: Medial patellofemoral ligament (MPFL) reconstruction improves radiographic measures of patella alta in children. Knee **21**, 1180–1184 (2014)
7. Greiwe, R.M., Saifi, C., Ahmad, C.S., Gardner, T.R.: Anatomy and biomechanics of patellar instability. Oper. Tech. Sports Med. **12**, 62–67 (2013)
8. Insall, J., Salvati, E.: Patella position in the normal knee joint. Radiology **101**, 101–104 (1971)
9. Marks, K.E., Bentley, G.: Patella alta and chondromalacia. J. Bone Joint Surg. 71–73 (1978)
10. Mesfar, W., Shirazi-Adl, A.: Biomechanics of the knee joint in flexion under various quadriceps forces. Knee **12**, 424–434 (2005)
11. Sanders, T.G., Loredo, R., Grayson, D.: Computed tomography and magnetic resonance imaging evaluation of patellofemoral instability. Oper. Tech. Sports Med. **9**, 152–163 (2001)

12. Schoettle, P.B., Zanetti, T.M., Seifert, B., Pfirrmann, C.W.A., Fucentese, S.F., Romero, J.: The tibial tuberosity-trochlear groove distance; a comparative study between CT and MRI scanning. Knee **13**, 26–31 (2006)
13. Teitge, R.A.: Plain patellofemoral radiographs. Oper. Tech. Sports Med. **9**, 134–151 (2001)
14. Tuna, B.K., Semiz-Oysu, A., Pekar, B., Bukte, Y., Hayirlioglu, A.: The association of patellofemoral joint morphology with chondromalacia patella: a quantitative MRI analysis. Clin. Imaging **38**, 495–498 (2014)
15. Waterman, B.R., Belmont, P.J., Owens, B.D.: Patellar dislocation in the United States: role of sex, age, race, and athletic participation. Knee Surg. **25**, 51–58 (2012)

Comparison of Rally Car and Passenger Car Safety Systems

Kamil Joszko, Wojciech Wolański[✉], Michał Burkacki, Sławomir Suchoń, and Marek Gzik

Department of Biomechatronics, Faculty of Biomedical Engineering, Silesian University of Technology, ul. F. D. Roosevelta 40, 41-800 Zabrze, Poland
{wojciech.wolanski,marek.gzik}@polsl.pl
https://www.polsl.pl/Wydzialy/RIB

Abstract. Safety systems in rally car are quite different than systems in passenger car. Differences arise from various factors including usage specifics and vehicles construction. In this paper authors presents comparison of conventional and rally safety systems. The basis parameters for evaluation were injury criteria determined for driver during frontal crash. For research authors used models developed in Madymo software. Results allowed to identify differences between common car and rally safety systems.

Keywords: Driver safety · Rally car · Injury criteria · Hans device · Frontal impact

1 Introduction

Major effort of automotive industry is focused on drivers and passengers safety [1,6]. There are plenty of safety system used in cars. They can be divided into two groups: active (e.g. ABS) and passive (e.g. seat belts). Active safety systems are not applied in rally car, because of rally discipline specifics. However passive safety systems in rally cars are used which have evolved and at this moment they are significantly different than common car protection. Whole car body is modified and enforced by safety roll cage. In place of seat there is bucket seat with multipoint harness. Crew wears fire resistant rally suit, helmet with head and neck support device (Fig. 1). Rally safety systems are designed especially to protect crew in case of accident with high speed [3,4,8] and focus on body fixation for reduction of displacement.

Technology migrates from rally and racing to commercial cars, for example: dual-clutch transmission or brake discs. The question is: Why not to use highly developed rally passive safety system in commercial cars? Putting aside user comfort, it is hard to tell if benefits overcome disadvantages.

The aim of presented studies is to determine advantages and disadvantages of using rally car safety systems compared to common car safety system. Factors chosen for assessment are injury criteria [2] obtained in selected scenarios. Authors decided to use Madymo software for conducting experiments which is designed to evaluate efficiency of safety systems [10].

© Springer International Publishing AG 2017
M. Gzik et al. (eds.), *Innovations in Biomedical Engineering*, Advances in Intelligent Systems and Computing 526, DOI 10.1007/978-3-319-47154-9_22

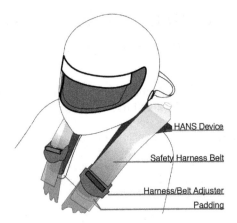

HANS Device

Safety Harness Belt

Harness/Belt Adjuster

Padding

Fig. 1. The attachment method of HANS head and neck support device with multipoint harness [5].

2   Numerical Models

Two numerical models of car interiors created with Madymo software were used. The first one as reference model representing common car from Madymo library *Frontal*, second one was interior of common car with implemented rally safety systems (*HANS*). As a reference model, generic model of front-left quarter of car interior with Hybrid III dummy in driver seat was used. This model was verified by Tass International. Second model (*HANS*) was created with the same interior model (dashboard, steering wheel etc.) and the same dummy model but with rally buckle seat, 5-point harness and HANS device (Fig. 2), which was verified i previous work [9]. The dummy set-up reflects rally driver position. Safety systems added to second model was verified by authors. Force-elongation characteristics of HANS tether were acquired with MTS Bionix strength test machine.

Helmet and head support device geometry was created basing on point cloud obtained through 3D scanning of real objects. These elements and buckle seat was made as multibody bodies with proper characteristics. Foam elements was represented by bodies with foam material properties. Seat belt, multipoint harness and head tether was created using finite elements. In both models contacts between dummy and interior were defined. Detailed boundary conditions and material properties were described in [9].

Authors have conducted scenarios during frontal crash with the following peak accelerations: 30 g, 45 g and 60 g for both models.

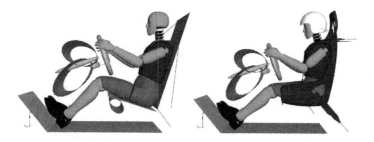

Fig. 2. On the left *Frontal* as reference model, on the right prepared model with rally systems - *HANS*.

3   Simulations Results

Simulations output data, besides animation (Fig. 4), includes waveforms from dummy sensors which give informations about accelerations, force and torque acting on dummy segments (Fig. 5). Basing on this values injury criteria for head and neck were determined (Fig. 3).

Highest resultant acceleration in thorax and head with 60 g impulse was obtained in *Frontal* model. The highest resultant acceleration of pelvis with 60 g impulse was observed in *HANS* model. Maximum shear force in upper and lower neck was acquired in *Frontal* model with 60 g input acceleration. Also flexion and extension torque in upper neck was highest with 60 g impulse for *Frontal*. Chest deflection was highest in every scenario for *Frontal* model.

Head Injury criterium HIC15 was highest for *Frontal* 60G. The limit for HIC15 was exceeded for *Frontal* 45 g and 60 g. Neck injury Criteria for NCF, NCE (Neck Compression-Flexion, Compression-Extension) was highest in 60G

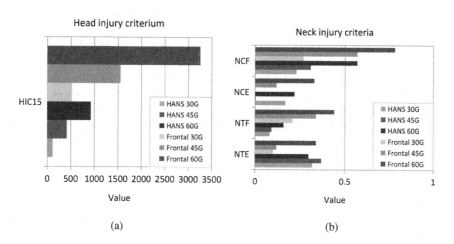

Fig. 3. Comparison of injury criteria with different decceleration impulses (a) Head injury criterium - HIC15, (b) Neck injury criteria.

for *Frontal* and NTF (Neck Tension-Flexion) was highest for *HANS* 45G. In all cases limit of neck injury criteria was not exceeded.

4 Discussion

Subject of modelling rally systems is not popular. Authors focus on vehicle structure FEM analysis [7,11,12] and also dynamic interactions in human body during common car crash [13]. The conducted research allowed to identify the differences between common car safety systems and rally safety systems. Results indicate that common car safety systems are less secure than rally systems during higher acceleration than 30 g, which corresponds to expectations of developing rally systems for higher accelerations. Safety belts and seat for *Frontal* are less rigid because of user everyday comfort which results in worse protection during high speed accidents.

Head acceleration in thorax is lower and more flattened than in every scenario of *Frontal* except 30 g simulation in which it is lower. Head acceleration and HIC15 parameter is higher for *Frontal*, because of more rapid contact with airbag during high accelerations. In this case it is recommended to keep greater distance from the airbag. Pelvis acceleration is similar in every scenario but the highest peak starts sooner for *HANS* because of more rigid seat. Thorax acceleration is highest for *Frontal* because of highest chest deflection, which is caused by smaller contact area of single belt with respect to 5-point belt system. Despite of user comfort, multipoint harness allows more firm body fixation which could also exclude possibility of lap belt slip. These kind of approach also grants symmetry during crash and reduces risk of hitting inertial objects.

Resultant force in lumbar spine is higher in every scenario of *HANS* because fixation of body is more firmer. However shear force in upper neck is smaller in every scenario for *HANS* model. It is also a consequence of excluding airbag. Application of HANS device reduces flexion and extension torque in upper neck and also head acceleration by transferring the load to shoulders and chest. High extension in lower neck was observed in *Frontal* especially in 60 g simulation (Fig. 6) which could cause neck injuries.

Presented models are conducted in isolated conditions, without taking into account the moment of braking, rotation of the vehicle during crash and many other factors that could affect injury assessment. However studies indicate that rally systems are more safe which should lead to develop safety systems for common cars which will derive innovative solutions reducing risk of injury during crash.

Advantages and disadvantages of analysed systems are presented in Table 1. In general conclusion: common cars safety systems are less secure for driver protection during high speed frontal impact with respect to rally systems. However modern active safety systems reduce probability of crash, it is recommended to use rally systems for not only professional teams but also during occasional rally events for amateurs.

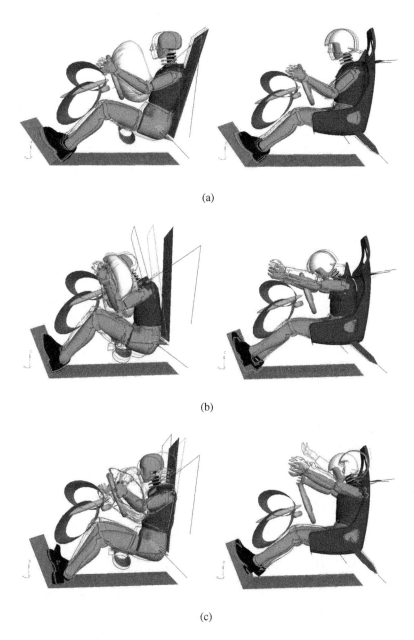

(a)

(b)

(c)

Fig. 4. Comparison of dummy kinematics with different decceleration impulses (left *Frontal*, right *HANS*): grey - 30 g, green contour - 45 g, red contour - 60 g; (a) at 30 ms, (b) at 90 ms, (c) at 160 ms. (Color figure online)

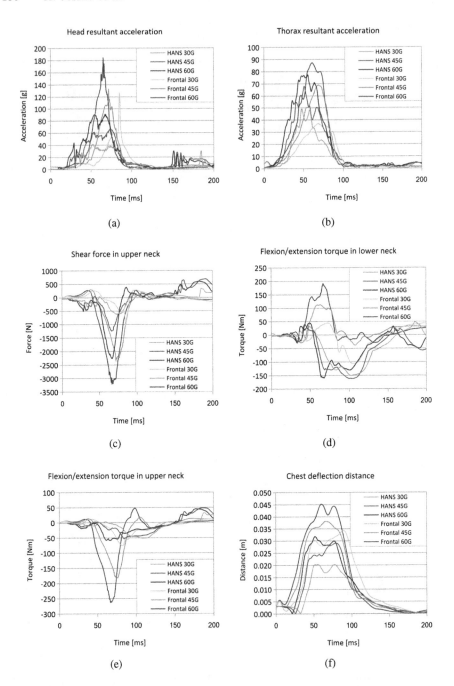

Fig. 5. Comparison of waveforms from dummy sensors: (a) head resultant acceleration, (b) thorax resultant acceleration, (c) shear force in upper neck, (d) flexion/extension torque in lower neck, (e) flexion/extension torque in upper neck, (f) Chest deflection distance.

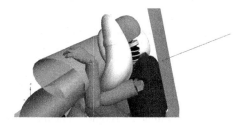

Fig. 6. Lower neck extension in *Frontal* during highest peak acceleration 60 g.

Table 1. Comparison of presented safety systems

	Common car	Rally car
Advantages	– More secure for normal speed frontal impact (<30 g)	– More secure for high speed frontal impact (>30 g)
	– Focusing on overall safety	– Preventing collision with interior by body fixation
	– More comfortable to use	– 5-point seat belt grants body symmetry during impact
Disadvantages	– Less secure for high speed frontal impact	– Focusing on head and neck safety
	– Is most efficient for 50-percentile human	– Less secure for normal speed frontal impact
	– Airbag could be harmful if user does not keep recommended distance	– Requires 5-point safety harness with buckle seat and helmet
		– Requires invidual setup

References

1. Bigi, D., Heilig, A., Steffan, H., Eichberger, A.: A comparison study of active head restraints for neck protection in rear-end collision. In: 16th International Technical Conference on the Enhanced Safety of Vehicles, Windsor, ON, Canada, DOT HS, vol. 808 (1998)
2. Eppinger, R., Sun, E., Bandak, F., Haffner, M., Khaewpong, N., Maltese, M., Zhang, A.: Development of Improved Injury Criteria for the Assessment of Advanced Automotive Restraint Systems-II (1999)
3. Gramling, H., Hodgman, P., Hubbard, R.: Development of the HANS head and neck support for formula one. In: Motor Sports Engineering Conference, Society of Automotive Engineers, paper no. 983060 (1998)
4. Gramling, H., Hubbard, R.: Sensitivity analysis of the HANS head and neck support. SAE Trans. **109**(6), 2488–2498 (2000)
5. HANS Device Quick Start Guide, HANS Performance Products (2014)

6. HEAD RESTRAINTS-Identification of Issues Relevant to Regulation, Design, and Effectiveness, National Highway Traffic Safety Administration Report (1996). http://www.nhtsa.gov/cars/rules/CrashWorthy/HeadRest/status9/status9. html#38. Accessed 21 Mar 2016

7. Heimbs, S., Strobl, F., Middendorf, P., Gardner, S., Eddington, B., Key, J.: Crash simulation of an F1 racing car front impact structure. In: 7th European LSDYNA Users Conference, Salzburg (2009)

8. Hubbard, R., Begeman, P., Downing, J.: Biomechanical evaluation and driver experience with the head and neck support. In: Motor Sports Engineering Conference, Society of Automotive Engineers, paper no. 942466 (1994)

9. Joszko, K., Wolański, W., Burkacki, M., Suchoń, S., Zielonka, K., Muszyński, A., Gzik, M.: Biomechanical analysis of injuries of rally driver with head supporting device, vol. 18(4) (2016). doi:10.5277/ABB-00633-2016-03

10. Joszko, K., Wolański, W., Gzik, M., Żuchowski, A.: Experimental and modelling investigation of effective protection the passengers. In: The Rear Seats During Car Accident "in polish", Modelowanie Inżynierskie, no. 42 (2012). doi:10.1016/j.xxx. 2015.08.007

11. Nassiopoulos, E., Njuguna, J.: Finite element dynamic simulation of whole rallying car structure: towards better understanding of structural dynamics during side impacts. In: 8th European LS-DYNA Users Conference, Strasbourg, May 2011

12. Njuguna, J.: The application of energy absorbing structures on side impact protection systems. Int. J. Comput. Appl. Technol. 40(4), 280–287 (2011)

13. Gzik, M.: Dynamic interactions in human cervical spine during car accidents. Adv. Transp. Stud. 3, 43–56 (2004)

Numerical Analysis of Blood Flow Through Artery with Elastic Wall of a Vessel

Wojciech Wolański[1(✉)], Bożena Gzik-Zroska[2], Kamil Joszko[1], Marek Gzik[1], and Damian Sołtan[1]

[1] Department of Biomechatronics, Faculty of Biomedical Engineering,
Silesian University of Technology, ul. F. D. Roosevelta 40, 41-800 Zabrze, Poland
{Wojciech.Wolanski,Kamil.Joszko,Marek.Gzik}@polsl.pl,
damian.soltan@gmail.com
[2] Department of Biomaterials and Medical Devices Engineering,
Faculty of Biomedical Engineering, Silesian University of Technology,
ul. F. D. Roosevelta 40, 41-800 Zabrze, Poland
Bozena.Gzik-Zroska@polsl.pl
https://www.polsl.pl/Wydzialy/RIB

Abstract. The main objective of the work was to prepare the analysis of blood flow through the arteries taking into account the mechanical properties of the vessel wall. The mechanical properties of the specimens were determined using a testing machine MTS Insight 2, and digital image correlation (DIC). The developed numerical model allowed the assessment of the state of stress and deformation of the walls while the blood flow through the physiologically correct aorta.

Keywords: Computational fluid dynamics (CFD) · Blood flow · Artery · Mechanical properties · Endurance tests

1 Introduction

In the twenty-first century, a growing number of people has been affected by cardiovascular disease. The results of many epidemiological studies have shown that arterial hypertension and cigarette smoking are two independent risk factors that predispose to pathological changes in blood [23]. However, the basic pathophysiological mechanism is an increase in blood pressure associated with arterial stiffness. Its late diagnosis can lead to death and that is why it is important to detect it early and start an appropriate treatment. Extensive research using computer modelling of the dynamics of blood flow (called Computational Fluid Dynamics - CFD) conducted in recent years in the models of the arteries showed that the initiator of pathological changes is a high level of wall shear stress (Wall Shear Stress - WSS) influencing the vascular nodes [14,17,18]. Changes in the values of shear stress acting on the vascular nodes of arteries lead to endothelial dysfunction and remodelling of its structure initiating formation of aneurysm, which was confirmed histologically [17].

© Springer International Publishing AG 2017
M. Gzik et al. (eds.), *Innovations in Biomedical Engineering*, Advances in Intelligent Systems and Computing 526, DOI 10.1007/978-3-319-47154-9_23

The question what determines the increase in wall shear stress on these vascular nodes remains unanswered. The results of experimental studies made by Ferguson, Roach and Scott give a partial answer to this question. They observed that with the increase of the division angle the risk of local disorders of blood flow increases, including turbulence around the apex of the division [3,19]. This suggests that the geometry of division of the vessel can substantially determine the hemodynamic load around the top division and influence its value.

Latest technological achievements and computer-aided engineering methods of modern medical diagnostics, to which scientists have access nowadays, allow for help in treating cardiovascular diseases by preoperative planning. Numerical simulations allow to specify the distribution of stresses and strains in the blood flow in the aorta, which can be valuable information for physicians [1,21]. Engineers are becoming more and more often co-creators of effective procedures of diagnosis and treatment, while doctors formulate their opinions in an increasingly objectified, formal and repeatable way, skilfully using the latest technology. On the basis of this cooperation, engineers develop new methods of functional diagnostics at the meeting point of the organ and technological system, they determine intervention activities in cases of organ dysfunction [9,13,24], simulate the operating procedures [10,15] and lay down the rules of optimal surgical procedures [8,25]. Therefore, the goal of this work is the development of a numerical model of the aorta and carrying out simulation studies of the influence of the stiffness of the vessel wall on the value of the intravascular pressure.

2   Materials and Methods

The process of preparing the analysis of blood flow through the artery included several steps. At the beginning of the modelling of the aorta, it was necessary to develop the geometry of the modelled system and the identification of mechanical properties of the mapped structures. Mimics software was used to build the model, because it allowed the segmentation of two-dimensional images of computed tomography (CT) and preparation of three-dimensional geometric model (Fig. 1a, b). The process of creating geometry began by importing CT images obtained during routine tests in the diagnostic process. The segmentation was performed by threshold method of homogeneous areas in terms of shades of grey in a previously pre-defined search area using a Hounsfield's scale. In the next step of modelling the vessel, discretization of the model was performed (Fig. 1c), which was next exported to the ANSYS program.

The most problematic and questionable in numerical modelling of the flow is to determine the boundary conditions. It is necessary to define in the model the parameters of the blood flow at the inlet and outlet of the vessel. In order to analyse the blood flow the following parameters of blood were used: the speed at the inlet of the artery - 0.5 m/s, the molecular weight - 18.02 kg/kmol, density - 1050 kg/m^3, the heat capacity - 4181.7 J/kg K, viscosity - 0.0035 Pa · s. Figure 1d shows the model of the aorta with marked boundary conditions. The speed of blood is obtained from Doppler ultrasound examination that was set to the surface of the inlet in the analysed vessel model. Other properties of the blood were taken from the literature [6,11,16]. They allowed to analyse the blood flow at 37 °C, at a reference pressure ratio of 1 bar. The results of numerical simulations made it possible to display the maps of blood flow and distributions of wall shear stress of the vessel.

After making numerical calculations, one received the values of pressure, WSS on the surface of the vessel caused by the flow and lines representing the flow rate (Fig. 3a, b, c). The results characterizing the distribution of pressure are particularly important, since they have been used in the next step to calculate the deformation of the arterial wall.

It is necessary to define the properties and thickness of the arterial wall [12] in the simulation of blood flow taking into account the deformation. Materials

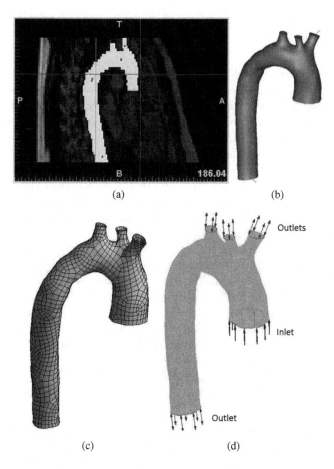

Fig. 1. The process of creating a model of the aorta: (a) segmentation of CT images, (b) geometric model, (c) discrete model, (d) model of the aorta with marked boundary conditions

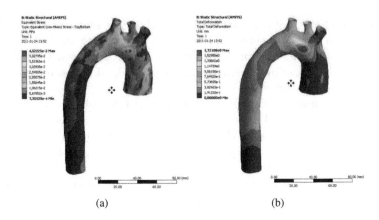

Fig. 2. The results of the strength analysis of the aorta: (a) equivalent stress according to Huber-Mises' hypothesis, (b) total deformation

data of the arterial wall needed to perform strength analysis (Static Structural) have been obtained from experimental studies that were conducted according to the methodology [5,7] with the use of digital image correlation and endurance machine MTS Insight 2. Previously prepared aorta samples were subjected to tensile test after placing their ends in the specially prepared clamps. The test was performed in a quasi-static conditions at a speed of 5 mm/min. Prior to performing the test the initial distance of the clamps and the thickness of the vessel were measured, and then it was stretched in the direction of the longitudinal axis. The head Q-400 from Dantec Dynamics was used for measuring displacements and deformations. It consists of two cameras in a stereoscopic system, light sources (LED) and ISTRA 4D software.

Mechanical properties of the aorta obtained from the experimental researches (Young's modulus - 2.3 MPa Poisson's ratio - 0.49) made it possible to analyse blood flow taking into account the deformation of the vessel wall. To this end, in the model of the aorta the pressure map, previously calculated in the first phase (Fig. 3b), was applied to its wall, whereas the edges of the inlet and outlet of the aorta were supported (Fixed Support). Next the calculation of stress analysis was prepared. Figure 2 presents the map of the stress reduced according to the Huber-Mises' hypothesis and the total deformation of the aortic wall. In the next part of the work the obtained results were used to make the analysis of the flow through the aorta taking into account the flexibility and the thickness of its walls.

All parameters concerning the blood property and the boundary conditions (initial) of the flow were the same as in the earlier analysis. What made this analysis different from of the previous one, was taking into consideration the deformation of the walls of the aorta induced by the flow. Figure 3d, e, f shows the results of the conducted analysis, which illustrate the total displacement of the aortic wall and pressure distribution.

3   Results

The results of the simulation of blood flow in the artery, including deformation of the vessel wall differ from the results of the analysis carried out in the absence of changes in the geometry of the aorta. The noticeable differences were observed between the distribution of pressure and tension, as well as between the velocities of blood flow through the vessel. The highest speed obtained for analysis of the deformable wall of the vessel is equal to 0.9 m/s, whereas in the absence of deformation of the vessel to 1.4 m/s (Fig. 3a, d). Furthermore, it was observed that the flow is less turbulent when the arterial wall is deformable.

A similar situation exists while comparing the distribution of blood pressure in the aorta (Fig. 3b, e). Higher values of the pressure are present in the artery when the vessel wall is rigid. In the presented case the maximum pressure was 537.5 Pa. Much lower pressure occurred in a vessel with a deformable wall, which amounted up to 418.3 Pa. It can therefore be concluded that the parameters of blood flow through the aorta are strongly influenced by the properties of the vessel wall. This is clearly evident on the example of distribution of WSS of the aorta (Fig. 3c, f).

The maximum value of the WSS of the aorta in the case of deformable vessel wall is much less than the average stress of rigid artery. The difference in those two cases is greater than 20 Pa and is almost four times greater than the maximum stress of the deformable vessel wall. WSS of the vessel without taking into account the properties of the artery may locally even reach 260 Pa, which can indicate maladjustment (no distortion) of the aorta to the parameters of blood flow. That is why it is so important in modelling the dynamics of blood flow (CFD) to take into account the properties of the vessel wall.

4   Discussion and Conclusions

The work presented in the research referred to the analysis of blood flow through the aorta. Computer simulations of blood flow dynamics (CFD) allow to specify a number of hemodynamic parameters which make it possible to assess of the state of the tension in the vessel. As it is known one of the factors contributing to the damage of the artery is hypertension leading to local increases in the wall shear stress in the vessel. These may conduce to damage of the artery and to the formation of aneurysms. Therefore, in the prediction and prevention of the formation of vascular lesions the above hemodynamic parameters are determined, in particular WSS. However, to be able to reliably estimate the risk of pathological changes, the simulation results and received values of these parameters must be as close as possible to the physiological (real) ones. The results of the simulation of blood flow through the aorta with a rigid wall, and taking into account the deformation of the vessel wall, have shown the differences in the blood flow in these two cases. The received results of hemodynamic parameters show that the properties of the vessels play a very important role in blood flow in the artery. Although the aorta is subject to constant physiological changes

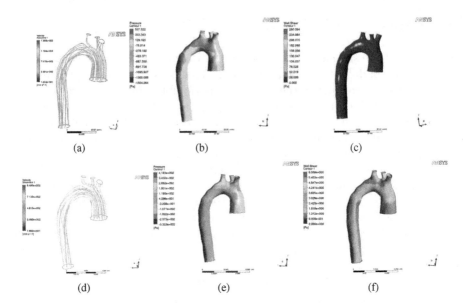

(a)   (b)   (c)

(d)   (e)   (f)

Fig. 3. Numerical results for models without taking into account the properties of the vessel wall - *top row* and taking into account the properties of the wall - *bottom row*: (a,d) velocities of the blood flow through the aorta, (b,e) the distribution of blood pressure in the aorta, (c,f) Wall Shear Stress (WSS) of the aorta

of the pressure, the blood flow is stable. This is so because of the elastic vessel wall, which thanks to deformations cause a reduction in pulsation. Therefore, it is important in the analysis of blood flow to take into consideration deformation of the vessel's walls. Values of hemodynamic parameters such as for example: pressure, stress (WSS) or the velocity of flow obtained during the analysis of the artery with non-deformable wall are larger than in case of the flexible vessels. Large values of these parameters may suggest the danger of damage to the vessel or aneurysm formation. However, in a situation close to physiological (the vessel with a deformable wall) these values are much lower, so there is no risk of the initiation of pathological lesions. Therefore, conclusion or prediction of artery damage should be based on the analysis of blood flow, taking into account the mechanical properties of the vessel wall, which is also confirmed by the researches of other authors [1, 22].

One method to obtain a higher arterial properties are experimental tests with the use of the endurance testing machine [7]. During the tensile test, we are able to determine the material properties of the vessel indispensable to analyse the flow. In this paper the authors, however, do not describe the DIC method used to determine the properties of artery, since this was not the aim of this study. However, one should be very careful so that the acquired properties of the vessels were close to the actual. This may be a problem in the case of preparing flow analysis for a particular patient. In this case it is impossible, or very dangerous for the patient, to obtaining samples of the vessels. In this situation one can use the properties of the vessels designated in advance, from the preparations done post-mortem (this is what the authors of this article have done), or taken from the literature [2,4,20]. However, when drawing conclusions based on such an analysis one should be cautious about the results.

Acknowledgements. The study was supported by the research grant Strateg Med 2/269760/1/NCBR/2015 of the National Centre for Research and Development.

References

1. Alishahi, M., Alishahi, M.M., Emdad, H.: Numerical simulation of blood flow in a flexible stenosed abdominal real aorta. Sci. Iran. B **18**(6), 1297–1305 (2011)
2. Azadani, A.N., Chitsaz, S., Mannion, A., Mookhoek, A., Wisneski, A., Guccione, J.M., Hope, M.D., Ge, L., Tseng, E.E.: Biomechanical properties of human ascending thoracic aortic aneurysms. Ann. Thorac. Surg. **96**, 50–88 (2013)
3. Ferguson, G.G.: Physical factors in the initiation, growth, and rupture of human intracranial saccular aneurysms. J. Neurosurg. **37**, 666–677 (1972)
4. Ferruzzi, J., Vorp, D.A., Humphrey, J.D.: On constitutive descriptors of the biaxial mechanical behavior of human abdominal aorta and aneurysms. J. R. Soc. Interface **8**, 435–450 (2011)
5. Fung, Y.C.: Elasticity of soft tissues in simple elongation. Am. J. Physiol. **213**, 1532–1544 (1967)
6. Fung, Y.C.: Biomechanics. Mechanical Properties of Living Tissues, 2nd edn. Springer, New York (1993)
7. Gzik-Zroska, B., Joszko, K., Wolański, W., Gzik, M.: Development of new testing method of mechanical properties of porcine coronary arteries. In: Information Technologies in Medicine: 5th International Conference ITIB 2016, vol. 2, pp. 289–297 (2016)
8. Gzik-Zroska, B., Wolański, W., Gzik, M., Dzielicki, J.: Engineer methods of assistance of toraco-chirurgical operation. In: Proceedings of the III ECCOMAS Thematic Conference on Computational Vision and Medical Image Processing, VipIMAGE 2011, pp. 307–310 (2011)
9. Gzik-Zroska, B., Wolański, W., Gzik, M.: Engineering-aided treatment of chest deformities to improve the process of breathing. Int. J. Numer. Method Biomed. Eng. **29**(9), 926–937 (2013)
10. Gzik-Zroska, B., Wolański, W., Kawlewska, E., Gzik, M., Joszko, K., Dzielicki, J.: Computer-aided correction of pectus carinatum. In: Manuel, J., Tavares, R.S., Natal Jorge, R.M. (eds.) Proceedings of VIPIMAGE 2013-IV ECCOMAS Thematic Conference on Computational Vision and Medical Image Processing, pp. 341–344. CRC Press/Balkema, Leiden (2013)
11. Holzapfel, G.A., Ogden, R.W.: Constitutive modelling of arteries. Proc. Roy. Soc. A: Math. Phys. Eng. Sci. **466**(2118), 1551–1597 (2010)
12. Humphrey, J.D., Holzapfel, G.A.: Review: Mechanics, mechanobiology, and modeling of human abdominal aorta and aneurysms. J. Biomech. **45**, 805–814 (2012)
13. Kajzer, A., Kajzer, W., Gzik-Zroska, B., Wolański, W., Janicka, I., Dzielicki, J.: Experimental biomechanical assessment of plate stabilizers for treatment of pectus excavatum. Acta Bioeng. Biomech. **15**(3), 113–121 (2013)

14. Kulcsar, Z., Ugron, A., Marosfoi, M., Berentei, Z., Paal, G., Szikora, I.: Hemodynamics of cerebral aneurysm initiation: the role of wall shear stress and spatial wall shear stress gradient. AJNR Am. J. Neuroradiol. **32**, 587–594 (2011)

15. Larysz, D., Wolański, W., Kawlewska, E., Mandera, M., Gzik, M.: Biomechanical aspects of preoperative planning of skull correction in children with craniosynostosis. Acta Bioeng. Biomech. **14**(2), 19–26 (2012)

16. Lasheras, J.C.: The biomechanics of arterial aneurysms. Annu. Rev. Fluid Mech. **39**, 293–319 (2007)

17. Meng, H., Wang, Z., Hoi, Y., Gao, L., Metaxa, E., Swartz, D.D., Kolega, J.: Complex hemodynamics at the apex of an arterial bifurcation induces vascular remodeling resembling cerebral aneurysm initiation. Stroke **38**, 1924–1931 (2007)

18. Miura, Y., Ishida, F., Umeda, Y., Tanemura, H., Suzuki, H., Matsushima, S., Shimosaka, S., Taki, W.: Low wall shear stress is independently associated with the rupture status of middle cerebral artery aneurysms. Stroke **44**(2), 519–521 (2013)

19. Roach, M.R., Scott, S., Ferguson, G.G.: The hemodynamic importance of the geometry of bifurcations in the circle of Willis (glass model studies). Stroke **3**, 255–267 (1972)

20. Sacks, M.S.: Biaxial mechanical evaluation of planar biological materials. J. Elast. **61**, 199–246 (2000)

21. Schulze-Bauer, C., Regitnig, P., Holzapfel, G.: Mechanics of the human femoral adventitia including the high-pressure response. Am. J. Physiol. Heart Circ. Physiol. **282**, 2427–2440 (2002)

22. Sharma, G.C., Jain, M., Kumar, A.: Performance modeling and analysis of blood flow in elastic arteries. Math. Comput. Model. **39**, 1491–1499 (2004)

23. Vlak, M.H., Rinkel, G.J., Greebe, P., Algra, A.: Independent risk factors for intracranial aneurysms and their joint effect: a case-control study. Stroke **44**, 984–987 (2013)

24. Wolański, W., Gzik, M., Kawlewska, E., Stachowiak, E., Larys, D., Rudnik, A., Krawczyk, I., Bazowski, P.: Preoperative planning the lumbar spine stabilization with posterior intervertebral systems. In: Manuel, J., Tavares, R.S., Natal Jorge, R.M. (eds.) Proceedings of VIPIMAGE 2013 - IV ECCOMAS Thematic Conference on Computational Vision and Medical Image Processing, pp. 345–348. CRC Press/Balkema, Leiden (2013)

25. Wolański, W., Larysz, D., Gzik, M., Kawlewska, E.: Modeling and biomechanical analysis of craniosynostosis correction with the use of finite element method. Int. J. Numer. Method Biomed. Eng. **29**(9), 916–925 (2013)

Informatics in Medicine

Signal to Noise Ratio in Intrauterine Environment During Acoustic Stimulation

Maria J. Bieńkowska[1]([✉]), Andrzej W. Mitas[2], Anna M. Lipowicz[3], and Agata M. Wijata[2]

[1] Faculty of Automatic Control, Electronics and Computer Science, Silesian University of Technology, Gliwice, Poland
`maria.bienkowska@polsl.pl`
[2] Department of Informatics and Medical Equipment, Faculty of Biomedical Engineering, Silesian University of Technology, Gliwice, Poland
[3] Institute of Anthropology, Wrocław University of Environmental and Life Sciences, Wrocław, Poland

Abstract. Acoustic stimulation in prenatal period is the issue that interest growing group of people. In this paper the ratio of maternal internal sounds (noise) and attenuated sounds from external environment (signal) is considered. There is indicated that only narrow range of frequencies is not drowned by internal sounds. The problem of a distance of sound source was also considered. It was noticed that the application of sound source on maternal abdomen does not increase the sound level in the uterus.

Keywords: Signal to noise ratio · Sound attenuation · Music therapy

1 Introduction

Acoustic stimulation in prenatal period which is used in order to induce positive impact in fetal development is an issue of a dual nature. On the one hand it arouses cognitive problems, but on the other it arouses willingness (at all costs) to stimulate the development of a child from the earliest moments of his/her life. However, knowledge about acoustic stimuli, that are registered by fetus brain (we cannot name it as recognition because of the lack of patterns for comparison and interpretation) is still insufficient and there is the lack of research.

The idea which is recommended and used by mothers is controversial. They use devices like headphones on the belly (anyway it is prohibited by experts [1]) or intravaginal speaker [2]. The main aim of such devices is (1) to isolate mother from perception of annoying or boring sounds or (2) to place the sound source as close as possible to fetal ear and brain. However, we should be critical to such acoustic stimulation on living organism without checking his/her behavioural state (fetus sleeps even 20 h per day). We can easy imagine "contentmen" of an adult man who is stimulated by Aida Triumphal March during his deep sleep.

© Springer International Publishing AG 2017
M. Gzik et al. (eds.), *Innovations in Biomedical Engineering*, Advances in Intelligent Systems and Computing 526, DOI 10.1007/978-3-319-47154-9_24

Movements of mother's and fetus' bodies, activity of internal organs or amniotic fluid generate sounds louder and closer to fetal ear than the sounds which come from the external environment. Basic problem is to determine the level an external signal height to the level of permanent noise from inside the body. This problem was the main issue, which was analyzed in this study. Moreover, purpose of the study was to evaluate the impact of the distance of the sound source from the recorder (in this case a hydrophone) and the appointment of attenuation characteristics of the mother's abdominal wall.

2   Hearing System Development

Development of a hearing system is a complex process that begins at early stage of pregnancy. It begins in third week, when otic placodes are formed. In the next stage, they grow and create two auditory vesicles. The vesicles divide into semicircular canals. It is considered that the inner ear ends its development in sixth pregnancy week. In the next step, in 8 week of pregnancy ossicles, eardrum and earlobe — the middle and outer ear are developed.

The nervous system begins to develop around the 17th day of fetal life. In the early development 3 stages: neural plate, neural groove and, finally, neural plate can be distinguished. The latter one is the base of the brain and the spinal cord. In 4th gestational week forebrain, midbrain and hindbrain appear. In 5th week 5 distinct parts: cerebrum, diencephalon, midbrain, secondary hindbrain, and myelencephalon can be discriminated. In the next weeks cerebral hemispheres develop. It is believed that in 7th week the brain of the fetus has configuration similar to the adult brain, and then it starts to fulfill its main role — coordination of the work of other organs [3,4].

The brain achieves full functionality, which allows to hear sounds, until 25th week of gestation. Since that moment the fetus can receive sound and respond to this stimuli. Hair cells in the cochlea are properly "tuned" to specific frequencies between 26th and 30th gestational week. In 30th week the auditory system is able to receive the entire sound bandwidth and distinguishes the particular phonemes (the smallest unit of the language system). The last feature is associated with the beginning of the speech and language development [5].

3   Attenuation of Sound Stimuli

The hearing system is completely developed in prenatal life, so fetus can hear sounds before his/her birth. However it is uncertain what exactly reach to the fetal inner ear. The sounds which have a source in external (from the fetus point of view) environment are distorted on a path to the uterus. At the beginning, sound from the source, for example sound speaker, has to reach to maternal body. Then it has to go through mother's clothes and her multilayer abdominal wall. At the end the sound is propagate through aquatic environment (amniotic fluid) and, finally, it can reach the fetal inner ear. The most significant is the barrier of maternal abdominal wall, which is complex and changes in time of pregnancy.

3.1   Layers of Maternal Abdominal Wall

Abdominal wall consists of several layers of various thicknesses. External layer is the skin (which include epidermis, dermis and subcutanecous tissue), underneath skin is subcutanecous fat. Then there are abdominal muscles and tendons and, finally, peritoneum. Also uterine wall should be considered. It should be underline that everybody has different body structure and, what is more, changes during pregnancy also vary in female population. Therefore, sound attenuation during acoustic stimulation is the complex process which changes in population and also for women with the same pregnancy stage. So the modelling of such process faces many difficulties and needs a careful approach.

3.2   Experiment

Even simplified model can indicate some features of sound attenuation in tissues. In our work we propose measurements of the sound attenuation in muscle tissue, which considered the impact of the sound source distance. Measuring system, which was used in the experiment, consisted of a hydrophone, amplifier, A/D converter, computer and speaker. Hydrophone was suspended on a stand to eliminate resonance of substrate. Then hydrophone was connected to other elements of the measuring circuit (Fig. 1). Muscle tissue of pregnant woman was simulated using a striated muscle tissue of beef 3 mm thick.

Acoustic stimulus consists of a few generated synthetic sinusoidal signals with frequency 100, 200, 500 and 1000 Hz separately. Acoustic signal was prepared using the Audacity. The experimental procedure involved registration the acoustic wave propagation in two environments:

- air,
- striated muscle tissue.

Hydrophone registered an acoustic signal, which has a source in a speaker placed in two distances:

- speaker close on the hydrophone,
- speaker at a distance of 40 cm.

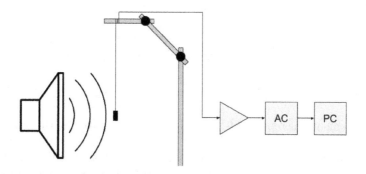

Fig. 1. The measuring system

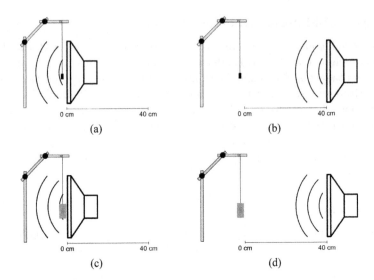

Fig. 2. The configuration of the environment and the distance

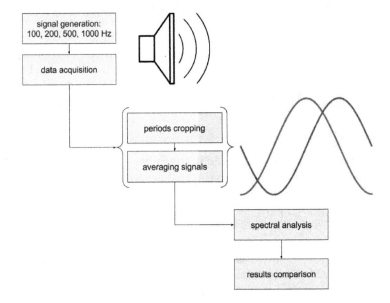

Fig. 3. The workflow

The measurement was repeated 5 times for each configuration of the environment and the distance (Fig. 2).

During analysis, for each frequency the fragment containing 10 complete periods was chosen. Data from 5 measurements of the same conditions were averaged. The same transformations were done for both cases — air and muscle tissue. Finally the averaged signals were compared (Fig. 3).

3.3 Results

Table 1 contains obtained results of attenuation of acoustic stimulus in two cases: a speaker near the hydrophone and at a distance of 40 cm. Sound stimulus after passing through striated muscle tissue was attenuated of 20–30 dB. Small changes of recorded values suggest little influence of close distance on sound attenuation.

Table 1. Change of sound intensity level in relation to the distance

Frequency, (Hz)	Sound intensity level (dB)	
	0 cm	40 cm
100	−29.62	−25.47
200	−33.15	−28.27
500	−26.70	−25.59
1000	−22.22	−22.48

4 Signal to Noise Ratio in Intrauterine Environment

The fetal sound environment does not consist only of external sounds but also of sounds which have a source in maternal body, so the level of both to assess resultant sounds in uterus should be taken into consideration.

4.1 Coefficients of Sound Attenuation

Abrams et al. and Gerhardt et al. [6,7] had conducted the experiments by the use of the hydrophone, which had registered the sound level in the sheep's uterus. There had been reported that low frequency sounds (250–300 Hz) were hardly attenuated and the attenuation had increased with the rate of 5 to 6 dB per octave reaching the value of 20 dB for 4 kHz. These data correspond to the characteristics of the first order low–pass passive filter. On this basis coefficients of sound attenuation for particular frequencies could be designated [8].

4.2 Background Sound Level in Uterus

Sounds produced by maternal body comes from her digestive, respiratory and cardiovascular systems and they are consisted of low frequency components. The lowest frequency reaches the level up to 90 dB [9], which for higher components is decreased to 40 dB [10,11].

The works of Abrams et al. and Gerhardt et al. [10–12] contain the diagrams of intrauterine sound pressure level which enabled us to prepare averaged characteristics of sound level in the uterus. It is presented in Fig. 4.

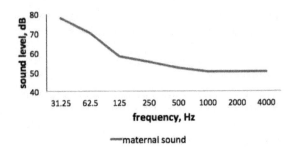

Fig. 4. Intrauterine sound level

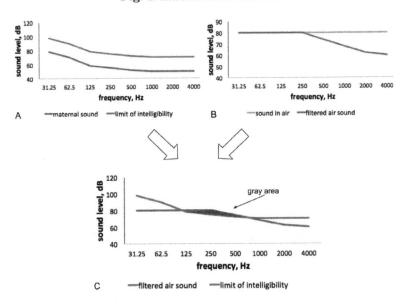

Fig. 5. Level of sound produced by maternal body (a), limit of intelligibility (a, c), base level of external sound (b) and filtered sound characteristics (b, c)

4.3 Signal to Noise Ratio

Sound intelligibility in noise environment are discussed in literature. They indicate that maximum acceptable level of background noise is 20 dB below the voice level [13,14].

According to these data information about limit of intelligibility was added in Fig. 4 — only sounds with level above blue curve had not been drowned by sounds of maternal digestive, cardiovascular and respiratory systems (Fig. 5a).

For this analysis level of external sounds at 80 dB was stated. This level corresponds to sounds of loud music. Then filtration of this sound using first order low–pass filter characterized in previous chapter was simulated. These data are presented in Fig. 5b.

Finally, curves of filtered air sound level and limit of intelligibility level were connected. During stimulation with external sounds at level 80 dB stimuli in very narrow range were intelligible in uterine environment. This range is marked in Fig. 5c with gray area.

5   Conclusions

In this research it was established that sound stimulation (for the fetus it is not music) close to maternal abdomen is not justified. Stimulation from a few feet distance is equally effective. What is more, sounds should be supplied at high level, which can exceed level of intrauterine noise. Only in such condition the distinction between signal and noise is possible (according to theory of signals). For acoustic wave at level 80 dB, transmission through maternal abdominal wall is an effective barrier. Only narrow range of remaining frequencies can carry residual information (including elements of music). The need of obtaining results without effort is an obvious stimulator for the development of civilization. However, during prenatal music therapy it is reduced to invasion in the environment of the developing fetus without consideration of his/her emotional state. Aside from the problem of children's right, it is worth to consider the possibility of extraction elements of music whose organized and predictable influence can be the background sound for relaxation of tension states of the mother and the fetus. Such research, which is a continuation of presented observations, is the main topic of the works of the authors' group.

Acknowledgements. The work has been partially financed by Polish Ministry of Science and Silesian University of Technology statutory financial support for young researchers BKM–508/RAu–3/2016.

References

1. Garven, S.N.: Sound and the developing infant in the NICU: conclusions and recommendations for care. J. Perinatol. **20**, 88–93 (2000)
2. López-Teijón, M., García-Faura, A., Prats-Galino, A.: Fetal facial expression in response to intravaginal music emission. Ultrasound **23**, 216–223 (2015)
3. Bartel, H.: Embriologia. PZWL, Warszawa (2012)
4. Ostrowski, K.: Embriologia człowieka. PZWL, Warszawa (1985)
5. McMahon, E., Wintermark, P., Lahav, A.: Auditory brain development in premature infants: the importance of early experience. Ann. N.Y. Acad. Sci. **1252**, 17–24 (2012)
6. Abrams, R.M., Griffiths, S.K., Huang, X., Sain, J., Langford, G., Gerhardt, K.J.: Fetal music perception: the role of sound transmission. Music Percept. **15**(3), 307–317 (1998)
7. Gerhardt, K.J., Abrams, R.M., Oliver, C.C.: The sound environment of the fetal sheep. Am. J. Obstet. Gynecol. **162**(1), 282–287 (1990)
8. Bienkowska, M., Mitas, A., Lipowicz, A.: Model of attenuation of sound stimuli in prenatal music therapy. In: Information Technologies in Medicine Advances in Intelligent Systems and Computing, vol. 471, pp. 421–432 (2016)

9. Gerhardt, K.J., Abrams, R.M.: Fetal hearing: characterization of the stimulus and response. Semin. Perinatol. **20**(1), 11–20 (1996)
10. Gerhardt, K.J., Abrams, R.M.: Fetal exposures to sound and vibroacoustic stimulation. J. Perinatol. **20**, 21–30 (2000)
11. Abrams, R.M., Gerhardt, K.J.: The acoustic environment and physiological responses of the fetus. J. Perinatol. **20**, 31–36 (2000)
12. Abrams, R.M., Gerhardt, K.J., Griffiths, S.K., Huang, X., Antonelli, P.J.: Intrauterine sounds in sheep. J. Sound Vib. **216**(3), 539–542 (1998)
13. Bistafa, S.R., Bradley, J.S.: Reverberation time and maximum background-noise level for classrooms from a comparative study of speech intelligibility metrics. J. Acoust. Soc. Am. **107**(2), 861–875 (2000)
14. Bistafa, S.R., Bradley, J.S.: Optimum acoustical conditions for speech in classrooms. Vib. Worldw. **31**(9), 12–17 (2000)

Tumor Texture Analysis in PET: Relationship Between the Level of Uptake of Radio-Label at the Time of Treatment and the Level of Uptake of Radio-Label Before and After Treatment

Aleksandra Juraszczyk[1]([✉]), Kamil Gorczewski[2], and Damian Borys[3]

[1] Faculty of Biomedical Engineering, Silesian University of Technology,
Roosevelta 40, 41-800 Zabrze, Poland
aleksandra.juraszczyk@polsl.pl
[2] Department of PET Diagnostics, Maria Skłodowska-Curie Memorial Cancer Center
and Institute of Oncology, Gliwice Branch, ul. Wybrzeże AK 15,
44-100 Gliwice, Poland
[3] Institute of Automatic Control, Silesian University of Technology,
Akademicka 16, 44-100 Gliwice, Poland

Abstract. In this paper we present an analysis of relationship between the level of uptake of radio-label at the time of treatment and the level of uptake of radio-label before and after treatment. The analysis is based on correlation analysis of the tumor features. The patients had 3 examinations: before, during, and after the therapy within 1 month. The fusion of the examinations was performed and the tumors were designated. Then, 108 features were calculated. 3 features determine the tumor: maximum, minimum and average value of Standardized Uptake Value (SUV). 105 features are the texture indices indices based on histogram, histogram of sums, histogram of differences and co-occurrence matrix. The relationship between the features and the uptake levels was analyzed using the Pearson correlation. 29 features proved to be relevant for the correlation.

Keywords: PET/CT · Tumor characterization · Texture indices

1 Introduction

Contemporary oncology uses diagnostic imaging as a very important source of information about a patient's health and stage of the disease. Imaging reveals anatomical details as well as physiological processes. Medical images can be divided into images showing the morphology or metabolism of organs [7].

Morphological images show anatomical information by measuring physical properties of tissues. This can show whether a structure is growing or shrinking [7]. Metabolic images show processes undergoing in an organ or tissue. Cancer cells proliferate more rapidly than normal. Therefore, they consume

© Springer International Publishing AG 2017
M. Gzik et al. (eds.), *Innovations in Biomedical Engineering*, Advances in Intelligent
Systems and Computing 526, DOI 10.1007/978-3-319-47154-9_25

increased amounts of energy [7]. Metabolic images do not show the anatomy, which makes it difficult to determine the location of the tumor. Therefore, hybrid imaging methods, which allow for connection of morphological and metabolic images become useful. The most common example of a hybrid method is the fusion of images of PET/CT and SPECT/CT. The possibilities of connection of PET/CT/MR images are developed as well.

PET is performed after injecting of a biologically active radio-label into the patient's body. It is a chemical substance consisting of two major parts. The first one is the marker which is a specifically selected radioactive isotope. The second part is the carrier, which is a chemical compound with the ability to be accumulated in certain tissues normal or tumor cells [8]. Most commonly used radio-labels are:

- 18F-FDG,
- 18F-Choline,
- 68Ga-DOTA-TATE, 68Ga-DOTA-TOC.

18F-FDG is a very popular radio-label. Glucose (FDG) is the carrier distributed throughout the body. Rapidly proliferating cells, such as cells of heart, brain or tumors feature a greater demand for glucose. Therefore, they accumulate more isotope which, in this case, is flour (18F) [8].

68Ga-DOTATATE, 68Ga-DOTA-TOC are used in the diagnosis of neuroendocrine tumors (NET). 68Ga-DATATATE or 68Ga-DOTA-TOC connect easily with somatostatin receptors, which are common in NET [8].

90Y-DOTA is an octapeptide (which is a somatostatin analogue) labeled with yttrium (90-Y). During the decay, yttrium emits electrons of an energy of 2.28 MeV, which destroy cells in their environment. The octapeptide transports the isotope 90-Y to the tumor cells. Thus, most of the isotope is absorbed by tumor cells and destroyed then. 90Y-DOTA is used in radiotherapy, not for diagnosis in PET. During the therapy, the activity of 90-Y is high (1–2.5 GBq) and performing PET is possible [8].

Frequently calculated 18F-FDG PET image features are: a standardized uptake value (SUV) [1–4], the size of metabolic value (MV) [1–4], the total change in glucose [1,2,4], the texture indices calculated based on the co-occurrence matrix [1,2,4], matrix of gray levels [1] and matrix of gray level differences [1], the intensity histogram [2,4] and the matrix of differences of intensity in neighborhood pixels [2].

Texture is a representation of image properties such as directionality of a pattern or porosity. On this basis it is possible to distinguish between two images, as well as determine whether a region of interest satisfies certain conditions [6].

The analysis of image features is performed for different purposes, for example to determine the effect of changes in the characteristics of the various ways of segmentation of the tumor [1], finding the changes of parameters describing the tumor reaction for treatment [2,3] or the specific tumor type.

The aim of the study is to find a correlation between the level of uptake of 90-Y radio-label during treatment and the level of uptake of radio-label 68Ga-DOTA-TATE tests before and after therapy based on the calculated value of

SUV and texture indices. The study was performed among patients who were diagnosed with lung cancer [1,3], small intestine cancer [1], breast cancer [1] or the esophagus cancer [2].

2   Materials and Methods

2.1   Patients

In the study, 3 patients were included. Table 1 presents the patients' characteristics. All patients received the radiotherapy with 90-Y radio-pharmaceutical.

Table 1. The patients' characteristics.

	Age	Diagnosis	Number of lesions
Patient 1	54	Pheochromocytomas and paragangliomas adrenal neuroendocrine tumor of unknown starting	5
Patient 2	42	Point metastatic to the ovaries, lymph nodes in the neck, supraclavicular, mediastinal and numerous metastases to the spine and pelvis	18
Patient 3	53	Endocrine tumor of the small intestine	3

2.2   PET/CT Protocol

The study was conducted in the PET Diagnostics Department, Center of Oncology - Maria Sklodowska-Curie Memorial Institute, Branch in Gliwice. Each patient had 3 hybrid PET/CT examinations: before (examination 1), during (examination 2), and after (examination 3) the therapy within one month. All tests were performed on a hybrid camera PET/CT Siemens Biograph mCT. Examinations 1&3 provided two series: CT (size $512 \times 512 \times 300$) and PET (size $200 \times 200 \times 300$), which correspond to scanning the patient from mid-thigh to elbows (hands above his head). Examination 2 provided one series of CT (size $512 \times 512 \times 75$) and PET (size $200 \times 200 \times 75$), which corresponds to scanning the whole abdomen and part of the pelvis and the chest. PET scans during examinations 1&3 were performed after the injection of the radio-pharmaceutical 68Ga-DOTA-TATE. Examination 2 was performed using 90Y-DOTA.

2.3   The Fusion Study

To compare the examination result, the fusion of the images is necessary. The fusion is carried out on CT images. At the beginning, images CT were subsampled and aligned in a common space. Then Mutual Information, Nelder-Mead Simplex and Affine Transformation are performed. In contrast, the fusion of CT and PET require only interpolation and superimposing the images, as the images are made on the same apparatus at the same time and the position of the patient does not change. Figure 1 shows a block diagram of the fusion procedure. Figure 2 shows an example of fused PET/CT images.

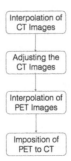

Fig. 1. Block diagram of the fusion procedure.

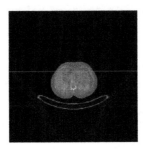

Fig. 2. Example of fused PET/CT images.

2.4   Tumor Segmentation

In order to designate all pathological changes in the PET examination, thresholding is employed. The threshold value is set to 41 % of maximum SUV value in the examination. Then, the expert has to approve the resulting images of tumors. Figure 3 shows an example of segmentation image.

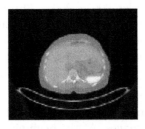

Fig. 3. Example of segmentation image.

2.5 Tumor Characterization

Characteristics (maximum, minimum and average value of SUV) are determined for each tumor. We also calculate the texture indices based on histogram, histogram of sums, histogram of differences and co-occurrence matrix. Histogram of sums and histogram of differences are calculated in four directions: top-down, bottom-up, left to right and right to left. Similarly, co-occurrence matrices are calculated in the directions of $0°$, $45°$, $90°$ and $135°$. Based on these matrices, 105 texture indices are calculated (Table 2). A total number of 108 tumor features are determined.

2.6 Correlation Analysis

The analysis of the correlation between uptake of radio-label in examination 2, and the ratio of uptake in examinations 1&3 was performed. The ratio indicates the tumor response to radiotherapy. Then, the results of the relationship and the feature values in examination 2 were normalized to the range 0-1 for each patient. The relationship was analyzed using the Pearson's correlation coefficient.

3 Results

The expert's verification confirmed, that the segmentation was successful for all tumors.

For each tumor 108 features were calculated (105 features were texture indices). Some features were invariable for all tests. These features included:

- energy and entropy calculated based on the histogram,
- average, moment of 2nd order and energy calculated based on the sum and difference histograms,
- average sum of rows and columns of the co-occurrence matrix.

The Pearson correlation coefficient analysis showed, that some features depend on others. Table 3 shows the features for which the correlation coefficient proves an existing relationship.

4 Discussion

The main aim of the research was to find a correlation between the level of uptake of radio-label in the examination during treatment and the level of radio-label uptake in examinations before and after the treatment, based on the calculated characteristics of the tumor. 29 features proved to be relevant for the analyzed correlation. It can be noted, that the texture indices calculated based on the histogram did not correlate with each other. Similarly it is with the SUV values. The greatest correlation was found between the texture indices calculated based on the co-occurrence matrix.

Table 2. List of indices calculated from texture matrices.

Matrix	Index
Histogram	Average
	SD
	Skewness
	Energy
	Entropy
Histogram of sums	Average
	Moment of 2nd Order
	Contrast
	Energy
Histogram of differences	Average
	Moment of 2nd order
	Contrast
	Energy
Co-occurrence matrix	Average sum of rows
	SD sum of rows
	Average sum of columns
	SD sum of columns
	2nd moment
	Contrast
	Correlation
	Variance
	Inverse differential moment
	Sum of average
	Entropy summation
	Variance summation
	Entropy
	Differential entropy
	Differential variance
	Correlation meter information
	Maximum correlation coefficient

The feature values calculated for the examination 2 are much smaller than for the examinations 1&3. For example, the maximum value of SUV for examinations 1&3 is about 20 and for the examination 2 is about 1. Such great differences are due to different radio-labels. Y-90 is usually used for treatment and not the diagnosis. Using the same radio-label for all studies could prove that more features are relevant for the correlation.

Table 3. List of indices for Pearson's correlation coefficient greater than 0.5 or less than −0.5.

Texture indices	Correlation coefficient
Histogram sums - bottom to top: contrast	0.5
Histogram sums - bottom to top: energy	−0.5
Co-occurrence matrix 0°: SD sum of rows	0.97
Co-occurrence matrix 0°: SD sum of columns	0.97
Co-occurrence matrix 0°: contrast	0.58
Co-occurrence matrix 0°: variance	0.58
Co-occurrence matrix 0°: differential variance	0.72
Co-occurrence matrix 45°: SD sum of rows	0.96
Co-occurrence matrix 45°: SD sum of columns	0.96
Co-occurrence matrix 45°: 2nd moment	0.96
Co-occurrence matrix 45°: contrast	0.57
Co-occurrence matrix 45°: variance	0.57
Co-occurrence matrix 45°: entropy summation	−0.59
Co-occurrence matrix 45°: variance summation	0.75
Co-occurrence matrix 45°: entropy	−0.97
Co-occurrence matrix 45°: correlation meter information	−0.52
Co-occurrence matrix 90°: SD sum of rows	0.59
Co-occurrence matrix 90°: SD sum of columns	0.59
Co-occurrence matrix 90°: contrast	0.66
Co-occurrence matrix 90°: variance	0.66
Co-occurrence matrix 90°: inverse differential moment	−0.98
Co-occurrence matrix 90°: entropy	−0.96
Co-occurrence matrix 135°: SD sum of rows	0.96
Co-occurrence matrix 135°: SD sum of columns	0.96
Co-occurrence matrix 135°: 2nd moment	0.64
Co-occurrence matrix 135°: contrast	0.75
Co-occurrence matrix 135°: variance	0.75
Co-occurrence matrix 135°: entropy	−0.65
Co-occurrence matrix 135°: correlation meter information	−0.55

5   Conclusion

It has been demonstrated that the SUV and texture indices are not correlated with the uptake of the radio-label. Therefore, the therapy effectiveness cannot be determined based on these features. In contrast, texture indices calculated based on the co-occurrence matrix are correlated with the uptake levels. They can be used to determine the effectiveness of radio-pharmaceutical therapy using

Y-90. In the future, the experiments have to be performed on a larger number of cases.

References

1. Orlhac, F., et al.: Tumor texture analysis in 18F-FDG PET: relationships between texture parameters, histogram indices, standardized uptake values, metabolic volues, and total lesion glycolysis. J. Nucl. Med. **55**(3), 414–422 (2014)
2. Tixier, F., et al.: Intratumor heterogeneity characterized by textural features on baseline 18F-FDG PET images predicts response to concomitant radiochemotherapy in esophageal cancer. J. Nucl. Med. **52**(3), 369–378 (2011)
3. Cook, G.J.R., et al.: Are pretreatment 18F-FDG PET tumor textural features in non-small cell lung cancer associated with response and survival after chemoradiotherapy? J. Nucl. Med. **54**(1), 19–26 (2013)
4. Tixier, F., et al.: Reproducibility of tumor uptake heterogeneity characterization through textural feature analysis in 18F-FDG. J. Nucl. Med. **53**(5), 693–700 (2012)
5. Cheebsumon, P., et al.: Impact of 18F-FDG PET imaging paramaters on automatic tumour delineation: need for improved tumour delineation methodology. Eur. J. Nucl. Med. Mol. Imaging **38**(12), 2136–2144 (2011)
6. Snitkowska, E.: Analiza tekstur w obrazach cyfrowych i jej zastosowanie do obrazow analogowych. Ph.D. Thesis, Politechnika Warszawska (2004)
7. Tadeusiewicz, R., Augustyniak, P., et al.: Podstawy Inzynierii Biomedycznej. Krakow: Wydawnictwo AGH (2009)
8. Krolicki, L., Kunikowska, J., Maczewska, J.: Metoda pozytonowej tomografii emisyjnej w medycynie. Zaklad Medycyny Nuklearnej, Warszawski Uniwersytet Medyczny. http://www.instytucja.pan.pl/index.php/component/content/article?id=1892:metoda-pozy. Accessed 04 June 2015

Optimization Analyses of Functional MR Imaging of Motor Areas in Preoperative Patients

Ilona Karpiel[1,2](✉), Zofia Drzazga[1,2], Patrycja Mazgaj[1,2], Paweł Ulrych[3], and Aldona Giec-Lorenz[3]

[1] Department of Medical Physics, Institute of Physics, University of Silesia, Uniwersytecka 4, 40-007 Katowice, Poland
ilona.karpiel@smcebi.edu.pl
[2] Silesian Center for Education and Interdisciplinary Research, 75 Pułku Piechoty 1, 41-500 Chorzów, Poland
[3] Laboratory of Magnetic Resonance Imaging, Helimed Diagnostic Imaging Sp. z o.o., Medyków 14, 40-752 Katowice, Poland
http://fizmed.us.edu.pl

Abstract. Increasingly, fMRI is used for preoperative diagnosis of patients. This method gives the possibility to locate the relevant functional areas of the brain responsible for movement, sensation and speech, which are often adjacent to the tumor. The ultimate success of any experimental fMRI depends not only on the quality of the collected image data but also appropriate selection of the parameters (Gaussian kernel, level of significance, extent threshold) so as to maximize statistical power. Our fMRI analysis carried out in SPM 12 package for the 5 patients with lesions have shown that increasing the value of clinical diagnosis requires an individual approach taking into account a given pathology and the possible implications for surgical intervention. The values of parameters which could be taken as preliminary to analyze of activations of motor cortex - primary (M1) and supplementary (SMA) are discussed.

Keywords: fMRI · Preoperative · Motor cortex · Optimization · Human brain

1 Introduction

Currently increasingly used, non-invasive method of mapping brain activity is functional magnetic resonance imaging. fMRI based on the fact, that the local intensity of the blood flow is closely related to the activity of the brain region [1]. The most commonly used sequence is BOLD [2,3], although diffusion sequence is also applied. Especially important application of fMRI examination seems to be used to pre- and postoperative diagnostics, because it allows to checking whether the location of functionally important structures adjacent to tumor or other pathology.

© Springer International Publishing AG 2017
M. Gzik et al. (eds.), *Innovations in Biomedical Engineering*, Advances in Intelligent Systems and Computing 526, DOI 10.1007/978-3-319-47154-9_26

The fMRI imaging of preoperative patients allows to more accurate planning neurosurgeries in order to save functionally important structures and reduce postoperative neurological deficits resulting from medical procedures. On the other hand, studies of postoperative patients allow for postoperative control and monitoring the effects of further treatment. Functional magnetic resonance imaging may contribute to the explanations of neurological disorders and can aid in further diagnostic or neurological rehabilitation [4].

Functional neuroimaging studies are highly specialized medical imaging procedures, which not only require close cooperation between medical staff during examination, but also earlier preparation of individual paradigms, which consider localization of lesions and neurosurgical interventions. In our studies we focused on activations of motor cortex - primary (M1), premotor (PMA) and supplementary (SMA) [5], which are important in terms of life quality - ability of movement and process of speech. Brain movement areas known as a Brodmann Areas (BA) 1–4,6,8, are located in frontal lobe and parietal lobe [6], which are connected with cerebellum. These areas are responsible planning, making exercise, controlling and coordinating of movements. There are also area related with motor cortex, which are responsible for motor imagery and learning, saccadic movements, inhibition of blinking and executive control of behavior. Paradigms such as finger tapping, ankle dorsiflexion and ankle plantar flexion and also tongue movement are generally used for activation motor cortex ([2,7,8] and references inside).

The fMRI study depends on the number of used paradigms and usually last about one hour, so it is relatively long and also costly. Description of results requires accomplish a specialized analysis using SPM software (Statistical Parametric Mapping [9]) frequent updates. It is known, that all steps of fMRI study: proper preparation patient to the study, appropriate selection of paradigm, processing of acquired data are important. Results of SPM analysis depend on the used parameters [10] such as: fixed Gaussian kernel (σ), level of significance (p) and also the number of analysed voxels. Therefore in this paper we draw attention to the optimization of fMRI in preoperative patients considering the duration of measurements and analysis as well as diagnostic value of clinical study.

2   Materials and Methods

2.1   Subjects and fMRI Data Acquisition

Five preoperative patients with different lesions were included in the study, comprising 3 females of age ranging 24.3 ± 4.7 years and 2 males (a mean age 37 ± 4 years)) which listed in Table 1. For comparison healthy 24 years old volunteer has been included in experiment. Brain imaging studies were performed with 1.5T MAGENTOM Aera scanner (Siemens, Erlangen, Germany), equipped with a 20-channel head-neck coil in Helimed Diagnostic Imaging Center in Katowice as part of normal clinical work. Ultrafast Gradient Echo 3D sequence (3D T1-MPRAGE) [TR = 1900 ms, TE = 2.67 ms, TI = 1100 ms, slice thickness 1.0 mm, FOV = 250 mm × 250 mm, matrix size = 256 × 256] and axial EPI

SE sequence [TR = 3140 ms, TE = 50 ms, TI = 1100 ms, slice thickness 4.0 mm, FOV = 1320 mm × 1320 mm, matrix size = 384 × 384] are applied. Scanner software containing syngo.MR Neuro 3D Engine allowed to preview the results of the study (activation) in real time [11].

2.2   Experimental Paradigm

Paradigms with classic blocked design, which means, that the "active" and "rest" blocks emerge alternately were prepared in PsychoPy software [12]. Nonetheless, human brain works continuously, so "rest block" means here the part of paradigm when the task not displayed. Created paradigm to stimulate the motor cortex composed of 4 active and 5 rest blocks - collected 90 volumes. For activation motor cortex we used paradigms finger tapping and ankle flexion (dorsiflexion and plantar flexion) using a computer coupled projector. For all preoperative patients both hands finger tapping tests were performed. Additionally in two cases ankle flexion paradigm was used.

2.3   Data Analysis

Analysis of brain activations based on EPI SE sequence was performed in SPM12 package in MATLAB (MathWorks, Inc.) environment. The steps of data analysis process consisted of spatial pre-processing: 'realignment', 'coregistration' and 'spatial smoothing'. Realignment was used to reduce the misalignment between images in an fMRI time series, which were resulting of head movement during fMRI session. This step is also known as motion correction technique is realized using a rigid body transformation. This implies, that spatial transformation model based on six parameters: three related with translation (along x, y and z axis) and three with rotation (around x, y and z axis) and assumed that the effects of motion did not change the shape of the brain. Only position and orientation can change. All images were realignment to the first image according these six parameters [10,13]. Coregistration was performed to maximizing the mutual information between anatomical and functional MRI scans. It is necessary, because EPI images have low resolution and geometric distortion, while activated brain areas should be indicated on the anatomical images. This step is slow because a function has to be found, which measures a difference between these images [13]. Finally the, data has to be smoothed. Smoothing is a convolution operation, therefore it relies on multiplying each voxel intensity time-series data with a Gaussian kernel of a specified width at half maximum (FWHM). As a result each voxel's signal takes the averaged within neighbourhood values. The step is needed to be performed because of two particular reasons. First, to suppress the noise and make the data having distribution closer to normal for statistical reasons. Second, to facilitate the inter-subject analysis by data unification [14–16].

The goal of fMRI statistical analysis is to define those brain regions that show significant activation. The most popular statistical approach assume that dependence of the signal and stimulus is linear. This is described by so called

General Linear Model. For its purpose, a model of expected response is at first created and then estimated. In these analyzes we used model based on the T-statistic, where selected significance level (p) defined probability, that exist a difference between active and rest phases. The smaller value of p, the threshold level (T-threshold) increase. The T-threshold is the T-value in a T distribution with number of degrees of freedom that corresponds to the given significance level (p) [17].

In order to obtain the optimal highlighted active area analysis of fMRI measurements was performed for different parameters such as: fixed Gaussian kernels with various widths (FWHM of 0, 2, 4, 6 and 8 mm), significance level ($p < 0.001$ and $p < 0.01$) and extent threshold: 0 and 10 voxels (extent threshold ie. selection the number of voxels to restrict the minimum cluster size, where 0 means including single voxel clusters ('spike' activations)) [18]. Localization of active areas were made using functional atlases [19–22] and Talairach Client [23].

3   Results

3.1   Movement Activations

Figure 1 shows activations in M1 and SMA induced both hands finger tapping for healthy volunteer after normalization. Activation of BA 1–4 located in primary motor cortex (prefrontal gyrus) and activations of supplementary motor cortex (BA 6,8) located in midline surface of the hemisphere anterior to the M1 [24] were obtained in line with expectations. Reference regions of activation of motor cortex reveal high space resolution and are symmetrical.

For preoperative patients different disturbance of motor cortex activity in comparison with healthy men were observed. First of all, it is important to check the placement of pathologies in relation to the expected areas of motor activity. The obtained activities as a function of the estimated distance from the pathology are collected in Table 1. One can see that activations induced by finger tapping in patients no. 1–4 occurred in the near and in direct adhesion to the pathology for both M1 and the SMA. Only for patient no. 5 activations were symmetrical and far away from the lesion. In order to deepen the analysis of the cases in which the areas of physical activity are located near the pathology indicated was the use of the second test (unless there are medical contraindications e.g. pregnancy). The paradigm "ankle flexion" confirmed in two patients occurrence of activations directly adjacent to the pathology.

Figure 2 displays results of fMRI study for preoperative patient (no. 2) with an expansive lesion on the left side of hemisphere where activations in M1 and SMA areas are in the direct adhesion to the brain pathology or even overlap partly with potential regions of activation. It should be noted that this expansive lesion on the left side of hemisphere caused paresis of right upper. In other cases a shift activation were observed because of due to the proximity of pathology (not shown in this paper).

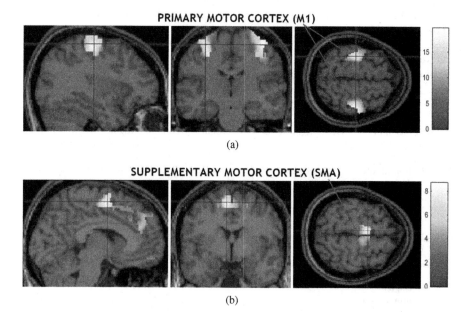

(a)

(b)

Fig. 1. Activations in primary (a) and supplementary (b) motor cortex in healthy volunteer. Applied paradigm: both hands finger tapping. Parameters: kernel 5, 10 voxels, $p < 0.001$.

3.2 Effect of Parameters (σ, p) on Motor Cortex Activation

Using different values of parameters in analysis SPM causes usually influences on size and shape of activated regions which may vary across the brain leading to images of different quality [25]. An effect of Gaussian kernel and level of significance on motor activations is presented in Fig. 3. The analysis shows, that activations induced by hands finger tapping are achieved in similar locations. However, for $p < 0.001$ areas of activations have better resolution than for $p < 0.01$, especially in the primary motor cortex. Nevertheless, it should be also noted that the small activation occurring in areas SMA may go unnoticed during the analysis with $p < 0.001$ unlike $p < 0.01$. Nonetheless, it seems that the analysis with the lower significance p-value ($p < 0.01$) can be helpful in preliminary imaging as well as finding the weak activations.

It follows from our analyses (Fig. 3) that Gaussian filter changing in 0–8 mm range has no a significant effect on activation images which is also confirmed by the similar value of T-value. However using higher kernels (not shown in this paper) leads to the expansion of the activation area and its blur which was reported earlier [25 and references inside].

The dependence of motor activity regions on extent threshold (10 and 0 voxels) for a patient.

Figure 4 shows that results of the analysis for extent threshold 0 and 10 (kernel 6, $p < 0.001$) differ substantially. Activities in SMA are displayed with

Table 1. Activities in M1 and SMA as a function of the estimated distance from pathology in both hemispheres (left (L) and right(P)) for finger tapping and ankle flexion. "+"/"−" (activity/no activity in the hemisphere) locations marked with these signs were not taken for further analysis but these activations were not relevant from the point of view medical diagnostic.

ID	Localization of pathology\Activity	Finger tapping				Ankle flexion			
		SMA		M1		SMA		M1	
		Left	Right	Left	Right	Left	Right	Left	Right
1	Right frontal lobe brain tumor	+	Adjacent	+	~1.5 cm	+ c	Adjacent	−	−
2	Expansile lesion of left parietal lobe	−	−	Adjacent	+	Adjacent	+	Adjacent	+
3	Right frontal lobe brain tumor	+	~2 cm	+	Adjacent	No paradigm		No paradigm	
4	Cavernous malformation in the left frontoparietal lobe	+	~1.5 cm	−	Adjacent	No paradigm		No paradigm	
5	Expansile lesion of left hemisphere	~4 cm	+	~4 cm	+	No paradigm		No paradigm	

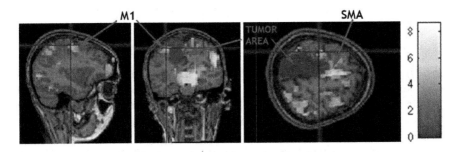

Fig. 2. Activations of M1 and SMA in direct adhesion to the lesion in preoperative patient. Applied paradigm: both hands finger tapping. Parameters: kernel 6, 10 voxels, p < 0.001.

better space resolution for 10 voxels than 0 probably because of omissions 'spike' activations present in 0 voxel analysis. Moreover analysis in the Talairach Client includes 32 statistically important areas for 10 voxels while for 0 voxel - 84 areas. The similar effect can be noted in M1.

4   Discussion

Preoperative fMRI studies allow to more accurate surgery planning, therefore it is possible to reduce not only the resection nearby the motor cortex but also other

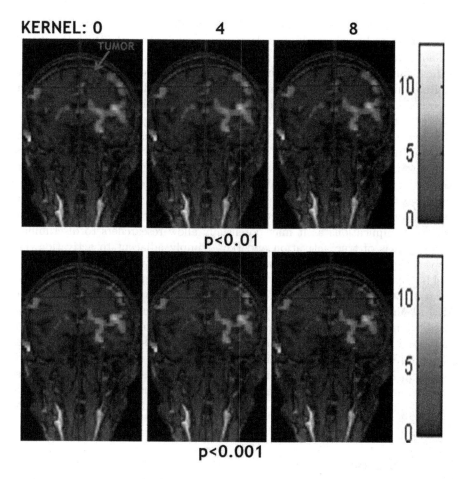

Fig. 3. Imaging of activations on SMA application for kernel, significance level for 10 voxels. Used paradigm: both hands finger tapping.

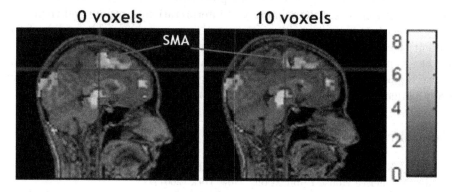

Fig. 4. Activity areas induced by right ankle flexion focused on SMA (coordinates: −8, −7, 58) for voxels 0 and 10, p < 0.001.

neurological injuries. It is essential to draw attention to appropriate selection of parameters i.e.: kernel, significance level and number of voxels. With the change of Gaussian filter, significance level (p) as well as extent threshold may increase medical value of functional imaging. Modification of these parameters can lead to situations where certain regions are under-smoothed, while others are over-smoothed – hence the necessity of methodology optimization. Choosing a low value we get false positive results, for the high we omit significant activations [27]. Moreover, to shorten the time and reduce the cost of measurement is possible to perform studies fMRI for reduced number of slices [26] covering the selected area instead of the whole brain, which can be especially useful for small lesions or in need of more accurate imaging of the selected brain area. Problem of adopted statistical techniques is not new subject, but still breaks the neuroscientists environment. An appreciate selection of parameters in the analysis of SPM has important implications as it may potentially allow researchers to discriminate between areas of true activation and those simply adjacent to activation. For analysis of preoperative patients we recommend to use two values of significance level because $p < 0.01$ seems to be suitable for display supplementary motor area and $p < 0.001$ for primary motor cortex. However, preoperative diagnosis using fMRI requires an individual approach taking into account pathologies as well as possible implications for surgical intervention. Method of examination as well as analysis of the results with adaptive parameters allows to obtain images with appropriate spatial resolution which is important from the point of view of the operation. However in our opinion personal approach is recommended because of individual variation among preoperative patients. Presentation of numerical results requires an increase in the number of cases in different pathologies in the future.

5   Conclusion

The fMRI is very helpful and a supportive tool for the diagnosis of preoperative brain. Is best to use two different procedures that application more than one paradigm increases the reliability of interpretation of results and their convergence with the medical descriptions and improve the quality of life of the patient. We suggest to perform a preliminary analysis using $p < 0.01$ and in a further steps to modify parameters in the analysis of SPM to yield a balance between smoothing the image and retaining detail in the activated regions for every patient individually taking into account his pathology.

References

1. Davis, K.D., Chudler, E.H. (eds.): New Techniques for Examining the Brain, pp. 37–38. Chelsea House Publications, New York (2007)
2. Tieleman, A., Deblaere, K., Van Roost, D., Van Damme, O., Achten, E.: Preoperative fMRI in tumour surgery. Eur. Radiol. 19(10), 2523–2534 (2009)

3. Smits, M.: Functional magnetic resonance imaging (fMRI) in brain tumour patients. Eur. Assoc. NeuroOncol. Mag. **2**(3), 123–128 (2012)
4. Filippi, M.: fMRI Techniques and Protocols. Human Press, New York (2009)
5. Tozakidou, M., Wenz, H., Reinhardt, J., et al.: Primary motor cortex activation, lateralization in patients with tumors of the central region. NeuroImage Clin. **2**, 221–228 (2013)
6. Trans Cranial Technologies: Cortical Functions, Reference. Trans Cranial Technologies Ltd. (2012)
7. Berns, G.S., Song, A.W., Mao, H.: Continuous functional magnetic resonance imaging reveals dynamic nonlinearities of "dose-response" curves for finger opposition. J. Neurosci. **19**(14), RC17 (1999)
8. Witt, S.T., Laird, A.R., Meyerand, M.E.: Functional neuroimaging correlates of finger-tapping task variations: an ALE meta-analysis. Neuroimage **42**(1), 343–356 (2008)
9. Penny, W., Friston, K., Ashburner, J., Kiebel, S., Nichols, T.: Statistical Parametric Mapping: The Analysis of Functional Brain Images, 1st edn. Academic Press, New York (2006)
10. Poldrack, R.A., Mumford, J.A., Nichols, T.E.: Handbook of Functional MRI Data Analysis. Cambridge University Press, Cambridge (2011)
11. Zimmers, J.: Neuro 3D - a clinical exam. RSNA Edition of MAGNETOM Flash **37**(3), 110–112 (2007)
12. Peirce, J.W.: PsychoPy–Psychophysics software in Python. J. Neurosci. Methods **162**(1–2), 8–13 (2007)
13. Nagata, T., Tsuyuguchi, N., Uda, T., Ohata, K.: Non-normalized individual analysis of statistical parametric mapping for clinical fMRI. Neurol. India **59**(3), 339–343 (2011)
14. Lindquist, M.: The statistical analysis of fMRI data. Stat. Sci. **23**(4), 439–464 (2008)
15. Ashburner, J., Henson, R., et al.: SPM manual, Welcome trust center for neuroimaging (2012)
16. Friston, K., Mapping, B.: Chapter 22, Statistics I: Experimental design and statistical parametric mapping. In: Toga, A.W., et al. (eds.) The Methods, 2nd edn. Elsevier, Amsterdam (2002)
17. http://www.ernohermans.com/wp-content/uploads/2011/11/spm8_startersguide.pdf
18. http://www.fil.ion.ucl.ac.uk/spm/doc/manual/results.htm
19. Tamraz, J., Comair, Y.: Atlas of Regional Anatomy of the Brain Using MRI: With Functional Correlations. Springer, Berlin (2005)
20. Orrison, W., Atlas, Jr.: funkcjonalny mózgu. PZWL, Warszawa (2010)
21. http://www.fmriconsulting.com/brodmann/Interact.html
22. http://braininfo.rprc.washington.edu/Default.aspx
23. http://www.talairach.org/client.html
24. Longstaff, A.: Neurobiologia, pp. pp. 285–288. PWN, Warszawa (2012)
25. Yue, Y.R., Loh, J.M., Lindquist, M.A.: Adaptive spatial smoothing of fMRI images. Stat. Interf. **3**, 3–13 (2013)
26. Król, A., Drzazga, Z., Klose, U.: Optimization of pulse-triggered fMRI measurement delay with acoustic stimulation. In: World Congress on Medical Physics and Biomedical Engineering, Toronto, Canada, pp. 103–106, 7–12 June 2015
27. http://prefrontal.org/blog/2010/11/paper-an-argument-for-proper-multiple-comparisons-correction/

Estimation of Pointer Calibration Error in Optical Tracking System

Bartłomiej Pyciński[✉]

Faculty of Biomedical Engineering, Silesian University of Technology,
Roosevelta 40, 41-800 Zabrze, Poland
bartlomiej.pycinski@polsl.pl

Abstract. This study presents methods of pointer calibration in optical tracking system. First, the problem of calibration is defined and algorithms solving this problem are described. Various input data are provided to assess the algorithms accuracy. If the process of calibration is performed carefully, a minimisation of algebraic linear equation system yields the smallest absolute error of calibration equal to 0.27 mm. If the procedure of calibration is disturbed, presented improvements of the algorithms allow to preserve error values below 1 mm.

Keywords: Image navigation system · Pivot calibration · Validation and evaluation

1 Introduction

Image navigation systems play important role in surgery nowadays. Especially, neurosurgeons or orthopaedists willingly make use of them, as they allow to fuse virtual model and the patient body during the surgery [1,2]. Elements, whose location and spatial orientation are tracked by the navigation system, are called "markers". A pointer is a specific type of marker, as it contains additional stylus whose tip allows to precisely mark points in the space.

Before a pointer can be employed by the navigation system, it has to be calibrated first. The process of pointer calibration is usually a first engineering procedure during image-guided surgery, it precedes image registration or segmentation [3]. Use of pointer is necessary to obtain the position of landmark points on the patient body.

There are several methods of pointer calibration. Usually they minimise an overdetermined system of linear equations or fit a sphere to a set of recorded marker positions. A wide review of calibration methods was performed recently by Yaniv [4].

The main goal of this paper is to assess the accuracy of the pointer calibration. The paper is organized as follows. Section 2 presents the navigation system and the calibration algorithms. Section 3 discuss the results. Section 4 concludes the study.

© Springer International Publishing AG 2017
M. Gzik et al. (eds.), *Innovations in Biomedical Engineering*, Advances in Intelligent
Systems and Computing 526, DOI 10.1007/978-3-319-47154-9_27

2   Materials and Methods

2.1   Optical Navigation System

Optical navigation system Polaris Spectra (Northern Digital Inc., ON, Canada) contains stereoscopic camera, which acquires infra-red image with maximum acquisition frequency equal to 60 Hz. Both camera lenses contain additional infra-red LEDs which beam the scene. The elements tracked by the system (i.e. markers) consist of three or four spheres of diameter equal to 10 mm rigidly fixed to cross-shape frame (Fig. 1). The spheres are covered by silver surface which intensively reflects IR-light, therefore they are presented as bright points at dark background (Fig. 2). The position and orientation (translation and rotation) of the markers are obtained by triangulation method using the images of both cameras [5].

Marker tracking accuracy is not worse than 0.25 mm, according to the manufacturer's note sheet [6]. The volume tracked by the camera ranges from 0.95 to 3 m (Fig. 3).

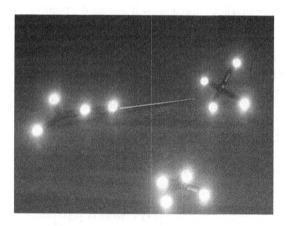

Fig. 1. Polaris navigation system markers

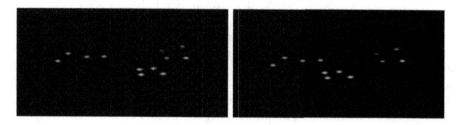

Fig. 2. Images of the markers from Fig. 1 recorded by both system cameras

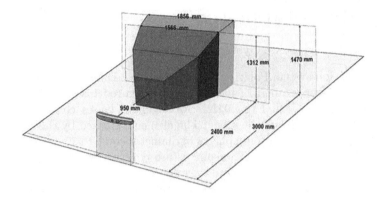

Fig. 3. Polaris spectra measurement volume. Orange colour denotes part with worse tracking accuracy [7] (Color figure online)

2.2 Pointer Calibration

A stylus tool with a marker attached to it is called "pointer" (Fig. 1, first from the left). Its goal is to get coordinates of arbitrary chosen points, touched by its tip.

Pointer calibration (also called "pivot calibration", Fig. 4) is a process of determining position of the pointer's tip in relation to the pointer marker's local coordinates frame $\mathcal{L}$ (denoted as $P^{\mathcal{L}}$). This position is constant regardless of pointer's movement in global space, as the pointer is a rigid body. The result of calibration ($P^{\mathcal{L}}$) is a homogeneous translation vector $[t_x, t_y, t_z, 1]^T$ of transformation matrix $M_{\mathcal{K}}^{\mathcal{L}}$, which transforms the tip to the marker's local coordinate frame $\mathcal{L}$. Rotation part of transformation matrix r_{ij} is irrelevant, because the position of the tip in global coordinates frame $P^{\mathcal{G}}$ depends only on the position of marker $M_{\mathcal{L}}^{\mathcal{G}}$ and the calibration vector $P^{\mathcal{L}}$:

$$
P^{\mathcal{G}} = M_{\mathcal{L}}^{\mathcal{G}} M_{\mathcal{K}}^{\mathcal{L}} P^{\mathcal{K}} = M_{\mathcal{L}}^{\mathcal{G}} \begin{bmatrix} r_{11} & r_{12} & r_{13} & t_x \\ r_{21} & r_{22} & r_{23} & t_y \\ r_{31} & r_{32} & r_{33} & t_z \\ 0 & 0 & 0 & 1 \end{bmatrix} \begin{bmatrix} 0 \\ 0 \\ 0 \\ 1 \end{bmatrix} = M_{\mathcal{L}}^{\mathcal{G}} \begin{bmatrix} t_x \\ t_y \\ t_z \\ 1 \end{bmatrix}. \tag{1}
$$

The calibration procedure involves fixation of the tip and rotation of the marker around the pivot point (Fig. 4) over the part of sphere. The frequency of circulation should not exceed 1 Hz to increase the accuracy of marker localisation. The higher the number of acquired positions is, the better accuracy is obtained [8]. In this study, the number of positions during calibration was equal to 200 in each experiment. The positions of the marker recorded in the global coordinate system $\left(M_{\mathcal{G}}^{\mathcal{L}}\right)_i$ are then used to determine the translation vector of transformation matrix $M_{\mathcal{L}}^{\mathcal{K}}$ (or, the coordinates of the tip in marker's coordinates system $P^{\mathcal{L}}$). Once the matrix is known, the global coordinates of the tip $P^{\mathcal{G}}$ are given on-line.

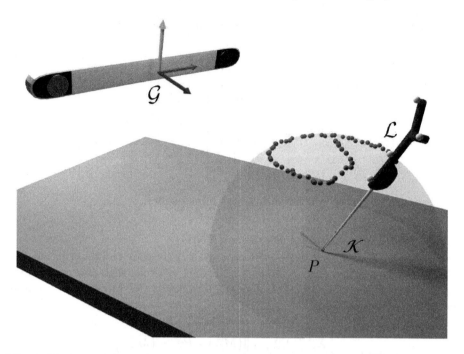

Fig. 4. Marker trajectory during calibration process. $\mathcal{G}$, $\mathcal{L}$ and $\mathcal{K}$ denotes coordinates system related to global camera, local marker and the pointer tip, respectively. P denotes position of the tip

2.3 Mathematical Formulations

The methods solving pivot calibration problem lead to the same result – the coordinates of translation vector $P^{\mathcal{L}}$. Algebraic basis of the employed methods are described below.

2.3.1 Algebraic Linear Equation System (ALES)

Assuming the tip of the pointer is fixed at one point and the pointer trajectory is spherical, the following equation is satisfied for all N positions:

$$\forall_{i \in \{1,...,N\}} P^{\mathcal{G}} = \left(M^{\mathcal{G}}_{\mathcal{L}}\right)_i \cdot P^{\mathcal{L}}. \tag{2}$$

Therefore single equation may be written:

$$\begin{bmatrix} x^{\mathcal{G}} \\ y^{\mathcal{G}} \\ z^{\mathcal{G}} \\ 1 \end{bmatrix} = \begin{bmatrix} (r_{11})_i & (r_{12})_i & (r_{13})_i & (t_x)_i \\ (r_{21})_i & (r_{22})_i & (r_{23})_i & (t_y)_i \\ (r_{31})_i & (r_{32})_i & (r_{33})_i & (t_z)_i \\ 0 & 0 & 0 & 1 \end{bmatrix} \cdot \begin{bmatrix} x^{\mathcal{L}} \\ y^{\mathcal{L}} \\ z^{\mathcal{L}} \\ 1 \end{bmatrix}, \tag{3}$$

which after some transformations leads to the following overdetermined equation system:

$$
\begin{bmatrix}
(r_{11})_1 & (r_{12})_1 & (r_{13})_1 & -1 & 0 & 0 \\
(r_{21})_1 & (r_{22})_1 & (r_{23})_1 & 0 & -1 & 0 \\
(r_{31})_1 & (r_{32})_1 & (r_{33})_1 & 0 & 0 & -1 \\
& \vdots & & & \vdots & \\
(r_{11})_N & (r_{12})_N & (r_{13})_N & -1 & 0 & 0 \\
(r_{21})_N & (r_{22})_N & (r_{23})_N & 0 & -1 & 0 \\
(r_{31})_N & (r_{32})_N & (r_{33})_N & 0 & 0 & -1
\end{bmatrix}
\cdot
\begin{bmatrix}
x^{\mathscr{L}} \\
y^{\mathscr{L}} \\
z^{\mathscr{L}} \\
x^{\mathscr{G}} \\
y^{\mathscr{G}} \\
z^{\mathscr{G}}
\end{bmatrix}
=
\begin{bmatrix}
(-t_x)_1 \\
(-t_y)_1 \\
(-t_z)_1 \\
\vdots \\
(-t_x)_N \\
(-t_y)_N \\
(-t_z)_N
\end{bmatrix}.
\tag{4}
$$

To minimize it, the LSQR method [9] was implemented.

2.3.2 Nonlinear Minimal Distance (NMD)

The method assumes that during the process of calibration the tool tip position $P^{\mathscr{L}}$ is invariant. Then root mean square distance between each pair of acquired tip positions is minimal [10]. Therefore the formula of cost function for minimisation is as follows:

$$
E(P^{\mathscr{L}}) = \sqrt{\frac{\Sigma_{i=1}^{N-1} \Sigma_{j=i+1}^{N} \left\| \left(M_{\mathscr{L}}^{\mathscr{G}}\right)_i \cdot P^{\mathscr{L}} - \left(M_{\mathscr{L}}^{\mathscr{G}}\right)_j \cdot P^{\mathscr{L}} \right\|^2}{\frac{1}{2}N(N-1)}}.
\tag{5}
$$

The formula above can be transformed into a simplified form:

$$
E(P^L) =
$$
$$
\sqrt{\frac{N\Sigma_{i=1}^{N}\left((x_i^{\mathscr{G}})^2 + (y_i^{\mathscr{G}})^2 + (z_i^{\mathscr{G}})^2\right) - (\Sigma_{i=1}^{N} x_i^{\mathscr{G}})^2 - (\Sigma_{i=1}^{N} y_i^{\mathscr{G}})^2 - (\Sigma_{i=1}^{N} z_i^{\mathscr{G}})^2}{\frac{1}{2}N(N-1)}},
\tag{6}
$$

where $[x_i^{\mathscr{G}}, y_i^{\mathscr{G}}, z_i^{\mathscr{G}}]^T = \left(M_{\mathscr{L}}^{\mathscr{G}}\right)_i P^{\mathscr{L}}$.

Minimisation of the cost function was performed with downhill simplex method (amoeba method, Nelder–Mead method) [11].

2.3.3 Sphere Fitting (SF)

A sphere, for which the sum of squares of the distances to the given points is minimal is referred to as "best fit". Determining the coordinates of the best fit sphere (i.e. radius, centre) is called as "sphere fitting". Given the positions of the pointer marker $M_i^{\mathscr{G}}$ during the calibration, if $P^{\mathscr{G}}$ denotes the centre (pivot point) and r denotes length of the radius, the formula of cost function for minimisation is as follows:

$$
E(P^{\mathscr{G}}, r) = \Sigma_{i=1}^{m}(\|M_i^{\mathscr{G}} - P^{\mathscr{G}}\| - r)^2.
\tag{7}
$$

Iterative minimisation method was implemented based on description presented in [12].

2.3.4   Power of Average Transformation Matrix (PATM)

PATM is an iterative method where a mean transformation matrix between consequent marker positions is created. Let

$$\widetilde{M} = \frac{1}{N} \Sigma_{i=1}^{N} M_{\mathscr{L}_{i-1}}^{\mathscr{L}_i}, \tag{8}$$

where $M_{\mathscr{L}_{i-1}}^{\mathscr{L}_i}$ is the transformation matrix between $i-1$ and i-th marker coordinate frame. It can be shown [13] that fourth column of consequent powers (i.e. $\widetilde{M}^N$) of the matrix gradually approximate the solution.

In the study the powers are computed until the exponent is equal to 5000 or the difference between last and previous translations is smaller than 10^{-6} mm.

2.4   Error Estimation

There are two approaches of estimating the error of the calibration. If ground truth (i.e. the real value of $P^{\mathscr{G}}$) is not known, then the error of calibration depends on the variation of tip position during the process of calibration [14]. Both root-mean-square error and mean error may be use to estimate the accuracy of calibration. If ground truth is known, then the error is simply the distance between it and the position computed during the calibration.

Let $\mathbf{E}$ is a vector of individual errors of all positions acquired during the calibration:

$$\mathbf{E} = \begin{bmatrix} \left\| P^{\mathscr{G}} - (M_{\mathscr{L}}^{\mathscr{G}})_0 \cdot P^{\mathscr{L}} \right\| \\ \vdots \\ \left\| P^{\mathscr{G}} - (M_{\mathscr{L}}^{\mathscr{G}})_N \cdot P^{\mathscr{L}} \right\| \end{bmatrix}. \tag{9}$$

2.4.1   Root-Mean-Square Error

($RMSE$) of vector $\mathbf{E}$ is defined as:

$$RMSE = \sqrt{\frac{1}{N} \Sigma_{i=1}^{N} \left\| P^{\mathscr{G}} - \left(M_{\mathscr{L}}^{\mathscr{G}}\right)_i \cdot P^{\mathscr{L}} \right\|^2}. \tag{10}$$

2.4.2   Mean Error

(ME) of vector $\mathbf{E}$ is defined as:

$$ME = \frac{1}{N} \Sigma_{i=1}^{N} \left\| P^{\mathscr{G}} - (M_{\mathscr{L}}^{\mathscr{G}})_i \cdot P^{\mathscr{L}} \right\|. \tag{11}$$

2.4.3   Absolute Error

(AE) is known only if real value of $P^{\mathscr{G}}$ is known. Let $P^{\mathscr{G}}_0$ is this ground truth, whereas $P^{\mathscr{G}}_{alg}$ is the result of current calibration algorithm. Then AE is defined as:

$$AE = \| P^{\mathscr{G}}_{alg} - P^{\mathscr{G}}_0 \|. \tag{12}$$

To be able to compute AE of all calibration procedures, P_0 was estimated by averaging $P^{\mathscr{G}}$ of five series having the smallest variation.

2.5   Modification of the Calibration Method

In this study, original ALES method was improved as follows:

1. After $P^{\mathscr{L}}$ value during calibration procedure had been obtained, a vector $\mathbf{E} = \{e_i\}$ containing all tip positions was computed:

$$e_i = \left(M_{\mathscr{L}}^{\mathscr{G}}\right)_i P^{\mathscr{L}}, \tag{13}$$

2. Mean value and standard deviation (*SD*) of the vector $\mathbf{E}$ was computed, and all positions, whose distances from the mean are greater than $3SD$, were rejected from further computations,
3. Vector $\mathbf{E}$ was divided into 8 parts and variation of each part was computed,
4. The elements of two parts with greatest variations were rejected from further computations,
5. The ALES algorithm was repeated with remaining input positions.

The goal of the above modifications was to reduce the impact of outliers – positions, that could be acquired inaccurately. Moreover, if during the calibration the global coordinate system was displaced (i.e. Polaris camera was shifted), the proposed procedure would allow to decrease the total error. In this study the modified algorithm will be denoted as ALES*.

3   Experiments and Results

3.1   Input Data

Input data consisted of two parts. First one contained trajectories recorded by Polaris camera during pointer calibration procedures. There were 47 independent calibrations, the numbers of acquired positions ranged from 214 to 286. Second part contained 33 artificially generated trajectories, each having 200 positions. Movement of the pointer during calibration was various. We can distinguish four different groups of pointer trajectories:

1. Precise circulatory movement on the sphere (Fig. 5a),
2. Precise movement on the sphere, but different paths: on one or two planes (Fig. 5b),
3. Movement on the sphere, but the tip was not fixed precisely and it slid on the surface (Fig. 5c),
4. Movement on the sphere, and the camera was shifting during the calibration (Fig. 5d).

Artificially generated trajectories were also divided into the following groups depending on type of added noise.

5. Points lying perfectly on the sphere (Fig. 5e),
6. Points on the sphere blurred by Gaussian or uniform noise (Fig. 5f),
7. Points on the sphere with the tip slided on the surface,
8. Points on the sphere with noise and 5 % of outliers.

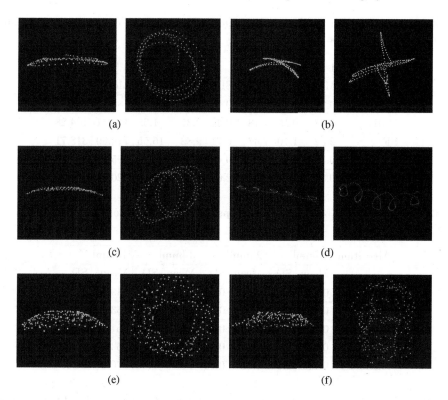

Fig. 5. Visualisations of pointer's marker positions from top and side view (left and right column, respectively). (a) to (d) Recorded trajectories, (e) and (f) Artificial trajectories

3.2 Results

In this study 47 series of calibration data were recorded and 33 series were generated. Four different algorithms and one modification were compared. Each algorithm was performed on each series of data.

Three types of errors defined in Sect. 2.4 were compared – AE, ME and RMSE. Dependencies between these errors were assessed. The values of mean values and standard deviations of the errors are given in Tables 1, 2 and 3.

Groups 3 and 4 of recorded data imitate a situation in the operating theatre, where there are disruptions during calibration procedure, such as sliding the tip of the pointer on the surface of operating table or the shifting of tracking camera. If there is no time to repeat the procedure, the algorithm should be as robust as possible [15].

Error values of ALES* algorithm are not significantly worse then the best results in groups 1 and 2, and in groups 3 and 4 its errors are the smallest.

Comparison of ME and RMSE with t-Student test ($p = 0.05$) indicates that in 1st and 2nd group of data RMSE is significantly higher than ME for algorithms

Table 1. Absolute errors [mm] of the algorithms performed on trajectories of four groups of recorded data

Algorithm	1 [mm]		2 [mm]		3 [mm]		4 [mm]	
	Mean	SD	Mean	SD	Mean	SD	Mean	SD
ALES	0.27	0.10	1.19	0.44	2.27	1.94	185.36	101.60
NMD	0.28	0.10	1.18	0.42	2.37	1.98	195.41	104.28
SF	2.52	1.70	7.47	6.71	9.83	16.55	716.69	318.71
PATM	0.29	0.12	1.12	0.45	2.29	1.81	195.74	108.27
ALES*	0.36	0.15	3.49	2.07	0.96	0.39	20.53	14.44

Table 2. RMSE [mm] of the algorithms performed on trajectories of four groups of recorded data

Algorithm	1 [mm]		2 [mm]		3 [mm]		4 [mm]	
	Mean	SD	Mean	SD	Mean	SD	Mean	SD
ALES	0.42	0.04	0.32	0.01	2.51	1.55	49.20	14.19
NMD	0.42	0.04	0.32	0.01	2.75	1.66	53.72	12.92
SF	0.99	0.40	0.88	0.80	3.89	3.20	157.84	60.66
PATM	0.42	0.04	0.32	0.01	2.76	1.66	53.82	12.97
ALES*	0.41	0.04	0.32	0.02	2.53	1.59	70.08	25.19

Table 3. Mean errors [mm] of the algorithms performed on trajectories of four groups of recorded data

Algorithm	1 [mm]		2 [mm]		3 [mm]		4 [mm]	
	Mean	SD	Mean	SD	Mean	SD	Mean	SD
ALES	0.39	0.03	0.29	0.01	2.29	1.45	45.52	13.77
NMD	0.39	0.04	0.29	0.01	2.41	1.47	49.12	12.35
SF	0.95	0.41	0.78	0.70	3.54	3.15	150.12	59.87
PATM	0.39	0.04	0.29	0.01	2.41	1.47	49.12	12.35
ALES*	0.37	0.03	0.29	0.02	2.33	1.52	59.13	21.08

ALES and ALES*. Additionally, in 2nd group this is true also for NMD and PATM. In 3rd and 4th group no significant differences is noticeable.

3.3   Estimation of Spatial Distribution of Absolute Error

Absolute error was defined as the distance between the real pivot point P_0 and the point yielded by the calibration algorithm P_{alg} (Sect. 2.4). Current study is the first approach to assess the direction of the 3D vector $[P_0 - P_{alg}]$ in the local marker coordinates system.

Table 4. Mean and standard deviations of absolute error distribution in space of four groups of recorded data

		1 [mm]		2 [mm]		3 [mm]		4 [mm]	
		Mean	SD	Mean	SD	Mean	SD	Mean	SD
ALES	X	0.18	0.13	0.47	0.42	0.18	0.51	37.15	30.49
	Y	0.13	0.09	0.61	0.59	0.85	0.69	176.77	99.79
	Z	0.09	0.05	0.68	0.31	0.07	2.13	30.64	17.46
NMD	X	0.18	0.13	0.48	0.43	0.18	0.48	38.40	31.05
	Y	0.14	0.10	0.61	0.56	0.73	0.61	185.53	102.89
	Z	0.09	0.05	0.68	0.31	0.07	2.21	35.72	20.95
PATM	X	0.19	0.14	0.46	0.38	0.21	0.57	41.78	37.47
	Y	0.16	0.07	0.56	0.54	0.72	0.51	183.33	107.43
	Z	0.10	0.06	0.68	0.31	0.06	1.95	35.64	25.20
ALES*	X	0.23	0.15	1.42	1.21	0.49	0.28	4.81	5.57
	Y	0.21	0.11	2.38	2.52	0.30	0.27	14.03	11.56
	Z	0.11	0.08	1.10	0.62	0.26	0.36	11.04	11.45

Results indicates that the distribution of the vector was symmetrical in all directions, as mean values did not exceed 0.05 mm in first group of trajectories.

If absolute values $[|P_{0x} - P_{alg_x}|, |P_{0y} - P_{alg_y}|, |P_{0z} - P_{alg_z}|]$ are taken into account, their means indicate the level of error variations in each direction (Table 4). The results show that in first group of recorded data there is no significant difference between the directions, although the values of mean and SD in Z-direction are always the smallest. This states that the tip localisation is the most accurate along Z axis.

4   Conclusion

In the paper, the study of pointer calibration error estimation has been presented. The results were obtained from recorded and artificially generated data. The latter proved correctness of the implemented algorithms.

For carefully performed calibration procedure, ALES method yielded the smallest errors, although there was no significant difference between its and NMD results. The values of AE were significantly smaller than RMSE and ME. Moreover, RMSE and ME might significantly differ, especially if these values were not large. This indicates, firstly, that RMSE and ME obtained during calibration process are in fact upper limits of the tip localisation inaccuracy and secondly, that two navigation system with different calibration error estimation (i.e. RMSE and ME) should not be compared directly.

If the process of calibration was disturbed, e.g. because of sliding the tip or shifting Polaris camera, improved algorithm ALES* (Sect. 2.5) yielded significantly better results – in group 3 AE was smaller than 1 mm, whereas values of other algorithms exceeded 2 mm, and in group 4 AE equalled to 20.53 mm, whereas others algorithms yielded values of AE higher than 180 mm.

There was no evidence that there were better pointer trajectories than circulating movements on the sphere.

Methods and algorithms described in this study are not limited to optical tracking systems. Other types of tracker (e.g. electromagnetic) could be freely used with presented algorithms.

Acknowledgement. This research is supported by Silesian University of Technology Grant No. 211926/E-367/M/2016.

References

1. Krysztoforski, K., Krowicki, P., Najwer, Ś.E., Będziński, R., Keppler, P.: Noninvasive ultrasonic measuring system for bone geometry examination. Int. J. Med. Robot. Comput. Assist. Surg. **7**(1), 85–95 (2011)
2. Juszczyk, J., Pycinski, B., Pietka, E.: Patient specific phantom in bimodal image navigation system. In: 2015 37th Annual International Conference of the IEEE Engineering in Medicine and Biology Society (EMBC), pp. 2908–2911 (2015)
3. Czajkowska, J., Badura, P., Piętka, E.: 4D segmentation of Ewing's Sarcoma in MR images. In: Pietka, E., Kawa, J. (eds.) Information Technologies in Biomedicine, Volume 2. AISC, vol. 69, pp. 91–100. Springer, Heidelberg (2010)
4. Yaniv, Z.: Which pivot calibration? In: Webster, R.J., Yaniv, Z.R. (eds.) Medical Imaging 2015: Image-Guided Procedures, Robotic Interventions, and Modeling. SPIE-The International Society for Optical Engineering, March 2015
5. Gremban, K., Thorpe, C., Kanade, T.: Geometric camera calibration using systems of linear equations. In: Proceedings of IEEE Conference on Robotics and Automation (ICRA 1988), vol. 1, pp. 562–567, April 1988
6. Wiles, A.D., Thompson, D.G., Frantz, D.D.: Accuracy assessment and interpretation for optical tracking systems. In: Proceedings of SPIE, Medical Imaging 2004: Visualization, Image-Guided Procedures, and Display, vol. 5367, pp. 421–432, May 2004
7. Northern Digital Inc.: Polaris measurement volume (2016). http://ndigital.com/medical/products/polaris-family/features/measurement-volume
8. Cleary, K., Zhang, H., Glossop, N., Levy, E., Wood, B., Banovac, F.: Electromagnetic tracking for image-guided abdominal procedures: overall system and technical issues. In: 27th Annual International Conference of the Engineering in Medicineand Biology Society, pp. 6748–6753. IEEE-EMBS 2005 (2005)
9. Paige, C.C., Saunders, M.A.: LSQR: an algorithm for sparse linear equations and sparse least squares. ACM Trans. Math. Softw. **8**(1), 43–71 (1982)
10. Zhang, H., Banovac, F., White, A., Cleary, K.: Freehand 3d ultrasound calibration using an electromagnetically tracked needle. In: Proceedings of SPIE, vol. 6141 (2006)
11. Nelder, J.A., Mead, R.: A simplex method for function minimization. Comput. J. **7**(4), 308–313 (1965)
12. Schneider, P.J., Eberly, D.: Geometric Tools for Computer Graphics. Elsevier Science Inc., New York (2002)

13. Onprasert, W., Ongwattanakul, S., Suthakorn, J.: Implementation on a new tool tip calibration method for biomedical applications. In: Qian, Z., Cao, L., Su, W., Wang, T., Yang, H. (eds.) Recent Advances in Computer Science and Information Engineering. LNEE, vol. 129, pp. 385–392. Springer, Berlin Heidelberg (2012)
14. Lasso, A., Heffter, T., Rankin, A., Pinter, C., Ungi, T., Fichtinger, G.: Plus: open-source toolkit for ultrasound-guided intervention systems. IEEE Trans. Biomed. Eng. **61**(10), 2527–2537 (2014)
15. Pycinski, B., Juszczyk, J., Bozek, P., Ciekalski, J., Dzielicki, J., Pietka, E.: Image navigation in minimally invasive surgery. In: Piętka, E., Kawa, J., Wieclawek, W. (eds.) Information Technologies in Biomedicine. AISC, vol. 284, pp. 25–34. Springer, Heidelberg (2014)

Contextual Database of Radiological Images: Liver Parameters

Paula Stępień[1]([✉]), Maria Bieńkowska[2], and Jacek Kawa[2]

[1] Faculty of Automatic Control, Electronics and Computer Science,
Silesian University of Technology, Gliwice, Poland
paula.stepien@polsl.pl
[2] Faculty of Biomedical Engineering, Silesian University of Technology,
Zabrze, Poland

Abstract. In this paper data from a contextual database of radiological images were analyzed in order to extract the parameters related to the volume and dimensions of the liver alongside with its intensity in the Magnetic Resonance Imaging (MRI) and Computed Tomography (CT). Pearson correlation of $P = 0.99$, $p < 0.01$ between mean value of pixels computed for the whole liver and for the biggest liver area in the 2D slice was obtained. High correlations ($P = 0.71$, $p < 0.001$) were received for the area of the largest 2D region of interest (ROI) and the overall volume of liver, independently of the image source. The results are even higher for CT studies only ($P = 0.79$, $p = 0.001$). The estimation of the whole liver parameters based on only one slice can significantly shorten the time needed for the preliminary diagnosis and help in the computer aided diagnosis (CAD) systems development.

Keywords: Medical imaging · Contextual database · Atlas · Liver · Segmentation

1 Introduction

It is estimated that approximately 29 million people in Europe suffer from various liver diseases. One of them, and the most dangerous is cirrhosis. The fatal outcome of the cirrhosis is the hepatocellular carcinoma which is the fifth most common cause of cancer in European countries and results in around 170 000 deaths per year [1]. The correct diagnosis of liver diseases and their suitable treatment is one of the main goals of modern medicine. The segmentation of the liver and the calculation of its features becomes an important issue. E.g. the liver size and volume is essential in the planning of the living-related donor liver transplant, split-liver transplantation and major hepatic resections [2,3].

The relationship between the body and the liver size has been examined for many years [4,5]. Several studies have been conducted in order to calculate the standard liver volume (SDL) [6]. For those purposes Computed Tomography (CT) as well as ultrasound have been used [7–9]. The ultrasound has become

© Springer International Publishing AG 2017
M. Gzik et al. (eds.), *Innovations in Biomedical Engineering*, Advances in Intelligent
Systems and Computing 526, DOI 10.1007/978-3-319-47154-9_28

the standard procedure because of the lower costs and the patient's safety. Still, the CT is the most reliable method determining the overall dimensions of the liver [10] due to various factors influencing the procedure.

A commonly used reference point for clinical assessment of liver size and localization in the ultrasound examination is the midclavicular line (MCL). It starts in the midpoint of the clavicle and extends downward over the trunk. The main disadvantage of the use of the midclavicular line is the reliance on the anterior surface of the body, which may vary from the interior body structure. The shift of the MCL can lead to the liver's volume under- or overestimation. In the study of Naylor et al. [11] the estimated distance from the midline to the MCL varied by up to 10 cm for 20 clinicians evaluating 3 subjects and was therefore called a *wandering landmark*. The error was independent from the patients build. The use of the body surface landmarks generates also the need to remove the clothes from the patients trunk which is another drawback. Therefore, despite the artifacts connected to the respiratory cycle, the CT scan seems to be a more approachable method in the evaluation of the liver volume. The reduction of the number of delineations needed to obtain the whole liver volume from the CT examination would be a step forward in the computed aided diagnosis systems (CAD).

Along with the CAD, the patient specific models (PSM) are an important innovation in the modern health care. Scientists design tools allowing the customization of the treatment of diseases and developing the branch of the minimally-invasive medicine. The obtained models can be used for guidance during laparoscopic operations, where the camera provides only a partial surface view of the organ to the surgeon [12]. Models simulate the deformations resulting from any kind of pressure or the respiratory cycle [13] and allow to construct patient specific phantoms [14].

The first step in obtaining a model is the collection of images and the segmentation of the selected organs. Still, the segmentation of the liver is a major issue that cannot be easily solved. The already published approaches involve a variety of methods from statistical shape models to granular computing [15]. The necessity to tackle this problem led to the organization of special events such as the MICCAI (Medical Image Computing and Computer Assisted Intervention) 2007 Grand Challenge workshop, where 16 research groups evaluated their liver segmentation algorithms on a set of 20 clinical images [16]. Already verified images (and delineations) can be indexed and arranged to form a database. Such databases (also known as atlases) were already implemented using lung radiograms and CT scans [17–20] as well as mammograms [21].

An appropriate atlas plays a crucial role in the assessment of algorithms and serves as a gold standard. In the current study, the existing radiological atlas [22] for patient specific model generation is extended to contain manual, expert delineations of selected organs (region of interests, ROI) and ROI-dependent features. One of the extracted parameters, the liver volume, is of our main interests.

In this paper we present the further work on a contextual database of radiological images. It focuses on the liver features. We present the correlations between the various parameters calculated from the 2D slice with the biggest ROI area and the whole generated volume. In the Sect. 2 we describe the data and the workflow of our research, the results are presented in the Sect. 3. The discussion in Sect. 4 concludes the paper.

2   Materials and Methods

2.1   Materials

The image database, partially indexed using radiological atlas, consists of 490 studies: 395 Computed Tomography (CT) and 95 Magnetic Resonance Imaging (MRI) examinations registered between years 2008 and 2013 using GE Light-Speed16 and GE Sigma HDxt 1.5T. The images are anonymized, evaluated and described by a physician.

Based on the radiological atlas, 41 CT and 6 MRI examinations of the abdominal were selected for delineation. The patients (17 women and 22 men) were born between 1927 and 2006. Twenty-one livers were tagged as healthy. Several pathologies were observed. Some of the examinations displayed more than one pathology (Table 1).

Table 1. Liver evaluation

Diagnosis	Number of cases
Normal	21
Enlarged	2
Steatosis	2
Cirrhosis	2
Focal lesions	4
Heterogenity	4
Cysts	14

2.2   Methods

The database presented in [22] was extended to contain manual, expert delineations of selected organs. The combination of raw data, expert delineations and descriptions made by a physician allowed the extraction of several parameters and their statistical analysis (Fig. 1).

Raw medical images in the DICOM format were imported into the open-source image viewer Horos[1] (macOS successor of OsiriX). Mac Book Air (13" screen) was used. The region of interest (ROI) was manually selected in 47 examinations in the traverse plane as seen in the Fig. 2. First, the series providing

---

[1] https://www.horosproject.org/.

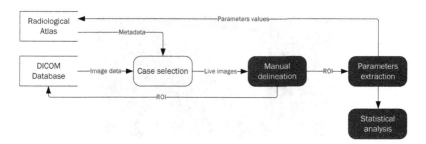

Fig. 1. Workflow

the best quality of the image was selected. Next, liver ROI was delineated in all relevant slices (frames). Finally, on the basis of the largest ROI in the series, several features were calculated:

- *area* – the area of the ROI outlined in the traversal plane,
- *mean* – the mean pixel intensities within the ROI,
- *standard deviation* – the standard deviation of pixel intensities belonging to the ROI,
- *sum* – the sum of the intensities of pixels belonging to the ROI,
- *min* – the minimum intensity value of pixels belonging to the ROI,
- *max* – the maximum intensity value of pixels belonging to the ROI,
- *length* – the length of the liver contour.

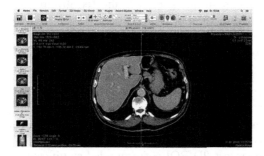

Fig. 2. 3D image of a healthy liver with manually delineated ROI

Using multiple 2D ROIs, a volume of interests was automatically generated (Fig. 3) and the parameters for the whole liver were obtained. The parameters were similar to those in the 2D space (for example the volume of the liver was calculated instead of area of the ROI).

The obtained features were collected in the database alongside the medical examination results and statistically analyzed.

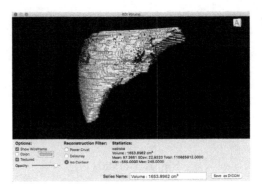

Fig. 3. 3D image of a healthy liver

3   Results

The obtained parameters were statistically analyzed. The modality-dependent parameters (signal intensity-based) were processed separately in MR and CT groups. Spatial parameters were processed together in both groups (CT and MR combined).

First, the distribution of the parameters was analyzed in the control group and groups featuring different pathologies. Selected parameters were shown to be statistically different. For example, volume of the liver was lower in the group of people with cyst, tumor (U Mann-Whitney test, $p = 0.014$), the liver perimeter was longer in the group with non-uniform liver density (U Mann-Whitney test). However, the number of subjects in each affected group was very low (over 30 patients in control group vs. 4 or 6 patients in tested groups).

Next, the correlation analyses was performed for all the subjects including extracted parameters only. High dependency was found between selected 3D parameters group and parameters computed over single slice with the largest ROI area:

1. Mean value of pixels computed in a whole liver volume and mean value computed in single slice was highly correlated (Pearson correlation $P = 0.99$, $p < 0.01$); CT studies (Fig. 4).
2. The area of the largest 2D ROI corresponded significantly to the overall volume of liver ($P = 0.79$, $p < 0.001$; CT studies only, and $P = 0.71$, $p < 0.001$ CT for and MR studies combined).
3. Maximum and minimum intensity values were related ($P = 0.79$, $p < 0.001$ and $P = 0.91$, $p < 0.001$, respectively; CT and MR studies combined).

4   Discussion

The outlining of ROIs is a laborious occupation. The precise delineation of liver borders in only one examination can consume up to one hour for more complex

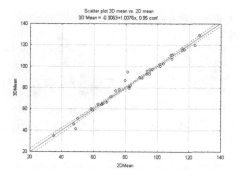

Fig. 4. Scatter plot 3D vs. 2D mean value of pixels

cases. The rendering of volumes based on data from several scans registered during one examination needs to be divided into consistent groups (one slice for one abdominal region). It this study the division was performed manually but for further research it should be automated.

The analysis of parameters distributed within control and pathology groups shows relationships between prevalence of selected diseases and some of the extracted parameters. Interestingly, despite MRI being considered more sensitive to the changes in the liver tissue than CT, the results seem to be independent of the modality or acquisition protocol (admission or lack of contrast agent, used phase, etc.). However, the number of subjects in affected groups is insufficient for statistically relevant inference and so is the number of cases for each acquisition protocol. The detected relationships shall not be considered valid until further research. One of the most important aims of the future studies will be finding the correlation of the parameters connected with cirrhosis in the 2D (Fig. 5) and 3D (Fig. 6) space. For this reason, more examinations concerning this fatal condition need to be gathered and analyzed.

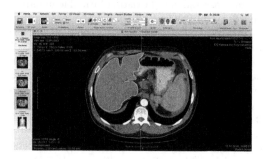

Fig. 5. 2D image of a liver diagnosed with cirrhosis

However, the impact of the 2D and 3D parameters dependency analysis seem to have practical implications. In selected cases, tedious 3D segmentation can

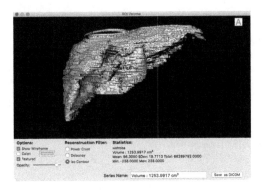

Fig. 6. 3D image of a liver diagnosed with cirrhosis

be replaced by 2D segmentation of the largest liver slice in both CT and MRI series. Reduction of the processing time, especially involving manual outlining, can be a significant factor on a way to fast diagnosis.

Acknowledgements. The work has been partially financed by Polish Ministry of Science and Silesian University of Technology statutory financial support for young researchers BKM-508/RAu-3/2016.

References

1. Blachier, M., Leleu, H., Peck-Radosavljevic, M., Valla, D.C., Roudot-Thoraval, F.: The burden of liver disease in europe: a review of available epidemiological data. J. Hepatol. **58**(3), 593–608 (2013)
2. Urata, K., Kawasaki, S., Matsunami, H., Hashikura, Y., Ikegami, T., Ishizone, S., Momose, Y., Komiyama, A., Makuuchi, M.: Calculation of child and adult standard liver volume for liver transplantation. Hepatology **21**(5), 1317–1321 (1995)
3. Chandramohan, A., Eapen, A., Govil, S., Govil, S., Jeyaseelan, V.: Determining standard liver volume: assessment of existing formulae in indian population. Indian J. Gastroenterol. **26**(1), 22 (2007)
4. DeLand, F.H., North, W.A.: Relationship between liver size and body size 1. Radiology **91**(6), 1195–1198 (1968)
5. Vauthey, J.N., Abdalla, E.K., Doherty, D.A., Gertsch, P., Fenstermacher, M.J., Loyer, E.M., Lerut, J., Materne, R., Wang, X., Encarnacion, A., Herron, D., Mathey, C., Ferrari, G., Charnsangavej, C., Do, K.A., Denys, A.: Body surface area and body weight predict total liver volume in western adults. Liver Transplant. **8**(3), 233–240 (2002)
6. Heinemann, A., Wischhusen, F., Püschel, K., Rogiers, X.: Standard liver volume in the caucasian population. Liver Transplant. Surg. **5**(5), 366–368 (1999)
7. Heymsfield, S.B., Fulenwider, T., Nordlinger, B., Barlow, R., Sones, P., Kutner, M.: Accurate measurement of liver, kidney, and spleen volume and mass by computerized axial tomography. Ann. Intern. Med. **90**(2), 185–187 (1979)
8. Niederau, C., Sonnenberg, A., Müller, J.E., Erckenbrecht, J.F., Scholten, T., Fritsch, W.P.: Sonographic measurements of the normal liver, spleen, pancreas, and portal vein. Radiology **149**(2), 537–540 (1983)

9. Fritschy, P., Robotti, G., Schneekloth, G., Vock, P.: Measurement of liver volume by ultrasound and computed tomography. J. Clin. Ultrasound **11**(6), 299–303 (1983)

10. Wolf, D.C.: Evaluation of the size, shape, and consistency of the liver. In: Walker, H.K., Hall, W.D., Hurst, J.W. (eds.) Clinical Methods: The History, Physical, and Laboratory Examinations, vol. 94, 3rd edn. Butterworths, Boston (1990)

11. Naylor, C.D., McCormack, D.G., Sullivan, S.N.: The midclavicular line: a wandering landmark. Can. Med. Assoc. J. CMAJ **136**(1), 48 (1987)

12. Plantefève, R., Peterlik, I., Haouchine, N., Cotin, S.: Patient-specific biomechanical modeling for guidance during minimally-invasive hepatic surgery. Ann. Biomed. Eng. **44**(1), 139–153 (2016)

13. Rohlfing, T., Maurer, C.R., O'Dell, W.G., Zhong, J.: Modeling liver motion and deformation during the respiratory cycle using intensity-based nonrigid registration of gated MR images. Med. Phys. **31**(3), 427–432 (2004)

14. Juszczyk, J., Pyciński, B., Pietka, E.: Patient specific phantom in bimodal image navigation system. In: 2015 37th Annual International Conference of the IEEE Engineering in Medicine and Biology Society (EMBC), pp. 2908–2911, August 2015

15. Juszczyk, J., Pietka, E., Pyciński, B.: Granular computing in model based abdominal organs detection. Comput. Med. Imaging Graph. **46**(Part 2), 121–130 (2015). Information Technologies in Biomedicine

16. Heimann, T., et al.: Comparison and evaluation of methods for liver segmentation from CT datasets. IEEE Trans. Med. Imaging **28**(8), 1251–1265 (2009)

17. Shiraishi, J., Katsuragawa, S., Ikezoe, J., Matsumoto, T., Kobayashi, T., Komatsu, K.I., Matsui, M., Fujita, H., Kodera, Y., Doi, K.: Development of a digital image database for chest radiographs with and without a lung nodule: receiver operating characteristic analysis of radiologists' detection of pulmonary nodules. Am. J. Roentgenol. **174**(1), 71–74 (2000)

18. Clark, K.W., Gierada, D.S., Moore, S.M., Maffitt, D.R., Koppel, P., Phillips, S.R., Prior, F.W.: Creation of a CT image library for the lung screening study of the national lung screening trial. J. Digital Imaging **20**(1), 23–31 (2007)

19. Reeves, A., Biancardi, A., Yankelevitz, D., Fotin, S., Keller, B., Jirapatnakul, A., Lee, J.: A public image database to support research in computer aided diagnosis. In: 31st Annual International Conference of the IEEE Engineering in Medicine and Biology Society, pp. 3715–3718 (2009)

20. Armato III, S.G., McLennan, G., Bidaut, L., McNitt-Gray, M.F., Meyer, C.R., Reeves, A.P., Zhao, B., Aberle, D.R., Henschke, C.I., Hoffman, E.A., et al.: The lung image database consortium (LIDC) and image database resource initiative (IDRI): a completed reference database of lung nodules on CT scans. Med. Phys. **38**(2), 915–931 (2011)

21. Heath, M., Bowyer, K., Copans, D., Moore, R., Kegelmeyer, P.: The digital database for screening mammography, digital mammography. In: IWDW 2000 5th International Workshop on Digital Mammography, pp. 212–218 (2000). http://marathon.csee.usf.edu/Mammography/Database.html

22. Kawa, J., Juszczyk, J., Pyciński, B., Badura, P., Pietka, E.: Radiological atlas for patient specific model generation. In: Pietka, E., Kawa, J., Więcławek, W. (eds.) Information Technologies in Biomedicine, Volume 4. AISC, vol. 284, pp. 69–84. Springer, Heidelberg (2014)

Digital Watermarking in Telemedicine an Example from ECG - Review of Challenges, Methods and Applications

Agnieszka Świerkosz[✉]

AGH University of Science and Technology, Kraków, Poland
aswierk@agh.edu.pl

Abstract. Despite fast growth of scope and availability of telemedicine, the concern of data security still remains one of crucial unresolved problems. This paper presents a review of solutions applied to ECG watermarking in both: local area and wide area networks. Digital watermarking provides a simple yet effective way of data protection against unauthorized access and modification, authentication of the sender and secret data containers for additional data. Thanks to a thorough, cardiology-oriented data analysis, all this is possible without alteration of medical content of the record. The review is followed by a discussion of their features and hierarchy in aspect of personalized telemedicine of cardiovascular diseases. It is possible to code in this transmission any other information. Why not to invent a new way of watermarking? This paper shows selected results of the work about this topic.

Keywords: Watermarking · ECG · Digital watermarking · Secret · Security · Secure communication · Authentication · Image retrieval · Medical data protection

1 Introduction

In medicine it is very important to get a good ECG signal without distortion. Now a doctor can send the data to his or her colleague to have another opinion about the illness.

Watermarking is a process by which a discrete data stream (watermark) is hidden. Information hiding techniques were primarily developed for data copyright protection. They can be also quite suitable for biomedical signal authentication. In these techniques the embedded data has been 'invisible' to maintain the quality of the host data. In present time, healthcare systems are expected to experience a drastic change in its structure and organization. As the volume of health care data increases, more complex storage of medical information is necessary. One of the major technological and ethical issue is data privacy. Protection from unauthorized access on medical history data and personal patient data is very important and should have a good quality. Watermarking has been

© Springer International Publishing AG 2017
M. Gzik et al. (eds.), *Innovations in Biomedical Engineering*, Advances in Intelligent Systems and Computing 526, DOI 10.1007/978-3-319-47154-9_29

implemented on digital audio, images or video data by using different methods like Fourier transform, wavelet transform and a scheme based on independent component analysis [3].

Digital watermarking is an adaptation of paper watermarks to the digital data carriers. Digital watermarking describes methods and technologies for hiding information in a digital carrier. There are several properties that a watermark should have [6]:

1. Imperceptibility,
2. Readability,
3. Low Complexity,
4. Security.

Digital watermarking allows to have information cross linked on the document, so as some parts are redundant. The name of a passport owner is printed in an open text and is also hidden as an invisible watermark in the owners photo. If anyone would try to counterfeit the passport by replacing the photo, it would be possible to detect the change in the way of scanning the passport and verifying the name hidden in the photo. In that case, it is also embedded patient's identification in two different ways [6].

Body area networks (BANs) are networks of wireless medical sensors, deployed on a person, for enabling pervasive, individualized, and real-time health management. As BANs deal with personal health data, securing them, especially their communication over the wireless link, is very important. Lack of adequate security measures may not only lead to a breach of patient privacy, but also potentially allows adversaries to compromise patient safety by modifying actual data resulting in wrong diagnosis and treatment [3].

2   Considered Methods

2.1   Digital Watermaking of ECG Data for Secure Wireless Communication

An interesting method for watermarking of the ECG signal, first proposed by [6] uses the 8-bit chirp signal. In that scheme, the chirp used is 'quadratic', where instantaneous frequency sweep $\phi(t)$ is given by:

$$f_1(t) = f_0 + \beta t^2 \tag{1}$$

where

$$\beta = (f_1 - f_0)t_1^{-2} \tag{2}$$

Each sample of ECG is quantized using 10 bits. The ECG signal is divided into frames using a rectangular window of a size equal to length of the chirp signal [3]. To each bin of the ECG signal a modulated chirp signal is added. The chirp signal is modulated according to the 'patient ID' which is exclusive for each individual

$$y_{chirp,mod} = y_{chirp} * f(b_j) \tag{3}$$

where b_j is the j-th bit of the patient ID in binary format:

$$f(x) = \begin{cases} 1 \text{ where } x = 1 \\ -1 \text{ where } x = 0 \end{cases} \tag{4}$$

y_{chirp} is the chirp signal and $y_{chirp,mod}$ is modulated chirp according to b_j.

For embed the bit of value '1' the added chirp is in same phase and for '0' - in opposite phase to the ECG signal. In order to make the system less vulnerable to errors, the 'patient ID' is spread to a certain factor u. It is defined as the number of times each bit of the watermark is embedded (for example - if $u = 3$ then three in phase chirps will be embedded for the bit '1' and three opposite phase chirps will be embedded for the bit '0'). Spreading factor is chosen to exploit the maximum payload capacity. The watermark sequence is a binary stream, dependent on patient's personal data which is unique. Now, to balance between the recovery capability of the watermark and its perceptibility, a 'k factor' is included to represent the required signal to chirp ratio (SCR) (5). The modulated chirp is multiplied with window-dependent k and then added to the ECG signal, resulting in the watermarked ECG signal with each sample of 11-bits.

$$SCR_{desired} = 10log\left(\frac{P_i}{k_i * P_{chirp}}\right) \tag{5}$$

where, P_i is ECG signal power of i-th window and P_{chirp} is the power of the chirp signal.

Each sample of the final signal is of 16-bit with first 11-bits representing the watermarked signal and in the remaining 5-bits the value of k and ID are embedded. This makes it a zero distortion watermark embedding scheme i.e. at the receiver one can separate the watermark, hence the patient's ID and the original ECG signal.

From the received signal the bits of 'k' and ID are extracted. The extracted ID facilitates in the detection of any alteration in the received ECG signal. The extracted k is used to get the replica of original signal at the receiver side. These bits are removed to get the 'watermarked signal'. It is then correlated with the chirp signal of same specifications as in encryption to find the ID. This ID is used to modulate the chirp signal using the same procedure as in encryption. It is then multiplied by extracted 'k' factor. To recover the original undistorted ECG signal, it is then subtracted from the obtained watermarked signal. The ID obtained from correlation is compared with extracted ID. This comparison enables the receiver for verification of the ECG signal. If they are not equal then it indicates that some tampering has been done [6].

2.2   Usable and Secure Key Agreement Scheme for Body Area Networks

Another concept was introduced in [7] to secure the inter-sensors communication by cryptographic keys.

The purpose of PSKA is to facilitate secure intersensor communications between two sensors by enabling them to agree upon a pair wise symmetric key, using physiological signal-based features. The key agreement process works as follows: one of the two sensors (sender) generates a random symmetric key that is then hidden using a feature vector obtained from the physiological signal. This hidden key is sent over to the other node (receiver) that uses its own version of the feature vector and obtains the random key after compensating for the differences between its own feature vector and the one used by the sender.

The fuzzy-vault scheme is designed to lock (hide) a secret (S) in a construct called a vault using a set of values A. Once the vault has been locked, it can be unlocked only with another set of values B that has a significant number of values in common with set A. The construction and locking of the vault is described in [7]:

The key agreement is achieved as follows [7]:

1. Feature Generation: First, both the sender and the receiver obtain physiological-signal-based features,
2. Polynomial Choice,
3. Vault Creation,
4. Vault Locking,
5. Vault Exchange,
6. Vault Unlocking,
7. Vault Acknowledgement.

2.3   A Low Complexity High Capacity ECG Signal Watermark for Wearable Sensor Network Health Monitoring System

In recent years, much work has been done for telemonitoring. Such medical data need to be protected from changes, during its online transmission. Various image (X-ray, MRI, PET, ...) and signal (ECG, EKG, ...) modalities all having unique data properties and formats, need also to be watermarked in a wireless health care system [5].

In a typical wireless telemonitoring scenario, the patient wears wireless sensors capable of reading samples of ECG, temperature, blood pressure, etc. In general, these data streams are sent separately to the hospital. In this scenario, biomedical information of different kind is watermarked inside the ECG signal in a patient's PDA device. Consequently, they are sent wirelessly to a central server, which can check the watermarked signal and extract the meta-information hidden within the signal. The server is then distributing the received deassembled information to e-doctors (e.g. doctors who are roaming around with mobile devices) that can take quick action according to its priority [5].

In this scenario, the watermarking algorithm must preserve the main features of the ECG signal for a typical normal and abnormal ECG. Moreover, it must guarantee that correct diagnostic interpretation of the ECG signal can be done directly without removing the watermark. The watermark must thus ideally be invisible on a trace. The methodology is described in [5].

Comparison of the resulting watermarked signal with the original signal is performed using a simple Euclidean error-distance: the Percentage Residual Difference (PRD), in common use for ECG measurements, as shown in Eq. 5.

$$PRD = \sqrt{\frac{\sum_{i=1}^{N} (x_i - y_i)^2}{\sum_{i=1}^{N} x_i{}^2}} \qquad (6)$$

where x_i represents the original ECG signal, and y_i represents the watermarked signal [5].

2.4   Secure and Efficient Health Data Management Through Multiple Watermarking of Medical Images

Healthcare and medical data management has changed over last years and has a guest influence in patient's treatment. The personal data can be send in network sensor in real time. That is why physicians can get information about the diagnosis from specialist quickly and threat in right way. Very important is that the communication between sender and receiver should be safe. Intruder can not get any personal information about patient's data. Thats why watermarked is a great challenge in future. It is new area, which can discover new solutions. This scheme is used in images but it can also be used in ECG. Multiple watermarks are embedded in the image by applying a 4-level discrete wavelet transform (DWT) and a proper quantization of coefficients. For protection medical images, patient's data or integrity control physician can use a specific algorithms.

There are many kind of information. For example: images, personal data or ECG signal. Each of them can be incoding using different algorithm. Some of them are similar. If someone want to encode information he should have specific key. This section describes especially image watermarking.

There are a few kind of purpose-specific watermarks, which are detaily described in [4]:

1. A signature watermark comprising the physician's digital signature or identification.
2. An index watermark that contains keywords.
3. A caption watermark containing patient's personal examination data.
4. A reference watermark is embedded for data integrity control.

In [4] is presented an overview of medical data watermarking and based on wavelet transform (DWT) watermarking scheme. A reference watermark can for example add a diagnostically significant region of interest (ROI), which is inserted information using reference watermark. Manipulation in sending data by someone other in unacceptable. That is why right and correct algorithms with good complexity are so important.

The embedding procedure is based on image decomposition through DWT. The proposed method exploits this attribute in the quantization scheme used to insert the multiple watermarks in embeddable coefficients. According to the algorithm, any coefficient selected to cast a watermark bit, is assigned a binary value through the following quantization function [4]:

$$Q(f) = \begin{cases} 0 \text{ if } 2k * \Delta + s \le f < (2k+1) * \Delta + s \\ 1 \text{ if } (2k+1) * \Delta + s \le f < (2k+2) * \Delta + s \end{cases} \tag{7}$$

where k is an integer, s is a user defined offset for increased security, and, the quantization parameter, is chosen to be equal to 2lin order to exploit the dyadic rationality of Haar coefficients. The above quantization function can be equivalently rewritten as follows:

$$Q(f) = \begin{cases} 0 \text{ if } \lfloor f - s/\Delta \rfloor \text{ is even} \\ 1 \text{ if } \lfloor f - s/\Delta \rfloor \text{ is odd} \end{cases} \tag{8}$$

where is the floor function.

Nowadays telemedicine has a great potential. Many personel and image data are in digital bases. Patient's identification code can help to find information about archiving information treatment in simple way. That is why right incoding is so important.

In simple description the multiple watermarks embedding procedure includes the following steps [4]:

- Step 1: The image is decomposed through 4-level Haar wavelet transform in a coarse scale image approximation at the highest decomposition level and a sequence of detail images at each of the four levels.
- Step 2: The above quantization function is applied to each coefficient f that is to be watermarked.
- Step 3: The 4-level inverse wavelet transform is implemented to produce the watermarked image [4].

The wavelet coefficients to be watermarked are specified based on a random key and the region of interest (ROI) map. Initially, the key selects the embeddable coefficients of all levels and subbands; in the cases of the data watermarks (signature, index, caption) however, the wavelet domain ROI map determines which of the key-selected coefficients will finally be used for embedding, by not belonging to the ROI. The specific distribution of the watermarks is also in accordance with the robustness requirements; due to the fact that most of the energy is concentrated in the high decomposition levels. The energy is calculated using the following equation:

$$e_k = \frac{1}{N_k M_k} * \sum_i * \sum_j | I_k(i,j) | \tag{9}$$

where k denotes the approximation and the detail images at each of the decomposition levels, I_k are the coefficients of the subband images, and N_k, M_k are their corresponding dimensions.

Due to the generally resembling behavior of horizontal and vertical subbands, the image modification is very likely to affect them in a similar way. Therefore, the selection of vertical subbands for reference watermark embedding provides a reflection of the potential tampering of the image. For imperceptibility reasons, the coarse scale image approximation is leftintact by the embedding procedure, because of its crucial effect on image quality resulting from the large energy concentration. Besides, the first decomposition level, coefficients are used exclusively for reference watermarking and not for signature, index, and caption watermarks embedding, due to their minor effect on image quality that makes them susceptible to common image processing, compression, or attacks. In order to enable a comprehensive image distortion report, the reference watermark is embedded in selected coefficients of the other three decomposition levels as well; in this way, it can be extracted from specific frequencies and/or spatial regions, in order to reflect their potential tampering [4].

3 Discussion of Features Relevant for Personalized Healthcare

In Sect. 2.1, a simple technique for watermarking of biomedical signals (ECG) is presented. The scheme highlights on 'Blind Recovery' of the original signal from the watermarked signal. Through this method one can also conceal the information about the patient's ID which can further be used for detection of any corruption of the original signal. Another novelty of the proposed scheme is its ability to remove the watermark completely from the recovered ECG signal and display it to the clinicians without distortion [6].

In Sect. 2.2, the author presented a usable and secure key agreement scheme for BANs called PSKA. It allows two sensors to agree on a shared key, in an authenticated manner, without any form of initialization or setup. The security analysis of the PSKA protocol showed that physiological signals meet the design goals for key agreement namely, length and randomness, low latency, and distinctiveness. Future work includes an expanded in-field study of PSKA to better understand the distinctiveness and temporal variance properties of the scheme [7].

In Sect. 2.3, another technique of watermarking is presented. Because the ECG signal collected over long periods of time can be enormous in size, it can be used as a host to carry other biomedical information watermarked inside it. Therefore, a bandwidth preserving technique is presented, where has been demonstrated that changing some parts of the ECG signal will not affect the medical utility of the ECG signal. Watermarking can also be used to embed the information inside the ECG signal [1,2]. It can be implemented in real time monitoring systems and does not add to overall transmission bandwidth [5].

Section 2.4 discusses the perspectives of digital watermarking in health information management and proposes, a medical purpose-oriented wavelet-based multiple watermarking scheme. This scheme simultaneously embeds four types of watermarks into medical images, intending to enhance the protection of sensitive data, provides origin and data authentication capability, and allows efficient image archiving and retrieval [4].

4   Conclusion

The main purpose of this work is review of watermarking methods suitable for wirelessly transmitted digital ECG signal. A few results of the digital images and ECG data watermark were also presented in this paper, however they may easily be adapted to the one-dimensional data series. It is noteworthy that this area of science is recently developed by several lead in research centers in the World. The presented review lead the author towards new ideas of implementation of watermarking technique. To conclude the paper it is worth writing that watermarking may be efficiently implemented in transform domain (e.g. bijective wavelet transform), the host ECG signal can carry supplementary digital data of any type (e.g. personal, diagnostic, auxiliary) and the effective capacity of the host signal strongly depends on local ECG features.

Acknowledgements. This scientific work is supported by the AGH University of Science and Technology in year 2016 as a research project No. 11.11.120.612.

References

1. Augustyniak, P.: Analysis of ECG bandwidth gap as a possible carrier for supplementary digital data. Comput. Cardiol. **39**, 73–76 (2012)
2. Augustyniak, P.: Encoding the electrocardiogram details in the host record's bandgap for authorization dependent ECG quality. Comput. Cardiol. **41**, 465–468 (2014)
3. Frooq, O., Datta, S., Blackledge, J.M.: Blind tamper detection in audio using chirp based robust watermarking. WSEAS Trans. Sig. Process. **4**(4), 190–200 (2008)
4. Giakoumaki, A., Pavlopoulos, S., Koutsouris, D.: Secure and efficient health data management through multiple watermarking on medical images. Med. Bio. Eng. Comput. **44**, 619–631 (2006)
5. Ibaida, A., Khalil, I., van Schyndel, R.: A low complexity high capacity ECG signal watermark for wearable sensor-net health monitoring system. Comput. Cardiol. **38**, 393–396 (2011). ISSN 0276–6574
6. Kaur, S., Frooq, O., Singhal, R., Ahuja, B.S.: Digital watermarking of ECG data for secure wireless communication. In: International Conference on Recent Trends in Information. Tele-communication and Computing. IEEE Computer Society (2010)
7. Venkatasubramanian, K.K., Banerjee, A., Gupta, S.K.S.: PSKA: usable and secure key agreement scheme for body area network. IEEE Trans. Inf. Technol. Biomed. **14**(1), 60–68 (2010)

4 Conclusion

Signal Analysis

Bioheat Transfer Model with Active Thermoregulation: Sensitivity of Temperature Field on Tissue Properties

Piotr Buliński, Wojciech Adamczyk, and Ziemowit Ostrowski$^{(\boxtimes)}$

Biomedical Engineering Lab, Institute of Thermal Technology, Silesian University of Technology, Konarskiego 22, 44-100 Gliwice, Poland
ziemowit.ostrowski@polsl.pl
http://www.itc.polsl.pl/ostrowski

Abstract. Research on heat transfer and temperature distribution in human tissues is significant not only in thermal comfort but it is also applied in modern dermatology. Information about temperature gradients near skin lesions can assist diagnosis of malignant melanoma. The main purpose of this research was to study sensitivity of temperature field on metabolic heat production rate and artery temperature of numerical model of bioheat transfer with active thermoregulation in human forearm. The influence of blood temperature and metabolic heat source on temperature profile in tissues was examined. Numerical results were validated against measurement data. In experiment the cold brass compress was applied on human forearm. Temperature of skin after the mild cooling was measured using IR camera.

Keywords: CFD · Pennes equation · Active thermoregulation

1 Introduction

The study presented here is a part of wider research project targeted in investigating the possibility of early diagnosis of skin lesions, with special interest in early stage malignant melanoma identification. Not only numerical simulations are the aim of this project. Measurements of heat transfer and temporal temperature distribution can also be used as input in diagnostic tools and methods of skin lesions.

In previous numerical work of the research team [3] thermographic (IR camera) measurements of skin recovering from local cooling was used to validate the numerical model of passive thermoregulation. However, during above mentioned research, additional experimental possibilities were identified. In a follow up research [4] model validation was done employing skin–cooling compress interfacial heat flux measurements. New experimental setup, including custom design cuboid brass cooling compress, was proposed to measure and record transferred heat flux using differential thermopile sensor. Comparison of the numerical model

© Springer International Publishing AG 2017
M. Gzik et al. (eds.), *Innovations in Biomedical Engineering*, Advances in Intelligent Systems and Computing 526, DOI 10.1007/978-3-319-47154-9_30

response with experimental data showed that the model meets the *in vivo* measurements.

The main purpose of this study was sensitivity analysis of two crucial parameters: metabolic heat production rate and artery blood temperature. Both of these quantities are hard to measure *in vivo*, therefore it is indispensable to inspect its impact on temperature distribution in human tissues. Examined simulation model include bioheat transfer equation with vasoconstriction term. Computational results were then validated against measurement data within current study. In reference case the properties of human tissues were based on well-established literature sources.

2   Methodology

To perform numerical calculations of heat transfer in human tissue, the geometry of forearm was developed. Two symmetry planes were assumed, therefore only quarter of model was analyzed. Geometry was consisted of five concentric homogeneous layers corresponding with real tissues types (i.e. bone, muscle, fat, skin) and is presented in Fig. 1. Precise dimensions of layers are presented in Table 1. To simulate mild cooling small cylinder was introduced on the top of skin. The length of simulated arm was 200 mm which was enough to provide solution independence of the boundary condition applied on the external boundaries – zero temperature gradient (Neuman BC). For outer skin as well as for compress external walls Robin boundary condition was specified with convective heat transfer coefficient $5\,\text{W·m}^{-2}\text{·K}^{-1}$ and air temperature $23\,^\circ\text{C}$. For all symmetry planes Neumann BC was applied (temperature gradient equal to zero. Numerical discretization of geometry was performed in ICEM CFD (Ansys Inc., USA). To provide high quality of elements blocking scheme was applied. Mesh was refined in areas where high temperature was expected, especially in the skin layers underneath compress. Final grid had 825 k elements and is presented in Fig. 2.

In proposed mathematical model the set of differential equations of bioheat transfer proposed by Pennes [5] was solved for each tissue in multilayer model:

$$c_i \rho_i \frac{\partial T_i(\mathbf{r}_i, t)}{\partial t} = \nabla \left[k_i(T_i) \nabla T_i(\mathbf{r}_i, t) \right] + q_{m,i}(\mathbf{r}_i, t) + q_{p,i}(\mathbf{r}_i, t) \tag{1}$$

$$q_{p,i}(\mathbf{r}_i, t) = \beta_{0,i} \left[T_a - T_i(\mathbf{r}_i, t) \right] = \omega_{b,i}(\mathbf{r}_i, t) c_b \rho_b \left[T_a - T_i(\mathbf{r}_i, t) \right] \tag{2}$$

where: c_i, c_b – specific heat (tissue, blood); ρ_i, ρ_b – density (tissue, blood); T_i, T_a – temperature (tissue, perfusing (artery) blood), t – time, k_i – tissue heat conductivity, $q_{m,i}$ – metabolic heat production rate, $q_{m,i}$ – perfusion heat production rate, $\beta_{0,i}$ – blood perfusion energy equivalent, $\omega_{b,i}$ – tissue specific blood perfusion rate, $\mathbf{r}$ – vector coordinate, subscript i denotes the tissue type.

On the tissue layers interfaces, as well as on metal compress–outer skin interface, ideal contact (i.e. continuity of heat flux and temperature) was assumed.

Under non-neutral conditions metabolic and perfusion rates vary with the local tissue temperature. The influence of temperature on metabolism and perfusion is modelled according to the Q_{10} relation. It states that for every $10\,\mathrm{K}$ reduction (change) in the tissue temperature, there is a corresponding reduction (change) in the cell metabolism Δq_m and perfusion Δq_m by the factor $Q_{10} = 2$, as reported in [1,7,9]:

$$q_m = q_{m,0} \cdot 2^{(T-T_0)/10} \tag{3}$$

$$q_p = \left(\beta_0 \cdot \frac{1}{1 + \alpha_{cs,i} C_s} \cdot 2^{(T-T_0)/10} \right) (T_a - T) \tag{4}$$

where T_0 – basal temperature distribution (i.e., in thermoneutral conditions), $\alpha_{cs,i} = 0.1945$ – distribution factor for vasoconstriction and $C_s = 0.0695$ – vasoconstriction signal for forearm (according to [2]).

Simulations were carried out using ANSYS Fluent 14 commercial CFD package (ANSYS Inc., USA). The additional source terms of heat conduction equation arising in bioheat transfer Eq. (1) were introduced by means of UDF (user-defined function) functionality of the ANSYS Fluent code. First order upwind scheme was applied to solve differential equation. Transient computations were performed using 0.5 s time step. To introduce initial condition transient simulations were preceded by steady state calculations in which thermoneutral state was archived. Material properties of human tissue are presented in Table 1. Metabolic heat production rate and perfusion source term were applied only within three layers: inner skin, fat and muscle. These properties, hard to measure in vivo, are based on [1,6]. Properties of brass were examined during experimental research using Laser Flash Analysis (LFA) for thermal diffusivity and Differential Scanning Calorimetry (DSC) for heat capacity. According to results density of brass was set to $730\,\mathrm{kg\cdot m^{-3}}$, thermal conductivity to $51\,\mathrm{W\cdot m^{-1}\cdot K^{-1}}$ and specific heat to $475\,\mathrm{J\cdot kg^{-1}\cdot K^{-1}}$.

The proposed numerical model of skin cooling and rewarming processes was validated against experimental data collected from subjects examined in course

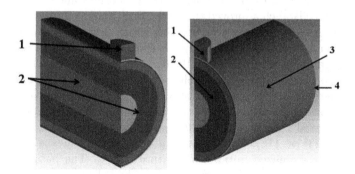

Fig. 1. 3-D geometrical model of computational domain with visible tissues layers: bone, muscle, fat, inner skin, outer skin (1 – cooling compress, 2 – symmetry planes, 3 – forehand outer skin, 4 – insulated walls - external boundary of the model)

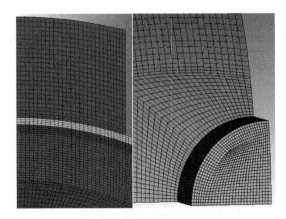

Fig. 2. Selected regions of numerical mesh: in symmetry plane (left) and seen from above the compress (right)

Table 1. Dimensions and properties of tissues and initial values of model variables (for steady state analysis) [1,6]

Tissue	Outer radius mm	Thermal conductivity $W \cdot m^{-1} \cdot K^{-1}$	Density $kg \cdot m^{-3}$	Specific heat $J \cdot kg^{-1} \cdot K^{-1}$	Perfusion rate s^{-1}	Metabolic heat production rate $W \cdot m^{-3}$
Outer skin	42.9	0.47	1085	3680	0	0
Inner skin	42.1	0.47	1085	3680	0.0011	631
Fat	41.1	0.16	850	2300	0.0000036	58
Muscle	35.3	0.42	1085	3768	0.000538	684
Bone	15.3	0.75	1357	1700	0	0

of pilot medical experiment (being part of wider research project). The medical ethical committee of Maria Skłodowska-Curie Memorial Cancer and Institute of Oncology Gliwice Branch approved the study. Each subject gave written consent prior to participation in the study. For the initial analysis at hand, the group of eight adult males was selected. Subject's characteristics (mean±SD) are: age 31.1±5.0, height 1.80±0.07 m, weight 102.0±10.4 kg. The studied skin sites were dorsal and ventral side of the left forehand halfway the wrist and inner side of the elbow. The subjects were asked to stay sited for 15 min prior to the measurements. The skin temperature history was recorded using PI160 (Optris GmbH, Germany) infrared camera (160 × 120 px, 120 Hz, LWIR, 7.5–13 μm detector, standard lens 23° × 17°). Cooling of skin was done by means of brass cooling compress at stabilized initial temperature 6–7 °C. The basal (thermoneutral) skin temperatures were measured by wireless iButton DS1922L (Maxim Integrated, USA) temperature data logger attached using adhesive tape near cooling zone (approx. 3 cm). Room temperature was measured using Almemo

2390-5 multifunction measuring instrument (AHLBORN, Germany) equipped with K-type thermocouple sensor.

3   Results

Numerical computations were performed in three steps: steady state (step #1), mild cooling (step #2) and recovery (step #3).

Step #1 In steady state run the same set of differential equations is solved, while the reference temperature (T_0) and initial temperatures are assumed to be uniform and (equal 37 °C) for all layers. Under this assumption, the transient simulation was performed long enough to obtain stationary temperature field (i.e. to mimic thermoneutral state = energy balance with environment). Resulting distributions of temperature, metabolic heat production rate as well as perfusion rates are then used as initial condition (state) for transient simulation of cooling (step #2) processes.

Step #2 Mild cooling was realized by means of cooled compress which was put on skin for 15 s. Ideal contact on skin-compress interface was assumed. The initial condition being result of step #1.

Step #3 Afterwards the compress was switched off and recovery stage was simulated for following 45 s, with initial state distributions being result of step #2.

Sensitivity analysis was executed for two most important material properties of tissues: metabolic heat production rate and artery temperature. In reference case blood temperature was set to 37 °C, for other cases it was decreased and increased by 1 K. The change of metabolic heat production rate was chosen to be ±10 % of basal value (cf. Table 1).

Step #1. Steady state simulation was performed not only to get an initial temperature distribution for step #2, but was used to tune model and obtain metabolic heat production rate q_m distribution and perfusion rates ω_b in the thermoneutral state (i.e. model in thermal equilibrium with environment). During this step type of volume representing cooling compress was turned off. Tissue properties, initial metabolic heat production rates and perfusion rates used in steady state calculations in reference case were presented in Table 1 after [1,6]. The temperature distribution being result of steady state analysis (shown in Figs. 3 and 4) is then prescribed as initial condition for further transient calculations. In addition, the resulting distributions of: temperature, metabolic heat production rate and perfusion rate are thereafter treated as:

- basal temperature distribution T_0,
- basal metabolic heat production rate $q_{m,0}$,
- basal blood perfusion rate $\omega_{b,0}$.

Sensitivity analysis of artery temperature revealed significant influence of that quantity on temperature distribution. In the bone region difference between temperature profiles is equal to 1 degree while for skin region it decreased to almost

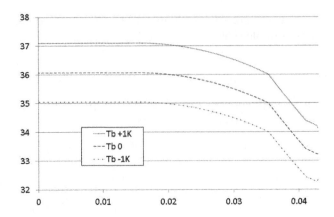

Fig. 3. Initial tissue temperature (in °C) distribution for transient analysis (step #2). Plot shows the radial distribution (bone-to-surface direction) in meters, plotted for three different artery temperatures

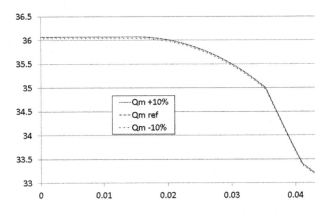

Fig. 4. Initial tissue temperature (in °C) distribution for transient analysis (step #2). Plot shows the radial distribution (bone-to-surface direction) in meters, plotted for three different metabolic heat production rates

half of degree. On the other hand, metabolic heat production rate changes indicate negligible effect on temperature distribution in forearm, which is confirmed in literature [8].

Step #2. Transient simulations were conducted to mimic the cooling procedure. The volume of compress was switched on and the uniform initial temperature of 7 °C was prescribed there. As reported in [3], application of ideal contact between compress and skin is irrelevant because of presence of hairs and limited allowable cooling compress pressure on skin therefore non-ideal contact was simulated. Contact resistance of $0.001 \, \mathrm{m^2 \cdot K \cdot W^1}$ was implemented on the skin-compress interface.

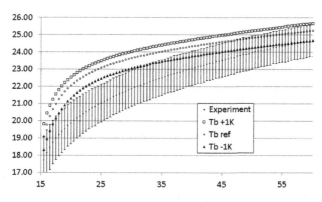

Fig. 5. Minimal outer skin temperature (in °C) vs. time (in s) for experiment (N = 14 samples) and CFD simulation for different artery temperature, presented results for time after cooling compress is removed

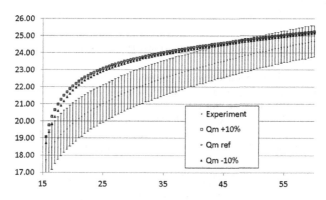

Fig. 6. Minimal outer skin temperature (in °C) vs. time (in s) for experiment (N = 14 samples) and CFD simulation for different metabolic heat production rate, presented results for time after cooling compress is removed

Step #3. After the cooling stage (15 s) the simulation of recovery was carried out. Compress volume was again switched off and 45 s of recovery process was examined and comparison of minimal skin temperature versus time was presented in Figs. 5 and 6.

Likewise in steady state computations the impact of metabolic heat production rate is insignificant on recovery temperature of skin, while artery temperature is crucial in prediction of that temperature. In comparison to experimental data none model predicted accurate skin temperature. It was noticed that the temperature in the beginning of recovery stage for numerical simulations was higher than in experiment which might mean that the contact resistance is improperly introduced.

4 Conclusions

Simulation of bioheat transfer with active thermoregulation in human forearm was conducted. The influence of artery temperature and metabolic heat production rate was examined. Artery temperature demonstrates significant influence in every stages of the cooling process, while the impact of metabolic heat production rate was minimal. In future computations it is necessary to check the influence of other material properties of human tissues which were based on literature.

Acknowledgements. This research was supported by host Institute within Ministry of Science and Higher Education (Poland) statutory research funding scheme. This help is gratefully acknowledged herewith.

References

1. Fiala, D., Lomas, K.J., Stohrer, M.: A computer model of human thermoregulation for a wide range of environmental conditions: the passive system. J. Appl. Physiol. **87**, 1957–1972 (1999)
2. Fiala, D., Lomas, K.J., Stohrer, M.: Computer prediction of human thermoregulatory and temperature responses to a wide range of environmental conditions. Int. J. Biometeorol. **45**, 143–159 (2001)
3. Ostrowski, Z., Buliński, P., Adamczyk, W., Kozołub, P., Nowak, A.J.: Numerical model of heat transfer in skin lesions. ZN PRz Mechanika **87**, 55–62 (2015)
4. Ostrowski, Z., Buliński, P., Adamczyk, W., Nowak, A.J.: Modelling and validation of transient heat transfer processes in human skin undergoing local cooling. Przegląd Elektrotechniczny **91**, 76–79 (2015)
5. Pennes, H.H.: Analysis of tissue and arterial blood temperatures in the rest-ing human forearm. J. Appl. Physiol. **1**, 93–122 (1948)
6. Severens, N.: Modelling hypothermia in patients undergoing surgery, Ph.D. thesis, Eindhoven University Press, Eindhoven (2008)
7. Severens, N., van Marken Lichtenbelt, W.D., Frijns, A.J.H., van Steenhoven, A.A., de Mol, B.A.J.M., Sessler, D.I.: A model to predict patient temperature during cardiac surgery. Phys. Med. Biol. **52**, 5131–5145 (2007)
8. Stańczyk, M., Telega, J.J.: Modelling of heat transfer in biomechanics a review. Part I. Soft tissues. Acta Bioeng. Biomech. **4**(1), 31–61 (2002)
9. Stolwijk, J.: A mathematical model of physiological temperature regulation in man, NASA contractor report CR-1855, NASA (1971)

Current Trends of Innovations in Microbiological Diagnosis by Light Diffraction

Igor Buzalewicz and Halina Podbielska[✉]

Bio-Optics Group, Faculty of Fundamental Problems of Technology,
Department of Biomedical Engineering,
Wrocław University of Science and Technology,
Wybrzeże Wyspiańskiego 27, 50-370 Wrocław, Poland
halina.podbielska@pwr.edu.pl

Abstract. Methods based on light diffraction on bacterial colonies create the new perspectives for innovations in microbiological diagnosis. Contrary to the conventional techniques, the proposed optical methods are non-contact and non-destructive. There is no requirement for any additional chemicals, immunological or fluorescence markers. The proposed methods are based on the images of light diffraction on bacterial colonies grown on solid nutrient media analyzed by statistical methods. The application of the digital holography can additionally facilitate and improve the efficiency of the microbiological examination.

Keywords: Optical diffraction · Digital holography · Bacterial colony · Bacteria identification

1 Introduction

The problem of rapid, sensitive and effective detection, as well as accurate identification of pathogenic bacteria is extremely important issue in many fields of life science, health safety and food protection (see [1]). Although the majority of microorganisms are able to coexist with humans, plants and animals with beneficial relations, many of them are pathogenic and can evoke some infectious diseases. There is a continuous increase of the bacteria resistance to the commonly used antibacterial chemicals (antibiotics, sterilization agents etc.), worldwide observed. In particular, the antibiotics resistance is widely analysed and discussed in the medical literature. The National Institute of Allergy and Infectious Diseases - NIAID warns that over 70 % of various bacteria species, most often causing hospital infections, are already completely resistant to at least one kind of antibiotics commonly used for their treatment (see [2]). In consequence, the therapeutics have a limited ability to fight infectious diseases and complications, quite common in patients undergoing chemotherapy, dialysis and surgery for that the treatment of secondary infections is crucial. The antibiotic therapy is one of the most important factors causing the antibiotic resistance around the world. It is assumed that up to 50 % of all prescribed antibiotics are

M. Gzik et al. (eds.), *Innovations in Biomedical Engineering*, Advances in Intelligent Systems and Computing 526, DOI 10.1007/978-3-319-47154-9_31

not necessary or are not effective as assumed. The effective diagnosis, essential for identifying bacterial species, enables appropriate therapeutic treatment by choice of antibiotic dedicated for specific bacteria species, what in consequence, will lead to reducing the use of broadspectrum antibiotics. According to the NIAID antibacterial resistance program (see [3]), the appropriate diagnosis is crucial in order to facilitate the use of narrow-spectrum therapeutics targeted to a specific pathogen. Therefore, some efforts are made towards the development of novel bacteria detection and identification techniques that can reduce the cost of analysis and quickly detect bacterial pathogens in food, water or in clinical samples.

2   The Current Problems and Challenges in Modern Microbiological Diagnosis

The most widely used techniques in microbiological laboratories to identify bacteria include biochemical, molecular, immunological or immunoassays and mass spectrometry methods (see [4]). The most commonly used in microbiology laboratories for bacterial identification are biochemical methods. Identification in this case is based on: the evaluation of bacterial colonies growth or its lack, the color change of the medium, the generation gas or a color reaction caused by the introduction into the medium of the reactant products generated by bacteria. The main disadvantage is that they rely on differentiating bacteria in terms of their certain biochemical properties, which can sometimes be common for the whole group of different bacteria species, and therefore obtained results can sometimes be ambiguous. The molecular methods involve amplification of the genes without cloning a DNA and the analysis is performed based on the polymerase chain reaction (PCR- Polymerase Chain Reaction) (see [5]). The fundamental disadvantage is the need to prepare the high quality samples containing only the genetic material to be tested, without any impurities. Typically, the initial stage of this technique include bacteria culturing on solid nutrient media and then only the representative colony is used for further analysis. In addition, it is necessary to obtain an appropriate amount of genetic material to ensure quantitative bacteria identification. Depending on the number of bacterial cells in the sample, as well as their rate of growth, the process of obtaining a suitable amount of genetic material of bacteria can take from 4 to 12 h. Although it is very sensitive, it is time-consuming according to hours needed for molecular analysis and it requires very pure samples, which additionally makes it expensive. Immunological or immunoassays methods are based on the reaction of bacterial antigens with antibodies directed against these antigens (see [6]). Currently, there is a large diversity of immunological tests, which differ only in the principals of detecting and visualization of immunological reaction. Despite the high effectiveness of this technique, which is based on a highly selective interaction of antibodies (or antigens), immunoassays are targeted for specific bacterial antigens. Therefore, it is necessary in conventional microbiological investigation to use a series of tests with different antibodies to identify different bacteria species/strains present in the sample. Moreover, these tests are not reusable, what additionally increases the cost of analysis. In recent years, the mass spectrometry is used, which is determining the ratio of the sample mass to the electric charge of sample ions. For the identification of the bacteria most commonly used type of mass spectrometry is the MALDI -TOF (Matrix - Assisted Laser Desorption - Ionization - Time Of Flight) (see [7]). This technique not only allows the identification of bacterial species, but also the analysis the relationship between the various bacterial strains of the same species. To conduct the test, samples containing at least 105 bacterial cells, are required. Thus, the process of initial sample multiplication procedures have to be included. Depending on the number of bacterial cells in the initial sample, this process can take up to 12–16 h. It should be pointed out, that described above methods, according to their costs and complicated procedure of measurements, are limited to the professional microbiological laboratories. The main disadvantages are the need of each time using chemical reagents, professional microbiological laboratory staff, high costs and relatively long duration of investigation. Therefore, some efforts are made towards the development of techniques that can reduce the cost of analysis and time of the bacterial pathogens detection. Optical biosensors are based on noninvasive and non-destructive detection, because in this case the amplitude and phase of light modulated by pathogens are examined, instead of pathogens themselves. Common optical techniques include infrared and fluorescence spectroscopy, flow cytometry, chromatography and chemi-luminescence analysis (see [8]). However, their main disadvantages include demanding and timeconsuming preparation of high quality samples and necessity to use an equipment with high sensitivity and spectral resolution according to need of single cells examination. The high percentage of false positives may be caused by e.g. similar pathogens fluorescence signature generated by non-biological objects existed in the examined sample. Over the past few year it was demonstrated that analysis of forward light scattering on bacteria colonies, mostly affected by diffraction effects, can be used for identification of different bacteria species (see [9–14]). Proposed by our group method is based on verified assumption that the diffraction patterns of bacterial colonies exhibit some specific features, which are suitable for bacteria species characterization and can be analyzed using scalar diffraction theory.

3   The Bacteria Identification by Light Diffraction

The fundamental concept of the proposed method is based on the already verified assumption that in case of bacterial colonies growing on the solid nutrient medium, the variation of the optical properties (as the refractive indices and transmission coefficients) and morphology properties (as the profile, size and shape the colony), are responsible for generating diffraction patterns that are unique for each bacteria species and strains. This identification system classifies the bacteria species/strains/serovars based on optical diffraction fingerprints or diffraction signatures of bacterial colonies. It is a new approach, which enables the preliminary examination on the first stage of bacteria sample preparation for other conventional bacteria identification methods. Our solution is a consequence of the collaboration of scientists from different fields of science and technology as: microbiology, biomedical optics, informatics and robotics.

3.1 The Optical System Configuration

The measurement setup is based on modified and developed optical system with converging spherical wave illumination, which was already described in (see [9–13]).

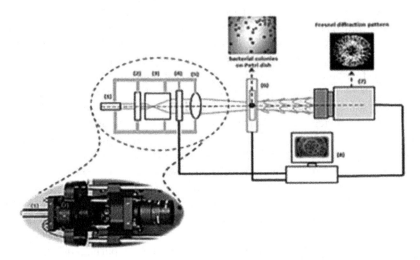

Fig. 1. The configuration of optical system for bacteria identification (description in the text)

This system configuration, which was not so far used for analysis of bacteria colonies diffraction patterns and significantly improves the process of investigation of light diffraction on bacteria colonies. The present setup was reconfigured and miniaturized and the main optical elements were integrated in cage-system (see Fig. 1). The proposed microbiological diagnosis system includes: (1) the laser diode module, (2) amplitude filters wheel, (3) beam expander, (4) iris diaphragm with automatically controlled diameter, (5) transforming lens, (6) sample of bacterial colonies in Petri Dish on automatic X-Y translation stage, (7) diffraction patterns recording CCD camera with imaging objective and a (8) computer. The modified optical system has cage configuration enables the automatic registration of diffraction patterns of bacterial colonies located on analyzed Petri dish.

3.2 The Methodology of Diffraction Patterns Analysis

The diffraction patterns for different bacteria species/strains exhibit the unique features observable under visual inspection, however to obtain the quantitative accuracy the image processing algorithms and statistical methods have to be applied (see [10–12]). Therefore, after recording of bacterial colonies diffraction pattern, edges and centers of pattern are marked. Next, each examined pattern is partitioned into 10 disjoined rings of equal thickness and, linear normalization algorithm is applied. Then, for each of the rings, numerical features denoting morphological and textural properties based on the central statistical moments, are calculated. Finally, the classification stage consists of building classification models QDA (Quadratic Discriminant Analysis) and SVM (Support Vector Machine).

3.3   The Exemplary Results Achieved by the Proposed Method

Measurements were performed on 13 bacteria species including: *Citrobacter freundii, Escherichia coli, Proteus mirabilis, Pseudomonas aeruginosa, Salmonella Enteritidis, Staphylococcus aureus, Staphylococcus intermedius, Klebsiella pneumoniae, Salmonella Typhimurium, Bacillus subtilis, Enterococcus faecalis, Listeria monocytogenes, Rahnella aquatilis* (two strains:x31N, x31E).

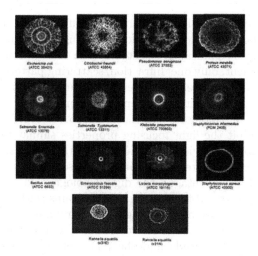

Fig. 2. The exemplary bacterial colonies diffraction patterns after 18 h of colony incubation

The bacteria samples were prepared according to the conventional microbiological procedures described in (see [9–14]). By fixing the parameters of the incubation process (nutrient medium, temperature and time of incubation etc.) and defined diameter of the colony, it is possible to perform the analysis of the differences between recorded diffraction patterns affected only by bacteria species/strain. These incubation and registration conditions have a significant influence on diffraction patterns and the classification accuracy what was reported in (see [9,11]). The exemplary diffraction patterns of bacterial colonies are presented on Fig. 2. It is shown that colonies diffraction patterns of different bacteria species and strains exhibit unique features and are suitable for bacteria identification. Performed statistical analysis of recorded diffraction patterns enabling the quantitative investigation have shown that it is possible to classify the bacteria species/strains with nearly 99 % accuracy. Obtained results have shown that the proposed technique based on optical signatures of bacterial colonies supported by statistical and image processing analysis enables bacteria classification and may be performed without professional laboratory equipments and highly qualified personnel. The developed method is appropriate for practical implementation for monitoring the bacteria presence in environmental samples with the differentiation on the level of the bacteria strains. It is possible to identify all bacteria genus, which diffraction signatures are collected in our reference database.

4   The Novel Perspectives on the Characterization of Species-Dependent Optical Signatures of Bacterial Colonies

Described above technique is based on the light diffraction in one selected direction and at a fixed distance from the colony, although the spatial distribution of diffraction patterns is significantly affected by the observation distance. During the single measurement, only one diffraction/scattering pattern can be recorded. Therefore, it is necessary to perform series of measurements in different distances from the colony, what is quite time consuming process. It should be pointed out, that the bacterial colonies being the continuously evolving in time biological structures, exhibit the light focusing properties similar to classical optical lenses (see [13]). This behavior significantly affects the possibility of recoding the series of diffraction patterns for different observation plane localizations. To eliminate above disadvantages, the digital holographic microscopic (DHM) technique was applied (see [14]). The digital holograms (DH) was recorded in inline configuration of the pointsource digital holographic microscope. From the recorded inline holograms of bacterial colonies, it was possible to reconstruct numerically both the amplitude and the phase of the incident optical fields diffracted on these analyzed biological objects. Obtained results have shown that the colonies of different bacteria species generate different holograms and reconstructed optical field amplitude and phase distribution inside the space occupied by bacterial colony (see [14]). Moreover, it was possible to reconstruct the optical field diffracted on bacterial colony in any desire observation plane based on single measurement-DH recording. Therefore, the DHM enables more effective performance of measurements focused on recording the series of diffraction patterns for different locations of observation plane. Presented patterns exhibit unique features associated with the morphological and optical properties of the bacterial species under study. Moreover, the obtained results have indicated high correlation between the numerically reconstructed DH of E. coli and

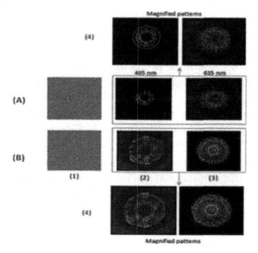

Fig. 3. Representative results of measurements for S. intermedius (A) and E. coli (B) bacteria. (1) Phase and (2) reconstructed intensity patterns of the optical fields, and (3) the representative diffraction patterns. (4) The wavelength-dependent differences between patterns of bacterial colonies reconstructed from digital holograms and recorded in our system (see [14])

S. intermedius colonies and previously recorded Fresnel patterns in optical system with converging spherical wave illumination (see Fig. 3).

The DHM creates new perspectives for the use of the light diffraction on bacterial colonies for their characterization and identification. The numerical reconstruction of DH enables to choose the most adequate amplitude patterns to classify different bacterial species without the need of time-consuming recording of diffraction patterns for different observation planes as in the classical optical system. The DHM enables the analysis of the reconstructed amplitude and intensity patterns that can be regarded as bacteria species classifiers and can be used for bacterial identification by choosing the diffraction patterns exhibiting many species-dependent features. Reported in (see [14]) results have shown, that DH, phase and amplitude patterns of optical field occupied by bacterial colonies, as well as from the desired observation plane location, can be used as species dependent optical signatures. The single DH hologram recording and its numerical reconstruction enables to obtain an additional reference bacterial diffraction signatures. In consequence, it is possible to extract the additional differentiating features, in contrast to the already proposed methods based on single scattering/diffraction patterns recorded in a fixed observation plane.

5   Conclusion

The optical diffraction on bacterial colonies have create new perspectives in microbiological diagnosis. The proposed methods enable nondestructive examination and offer significant facilities as no need for advanced and time-consuming sample preparation or the use of additional chemical reagents -fluorescence-immunological markers. Moreover, identification is reliable, fast, not expensive and what is extremely important it does not require any knowledge in advance. The automatization of the sample preparation process will enable the use of this method by non-professional staff. These techniques can significantly facilitate the increase of the common bacteria identification centers without the laboratory equipment on a much larger scale than conventional techniques. Therefore, the proposed techniques can contribute the facilitation of the use of narrow-spectrum therapeutics by enabling the use of therapeutics targeted to a specific pathogen. Currently, with the cooperation with the Bioavlee Ltd. (Wroclaw) the advanced works on the commercial device based on proposed technique of the diffraction patterns analysis, are conducted.

References

1. Wagar, E.: Bioterrorism and the role of the clinical Microbiology laboratories. Clin. Microbiol. Rev. **29**, 175–189 (2015)
2. ANTIBIOTIC RESISTANCE THREATS in the United States (2013). http://www.cdc.gov/drugresistance/pdf/ar-threats-2013-508.pdf
3. NIAID's Antibacterial Resistance Program: Current Status and Future Directions (2014). http://www.niaid.nih.gov/media/niaids-antibacterial-resistance-program-current-status-and-future-directions-2014
4. Morse, S.A., Butel, J.S., Brooks, B.G.F.: Medical Microbilogy. MacGraw-Hill, New York (2005)
5. Mackay, I.M.: Real-time PCR in the Microbiology laboratory. Clin. Microbiol. Infect. **10**, 190–212 (2004)
6. Schloter, M., Asmus, B., Hartmann, A.: The use of immunological methods to detect and identify bacteria in the environment. Biotechnol. Adv. **13**(1), 75–90 (1999)
7. Croxatto, A., Prod'hom, G., Greub, G.: Applications of MALDI-TOF mass spectrometry in clinical diagnostic Microbiology. FEMS Microbiol. Rev. **36**, 380–407 (2012)
8. Ivnitski, D., Abdel-Hamid, I., Atanasov, P., Wilkins, E.: Biosensors for detection of pathogenic bacteria. Biosens. Bioelectron. **14**, 599–624 (1999)
9. Buzalewicz, I., Wieliczko, A., Podbielska, H.: Influence of various growth conditions on Fresnel diffraction patterns of bacteria colonies examined in the optical system with converging spherical wave illumination. Opt. Express **19**, 21768–21785 (2011)
10. Suchwalko, A., Buzalewicz, I., Podbielska, H.: Statistical identification of bacteria species. In: Méndez-Vilas, A. (ed.) Microbial Pathogens and Strategies for Combating Them: Science, Technology and Education, pp. 711–721. Formatex Research Center, Badajoz (2013)
11. Suchwalko, A., Buzalewicz, I., Wieliczko, A., Podbielska, H.: Bacteria species identification by the statistical analysis of bacterial colonies Fresnel patterns. Opt. Express **21**, 11322 (2013)
12. Suchwalko, A., Buzalewicz, I., Podbielska, H.: Bacteria identification in an optical system with optimized diffraction pattern registration condition supported by enhanced statistical analysis. Opt. Express **22**, 26312 (2014)

13. Buzalewicz, I., Liżewski, K., Kujawinska, M., Podbielska, H.: Degeneration of Fraunhofer diffraction on bacterial colonies due to their light focusing properties examined in the digital holographic microscope system. Opt. Express **21**, 26493 (2013). OSA
14. Buzalewicz, I., Kujawinska, M., Krauze, W., Podbielska, H.: Novel perspectives on the characterization of species-dependent optical signatures of bacterial colonies by digital holography. PLoS ONE **11**(3), e0150449 (2016). doi:10.1371/journal.pone.0150449

Study of Structure-Cytotoxicity Relationships of Thiourea Derivatives Containing the 2-Aminothiazole Moiety

Anna Filipowska[1]([✉]), Wojciech Filipowski[1], and Ewaryst Tkacz[2]

[1] Faculty of Automatic Control, Electronics and Computer Science,
Silesian University of Technology, Gliwice, Poland
anna.filipowska@polsl.pl
[2] Department of Biosensors and Biomedical Signals Processing,
Silesian University of Technology, Zabrze, Poland

Abstract. In order to facilitate designing new drugs by means of the *in silico* method, it is necessary to first develop a model describing the influence of descriptors of a certain group of chemicals on their biological activity and cytotoxicity. For the purpose of this paper, the quantitative structure-cytotoxicity relationships have been determined for 11 thiourea derivatives containing the 2-aminothiazole moiety and demonstrating varied cytotoxicity against MT-4 cells. The statistical analyses were conducted by means of Multiple Linear Regression (MLR). This paper contains linear models of cytotoxicity depending on electronic, steric and lipophilic descriptors of the examined compounds containing the 2-aminothiazole moiety. The models have been validated by means of the Leave-One-Out Cross Validation (LOO CV).

Keywords: Structure-cytotoxicity relationship · Thiourea derivatives · 2-aminothiazole · Multiple linear regression

1 Introduction

The *in silico* method of drug design, i.e. theoretical design of new drugs utilizing computational systems in computer's virtual space, is developing very dynamically. One quite commonly used chemoinformatic method of drug discovery is the Quantitative Structure-Activity Relationships (QSAR) method [1], which entails determining mathematical relationships between chemical structure of compounds and theirs biological activity. This method is based on the assumption that the differences between particular compounds in terms of biological activity and physicochemical properties result from differences in their chemical structure. It is expected that compounds similar in structure are also similar in terms of biological activity [2]. In the case of this method, the physicochemical properties of compounds are described quantitatively by means of molecular descriptors that can be divided into several groups, e.g. hydrophobic, steric, electronic, electrostatic. The QSAR method is commonly used to find mathematical

© Springer International Publishing AG 2017
M. Gzik et al. (eds.), *Innovations in Biomedical Engineering*, Advances in Intelligent Systems and Computing 526, DOI 10.1007/978-3-319-47154-9_32

relationships between cytotoxicity and molecular descriptors [3,4]. Several relationships describing the influence of molecular descriptors for electronic properties (μ chemical potential, ω electrophilicity index, $HOMO$ the highest occupied molecular orbital energy, $LUMO$ the lowest unoccupied molecular orbital energy, E_E electronic energy, I_{C-C} core-core interaction) on cytotoxicity can be found in literature [5–7]. In the case of this research, after conducting an in-depth statistical analysis, models describing the influence of molecular descriptors on cytotoxicity of compounds containing the 2-aminothiazole moiety have been developed.

2   Experimental Works and Methods

Linear dependencies have been determined for all 11 compounds on Fig. 1 versus 7 molecular descriptors described on Fig. 2. Statistical analyses have been conducted for cytotoxicity expressed as log(1/MT-4) = –log(MT-4), where compound concentration (μM) required to reduce the viability of mock-infected MT-4 cells by 50 %, as determined by the MTT method. The measure of cytotoxicity described in this manner is characterized by nearly normal distribution. The first phase included statistical analysis for all 18 molecular descriptors described in the paper [8]. Statistically significant linear models have been obtained for 7 molecular descriptors: volume (V), surface area grid (SA_g), logarithm of the partition coefficient (log$P$), the highest occupied molecular orbital energy ($HOMO$), electronic energy (E_E), core-core interaction (I_{C-C}), chemical potential (μ) described by the following equation: $(LUMO + HOMO)/2$, electrophilicity (ω) described by the following formula: $\mu^2/(LUMO - HOMO)$. The statistical analysis was conducted using the STATISTICA 12 software [9]. The linear models of cytotoxic activity versus molecular descriptors proposed in the paper were determined by means of multiple linear regression (MLR) [10]. Cytotoxic activity log(1/MT-4) was the dependent variable, while the molecular descriptors were the independent variables. The statistical calculations were conducted at confidence level of 95 % (p <0.05). The analyses were conducted by means of multiple backward regression which entailed successively rejecting the least statistically significant molecular descriptors (molecular descriptors having the highest p value). Statistical parameters for the resulting regression equations: correlation coefficient (R), determination coefficient (R^2), adjusted determination coefficient for calibration (R^2_{adj}), a standard error of estimate (S_{EE}), determination coefficient of LOO validation (Q^2) are presented on Fig. 3.

The model has been validated by means of the *Leave-One-Out Cross Validation* (LOO CV). Successively one compound, utilized to validate the resulting model, was eliminated from the data set used as a basis for model ($n - 1$). The Q^2 validation coefficient was calculated from the formula [11]:

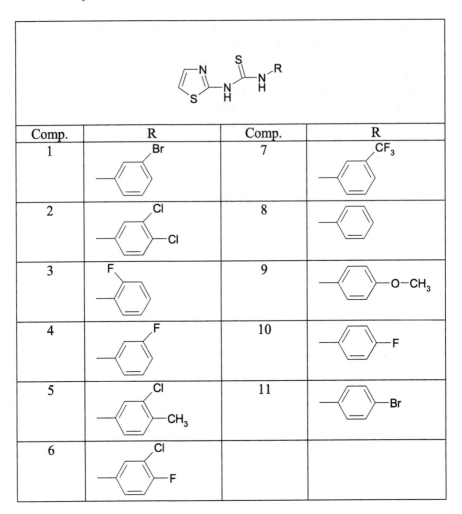

Fig. 1. Structures of thiourea derivatives used in the study

$$Q^2 = 1 - \frac{\displaystyle\sum_{i=1}^{n}(y_{exp,i} - y_{pred,i})^2}{\displaystyle\sum_{i=1}^{n}(y_{exp,i} - y_{ave,i})^2} \tag{1}$$

where: $y_{exp,i}$ - experimental output value for the i-th compound, $y_{pred,i}$ - predicted output value for the i-th compound, $y_{ave,i}$ - average value for the output variable without the i-th compound.

Comp.	log(1/MT-4)	μ [eV]	ω [eV]	HOMO [eV]	I_{c-c} [kcal/mol]	E_E [kcal/mol]	logP	V [Å^{-3}]	SA$_g$ [Å^{-2}]
1	-0.95424	-5.20	49.15	-8.84	277867	-335941	4.54	722.9	455.11
2	-0.95424	-5.20	48.36	-8.78	310801	-374979	4.78	740.53	464.01
3	-1.58546	-5.15	48.24	-8.79	286769	-346844	3.89	667.58	423.74
4	-1.03342	-5.22	49.53	-8.86	280663	-340740	3.89	670.34	424.83
5	-0.92942	-5.12	47.14	-8.72	313250	-373931	4.73	749.51	466.09
6	-0.89209	-5.26	49.93	-8.87	312569	-379595	4.40	711.68	446.71
7	-0.95424	-5.08	46.26	-8.66	391778	-474922	4.63	736.17	462.55
8	-1.69897	-5.08	46.66	-8.70	249185	-299463	3.75	661.34	414.73
9	-2.00000	-4.96	43.59	-8.50	313818	-374310	3.49	739.07	463.53
10	-1.03342	-5.19	48.75	-8.81	279104	-339181	3.89	669.83	425.68
11	-0.95424	-5.20	49.09	-8.83	276309	-334383	4.54	722.01	450.14

Fig. 2. Molecular descriptors of thiourea derivatives used in the study

Equation	R	R^2	R$^2_{adj}$	P<	S$_{EE}$	Q^2
log(1/MT-4)=)= -2.26(±0.66)·μ +0.51(±0.125)·logP-15.01(±3.23)	0.927	0.860	0.825	0.00038	0.162	0.796
log(1/MT-4)= -3.92(±0.76)·μ +0.0095(±0.0034)·SA$_g$-25.58(±4.5)	0.887	0.786	0.733	0.00209	0.201	0.543
log(1/MT-4)= -3.94(±0.76)·μ +0.0054(±0.0019)·V-25.32(±4.43)	0.888	0.788	0.735	0.00202	0.200	0.570
log(1/MT-4)= -3.89(±0.78)·μ +0.000004(±0.000001)·E$_E$-22.66(±4.19)	0.879	0.773	0.716	0.00265	0.206	0.694
log(1/MT-4)= -3.23(±0.62)·HOMO +0.018(±0.0035)·SA$_g$-34.67(±6.17)	0.887	0.788	0.734	0.00204	0.200	0.551
log(1/MT-4)= -3.26(±0.66)·HOMO +0.000006(±0.000002)·I$_{c-c}$-31.54(±6.0)	0.876	0.768	0.710	0.00289	0.208	0.721
log(1/MT-4)= 0.19(±0.038)·ω +0.000006(±0.000002)·I$_{c-c}$-11.92(±2.07)	0.878	0.771	0.714	0.00276	0.207	0.715
log(1/MT-4)= 0.185(±0.0362)·ω +0.012(±0.0035)·SA$_g$-15.03(±2.66)	0.886	0.784	0.730	0.00217	0.201	0.543

Fig. 3. Formulas describing the relationship of cytotoxicity against selected molecular descriptors

3 Results

Mathematical models of relationships between cytotoxicity and molecular descriptors have been determined as part of the research. They are presented in Figs. 4, 5, 6, 7, 8, 9, 10 and 11. The relationships were established by means of stepwise multiple regression. Figure 3 contains linear equations for two explanatory variables, so that the following condition is met: at least 5 compounds per one described parameter [12]. At least one explanatory variable in each equation is a descriptor describing electronic parameters of compounds. It is worth noting that electronic descriptors describe electron density distribution and, as a result, reactivity of a compound, i.e. the capability to interact electrostatically with the molecular target. On the other hand, steric descriptors describe molecular geometry, as well as general size and shape of a molecule. This makes it possible to consider the compatibility of the molecule with the molecular target. Lipophilic descriptor is another important descriptor worth mentioning. It describes the

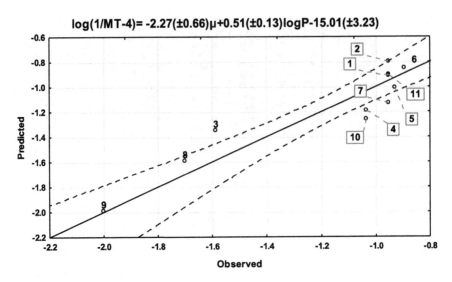

Fig. 4. Correlation of the cytotoxicity and μ, $\log P$

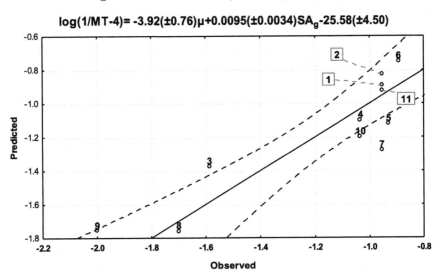

Fig. 5. Correlation of the cytotoxicity and μ, SA_g

compound's ability to permeate cell membranes, and therefore describes also transport and resorption parameters of the compound [13].

Four compounds 3, 10, 7 and 4, are outside the confidence interval for the relationship presented in Fig. 4. These compounds are different from the rest in terms of structure, as they contain fluorine atoms in different places (ortho, para and meta position) of the R substituent aromatic ring (Fig. 1). Compounds 3, 7,

log(1/MT-4)= -3.94(±0.66)µ+0.0055(±0.0019)V-15.32(±4.43)

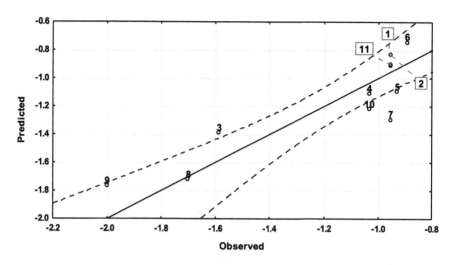

Fig. 6. Correlation of the cytotoxicity and μ, V

log(1/MT-4)= -3.89(±0.78)µ+0.000004(±0.000001)E$_E$-22.66(±4.19)

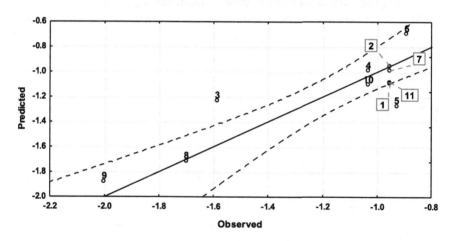

Fig. 7. Correlation of the cytotoxicity and μ, E_E

10 and 5 are outside the confidence interval for relationships presented in Figs. 5, 6, 8 and 11. Three compounds, 3, 7 and 10, contain fluorine atom in R substituent ring, and compound 5 contains chlorine atom in meta position and methyl in para position of the R substituent aromatic ring. Only two compounds, 3 and 5, are outside the confidence interval for the relationship presented in Figs. 7, 9 and 10. Compound 3 is outside the confidence interval for all relationships. It is

$$\log(1/MT\text{-}4) = -3.23(\pm0.62)HOMO + 0.012(\pm0.0035)SA_g - 34.67(\pm6.17)$$

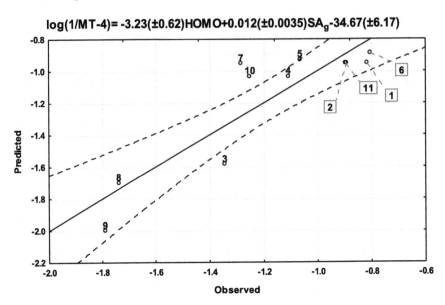

Fig. 8. Correlation of the cytotoxicity and $HOMO$, SA_g

$$\log(1/MT\text{-}4) = -3.26(\pm0.66)HOMO + 0.012(\pm0.0035)I_{c\text{-}c} - 34.67(\pm6.17)$$

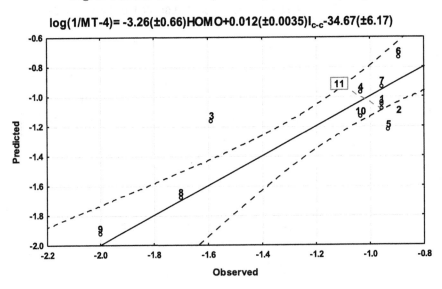

Fig. 9. Correlation of the cytotoxicity and $HOMO$, I_{C-C}

the only compound in the researched group in which the ortho position of the aromatic ring is occupied. All presented equations are statistically significant and meet the condition of acceptability for model $R^2 > 0.6$ and $Q^2 > 0.5$ [2,14], as well as coincidence condition.

$$\log(1/MT\text{-}4) = 0.18(\pm0.038)\omega + 0.000006(\pm0.000002)I_{c\text{-}c} - 11.92(\pm2.07)$$

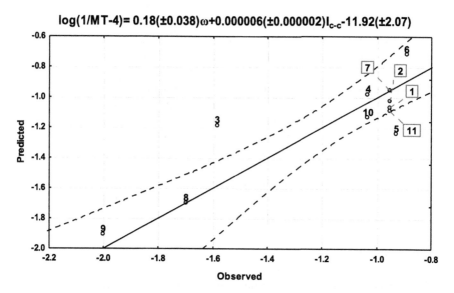

Fig. 10. Correlation of the cytotoxicity and ω, I_{C-C}

$$\log(1/MT\text{-}4) = 0.19(\pm0.036)\omega + 0.011(\pm0.0035)SA_g - 15.03(\pm2.66)$$

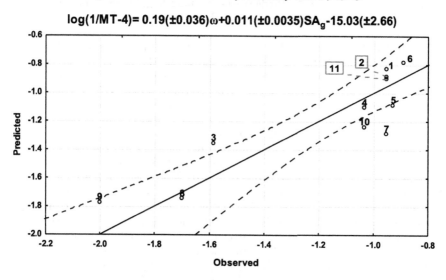

Fig. 11. Correlation of the cytotoxicity and ω, SA_g

4   Conclusion

As shown by conducted statistical analyses, cytotoxicity of the analyzed compounds is influenced by electronic descriptors such as μ, $HOMO$, ω, E_E, I_{C-C}, octanol/water partition coefficient log$P$, and steric descriptors V, SA_g. For all relationships on Fig. 3 a negatively correlated influence of electronic descriptors μ, $HOMO$ and positively correlated influence of all other electronic descriptors

ω, E_E, I_{C-C} on cytotoxicity of the analyzed compounds is noticeable. Steric descriptors (V, SA_g) and lipophilic descriptor ($\log P$) show a positively correlated influence on cytotoxicity of analyzed compounds. The best compatibility in terms of R^2 and Q^2 has been achieved for μ and $\log P$.

The presented models may be utilized to determine the influence of other atoms or molecules in R substituent aromatic ring on cytotoxicity of synthesized substances. When designing new compounds, the quantitative influence should be considered, and the type of influence (electronic, steric or lipophilic) on compound's cytotoxicity should be analyzed.

Acknowledgments. This work was partially supported by the Ministry of Science and Higher Education funding for statutory activities of young researchers of Faculty of Automatic Control, Electronics and Computer Science.

References

1. Winkler, D.A.: The role of quantitative structure-activity relationships (QSAR) in biomolecular. Brief. Bioinform. **3**, 73–86 (2002)
2. Golbraikh, A., Tropsha, A.: Predictive QSAR modeling diversity sampling of experimental data set and test set selection. J. Comput. Aided Mol. Des. **5**, 231–243 (2002)
3. Schultz, T.W., Cronin, M.T.D., Netzeva, T.I.: The present status of QSAR in toxicology. J. Mol. Struct. (Theochem) **622**, 23–38 (2003)
4. Kar, S., Roy, K.: QSAR modeling of toxicity of diverse organic chemicals to Daphnia magna using 2D and 3D descriptors. J. Hazard. Mater. **177**, 344–351 (2010)
5. Kupcewicz, B., Jarzęcki, A., Małecka, M., Krajewska, U., Rozalski, M.: Cytotoxic activity of substituted chalcones in terms of molecular electronic properties. Bioorg. Med. Chem. Lett. **24**, 4260–4265 (2014)
6. Pogorzelska, A., Sławiński, J., Brożewicz, K., Ulenberg, S., Bączek, T.: Novel 3-Amino-6-chloro-7-(azol-2 or 5-yl)-1,1-dioxo-1,4,2-benzodithiazine derivatives with Anticancer activity: synthesis and QSAR study. Molecules. **20**, 21960–21970 (2015)
7. Afantitis, A., Melagraki, G., Sarimveis, H., Koutentis, P.A., Markopoulos, J., Igglessi-Markopoulou, O.: A novel QSAR model for predicting induction of apaptosis by 4-aryl-4H-chromenes. Bioorg. Med. Chem. **14**, 6686–6694 (2006)
8. Stefanska, J., Nowicka, G., Struga, M., Szulczyk, D., Koziol, A.E., Augustynowicz-Kopec, E., Napiorkowska, A., Bielenica, A., Filipowski, W., Filipowska, A., Drzewiecka, A., Giliberti, G., Madeddu, S., Boi, S., La Colla, P., Sanna, G.: Antimicrobial and anti-biofilm activity of thiourea derivatives incorporating a 2-aminothiazole scaffold. Chem. Pharm. Bull. (Tokyo) **63**, 225–236 (2015)
9. StatSoft, Inc. (2014). STATISTICA (data analysis software system), version 12. www.statsoft.com
10. Dehmer, M., Varmuze, K., Bonchev, D.: Statistical modeling of molecular descriptors in QSAR/QSPR. Wiley-Blackwell **2**, 3–4 (2012)
11. Khaledian, S., Saaidpour, S.: Quantitative structure-property relationship modelling of distribution coefficients (logD7.4) of diverse drug by sub-structural molecular fragments method. Orient. J. Chem. **31**, 1969–1976 (2015)

12. Topliss, J.G., Edwards, R.P.: Chance factors in studies of quantitative structure-activity relationships. J. Med. Chem. **22**(10), 1238–1244 (1979)
13. Kuśmierz, E.: Synteza i badanie zależności pomiędzy strukturą a aktywnością w grupie pochodnych kwasów karboksylowych: mrówkowego, octowego, benzoesowego i difenylooctowego, Ph.D. thesis (2013)
14. Frimayanti, N., Yam, M.L., Lee, H.B., Othman, R., Zain, S.M., Rahman, N.A.: Validation of quantitative structure-activity relationship (QSAR) model for photosensitizer activity prediction. Int. J. Mol. Sci. **12**, 8626–8644 (2011)

QRS Complex Detection Based on Ensemble Empirical Mode Decomposition

Norbert Henzel[(✉)]

Institute of Medical Technology and Equipment ITAM,
Roosevelt'a 118, 41–800 Zabrze, Poland
`henzel@itam.zabrze.pl`

Abstract. The principal objective of this project was to investigate the detection of QRS complexes in noisy ECG signals. This study provides a novel approach to the construction of a QRS detector based on the Ensemble Empirical Mode Decomposition. The detection function is based on predicted probability that the current signal sample is a QRS fiducial point. The performances of the proposed method were verified on the MIT-BIH Arrhythmia Database. Results showed that this approach improves the QRS detection accuracy.

Keywords: ECG signal processing · QRS detection · Ensemble Empirical Mode Decomposition

1 Introduction

In the field of ECG signal processing, besides signal denoising [6,17,19,28], the concept of QRS complexes detection is of key importance. Almost all analysis and measurement performed on the ECG signal depend on correctly detected beat-by-beat QRS wave positions [8]. Classification of QRS complexes [16], fetal ECG signal processing [5,11], heart rate variability [2,27,30], and arrhythmia recognition [25,26] are some examples of application where the localization of QRS waves is a dominant feature.

The constant research in the area of software QRS detection methods for more than 40 years clearly indicate the great importance of this research topic. In this period, and particularly in the last twenty years, a multitude of new QRS detection methods have been presented in the literature. These methods use a vast range of different approaches: artificial neural networks, genetic algorithms, wavelet transforms, filter banks, matched filters, digital filtering and many others. A systematic review of classic QRS detection methods is presented in [12,24].

The quality of QRS detection is influenced mainly by two factors: the ECG signal noise and a vast spectrum of potential QRS shapes. In order to limit the influence of the first factor a noise attenuation techniques are applied [1,3,7,17, 21,28,34].

© Springer International Publishing AG 2017
M. Gzik et al. (eds.), *Innovations in Biomedical Engineering*, Advances in Intelligent
Systems and Computing 526, DOI 10.1007/978-3-319-47154-9_33

QRS detection and noise attenuation in case of the fetal ECG signals is much more complicated [13,15,18,31,32]. False detection of fetal QRS complexes may be caused not only by accidental interference signals, but also by other biophysical signals, whose power is often much higher than the useful signal power. Particularly complex procedure for verification of the fetal QRS detection methods has to be applied for the signals recorded for a twin pregnancy, where there are two sequences of uncorrelated events with similar amplitude characteristics [14].

Recently, a considerable literature has grown up around the theme of Empirical Mode Decomposition (EMD) [10] and Ensemble Empirical Mode Decomposition (EEMD) [33] and theirs applications in processing of non-linear and non-stationary signals. These methods were also applied in ECG processing for attenuation of baseline wander and powerline interference [1,3,21], as well as for QRS detection [22,23]. In the latter case the results of (E)EMD are used to construct a detection function, but the choice of a given model is often unclear.

The aim of this paper is to propose and evaluate a more systematic approach to construction of QRS detectors based on the Ensemble Empirical Mode Decomposition.

2   Method

The Empirical Mode Decomposition (EMD), proposed by Huang et al. [10], is a data-driven technique designed to process non-linear and non-stationary signals. This technique adaptively decomposes signals in terms of N intrinsic mode functions (IMFs)

$$x(t) = \sum_{i=1}^{N} c_i(t) + r(t) \tag{1}$$

where $x(t), c_i(t)$ and $r(t)$ denote the time-domain signal, the i-th IMF and the residual signal, respectively. The signals $c_i(t)$ are intrinsic to the signal $x(t)$ and represent different time-scale oscillations composing, together with $r(t)$, the entire signal. Every IMF is obtained in a recursive process called *sifting* and satisfies two conditions: (1) the number of extrema and the number of zero crossing must be equal or differ at most by one, and (2) the average value of the envelopes defined by the local maxima and the local minima should be equal to zero.

The main drawback of EMD is that oscillation with the same time scale could exist in different IMFs or one IMF may contain oscillation with different time scale. To overcome this mixing effect Wu and Huang [33] proposed an extended technique called Ensemble Empirical Mode Decomposition (EEMD). Figure 1 presents an example of ECG signal $x(t)$ decomposed into $N = 10$ IMFs and residual signal.

The higher the IMF number i is, the more lower time-scale oscillation the IMF contains. Using this property selective reconstruction of $x(t)$ could be performed. In order to attenuate low frequency components the following reconstruction, described by

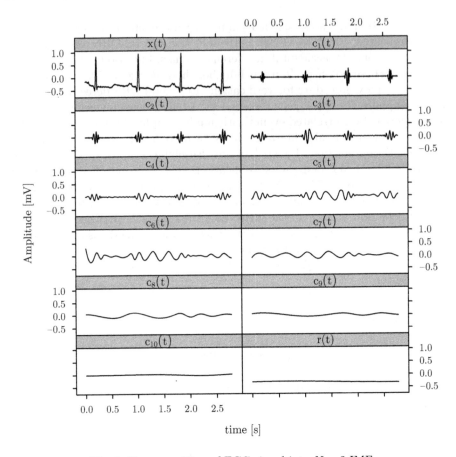

Fig. 1. Decomposition of ECG signal into $N = 3$ IMF

$$f2c_n(t) = \sum_{i=1}^{n} c_i(t) \tag{2}$$

may be used, where $n \leqslant N$. In the opposite case, when the high frequency signal components are undesired, more appropriate reconstruction is described by

$$c2f_n(t) = x(t) - f2c_n(t) = x(t) - \sum_{i=1}^{n} c_i(t). \tag{3}$$

Figure 2 presents the reconstruction signals $f2c_n(t)$ and $c2f_n(t)$, $1 \leqslant n \leqslant 6$ for IMFs presented in Fig. 1.

The $c_i(t)$, $f2c_n(t)$, $c2f_i(t)$ where $1 \leqslant i, n \leqslant N$ as well as their respective absolute values were used to create the feature set used to design the QRS detection function. For a given ECG signal, this function takes a value equal to 1 for maximum of each R-wave and 0 otherwise. The detection function, defined as

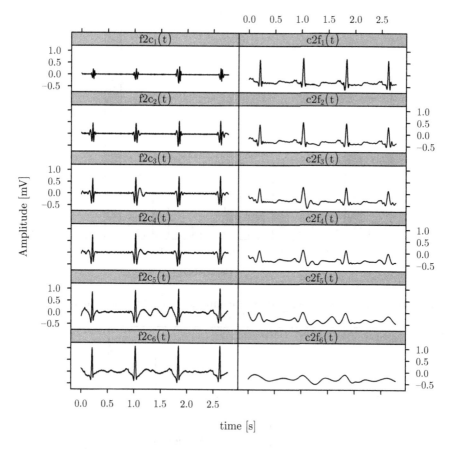

Fig. 2. Reconstruction signals $f2c_n(t)$ and $c2f_n(t)$, $1 \leqslant n \leqslant 6$ for IMFs presented in Fig. 1

$$\begin{aligned}
\mathscr{D} = {} & w_0 + w_1 c_1 + \cdots + w_N c_N + w_{N+1} f2c_1 + \ldots + w_{2N} f2c_N \\
& + w_{2N+1} c2f_1 + \cdots + w_{3N} c2f_N + w_{3N+1} |c_1| + \cdots + w_{4N} |c_N| \\
& + w_{4N+1} |f2c_1| + \cdots + w_{5N} |f2c_N| + w_{5N+1} |c2f_1| + \cdots + w_{6N} |c2f_N| \quad (4)
\end{aligned}$$

contains $6N + 1$ unknown parameters. In order to determine optimal parameter values, the Gradient Boosting with Component-wise Linear Models method developed by Buehlmann and Hothorn [4] was applied.

3   Experimental Results

The evaluation of the described above approach was performed using ECG signals from the easily available MIT-BIH Arrhythmia Database [9,20]. It contains 48, 30 minutes long, manually annotated ECG records, sampled at 360 Hz.

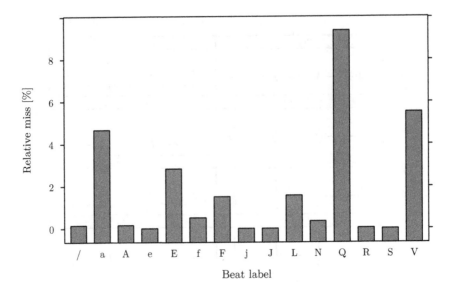

Fig. 3. Relative number of missed QRS complexes with different annotation labels.

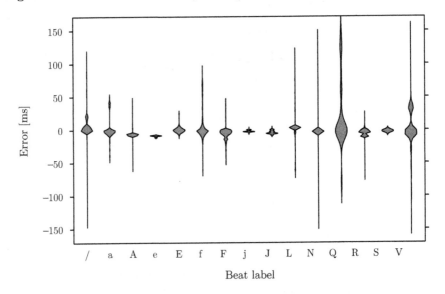

Fig. 4. Distributions of errors between instances when a QRS complex was detected and corresponding reference time

For each record in the database the values of $c_i, f2c_n, c2f_n, |c_i|, |f2c_n|, |c2f_n|$, $1 \leqslant i, n \leqslant N = 5$ were calculated. This data set was randomly divided into training (75 %) and testing (25 %) subset. The optimal parameters w_i were determined using 10-fold cross-validation on the training data. This procedure was repeated ten times and the results verified on the testing set. The reproducibility of the obtained results was verified by the detection accuracy (Ac), sensitivity (Se) and positive prediction value ($P+$). These values, calculated for all available data, attain, respectively, $Ac = 97.34\,\%$, $Se = 99.21\,\%$ and $P+ = 98.10\,\%$.

Figure 3 presents the relative number of missed QRS complexes with different annotation labels with respect to number of all QRS complexes with given label. The letters describing the different beat labels are standard symbols used in the MIT-BIH database annotations. The (relative) highest number of missed beats was for the following beat classes: Q (unclassifiable beat), V (premature ventricular contraction), a (aberrated atrial premature beat), E (ventricular escape beat), L (left bundle branch block beat) and F (fusion of ventricular and normal beat); the label N represents normal beat. This high relative miss error in many cases may be associated with small number of QRS complexes with given label, causing insufficient impact of this beats class during the learning process. A possible solution may be to develop a separate QRS detector branch for these "minority" cases.

The next figure, Fig. 4, presents distributions of errors between instances when a QRS complex was detected and corresponding reference time. The width of distribution corresponds to the number of result with given error value. For all beat classes, the large majority of obtained results is close to the corresponding reference values.

4   Summary

The purpose of the current study was to make a first step towards proposing a systematic approach to construction of QRS detectors based on the Ensemble Empirical Mode Decomposition. This approach does not require a separate noise attenuation step. The main obstacle to achieve very good detection rates seems to be the large diversity of QRS shapes and a small number of representative QRS shapes for less common QRS beats.

Acknowledgements. This scientific research work is supported by The National Centre for Research and Development of Poland (grant No. STRATEGMED2/ 269343/NCBR/2016).

References

1. Agrawal, S., Gupta, A.: Fractal and EMD based removal of baseline wander and powerline interference from ECG signals. Comput. Biol. Med. **43**, 1889–1899 (2013)
2. Akselrod, S., Gordon, D., Ubel, F.A., Shannon, D.C., Barger, A.C., Cohen, R.J.: Power spectrum analysis of heart rate fluctuation: a quantitative probe of beat to beat cardiovascular control. Science **213**, 220–222 (1981)
3. Blanco-Velasco, M., Weng, B., Barner, K.E.: ECG signal denoising and baseline wander correction based on the empirical mode decomposition. Comput. Biol. Med. **38**, 1–13 (2008)

4. Buehlmann, P., Hothorn, T.: Boosting algorithms: regularization, prediction and model fitting. Stat. Sci. **22**(4), 477–505 (2007)
5. Chourasia, V.S., Tiwari, A.K.: A review and comparative analysis of recent advancements in fetal monitoring techniques. Crit. Rev. Biomed. Eng. **36**(5–6), 335–373 (2008)
6. Chu, C.H.H., Delp, E.J.: Impulsive noise suppression and background normalization of electrocardiogram signals using morphological operators. IEEE Trans. Biomed. Eng. **36**(2), 262–273 (1989)
7. Fasano, A., Villani, V.: Baseline wander removal for bioelectrical signals by quadratic variation reduction. Signal Process. **99**, 48–57 (2014)
8. Friesen, G.M., Jannett, T.C., Jadallah, M.A., Yates, S.L., Quint, S.R.: A comparison of the noise sensitivity of nine QRS detection algorithms. IEEE Trans. Biomed. Eng. **37**, 85–98 (1990)
9. Goldberger, A.L., Amaral, L.A.N., Glass, L., Hausdorff, J.M., Ivanov, P.C., Mark, R.G., Mietus, J.E., Moody, G.B., Peng, C.-K., Stanley, H.E.: PhysioBank, physiotoolkit, and physionet: components of a new research resource for complex physiologic signals. Circulation **101**(23), e215–e220 (2000)
10. Huang, N.E., Shen, Z., Long, S.R., Wu, M.C., Shih, H.H., Zheng, Q., Yen, N.-C., Tung, C.C., Liu, H.H.: The empirical mode composition and the Hilbert spectrum for nonlinear and non stationary time series analysis. Proc. Roy. Soc. **454**, 903–905 (1998)
11. Jezewski, J., Matonia, A., Kupka, T., Roj, D., Czabanski, R.: Determination of the fetal heart rate from abdominal signals: evaluation of beat-to-beat accuracy in relation to the direct fetal electrocardiogram. Biomed. Eng. **57**(5), 383–394 (2012)
12. Kohler, B.U., Hennig, C., Orglmeister, R.: The principles of software QRS detection. IEEE Eng. Med. Biol. Mag. **21**(1), 42–57 (2002)
13. Kotas, M., Jezewski, J., Matonia, A., Kupka, T.: Towards noise immune detection of fetal QRS complexes. Comput. Meth. Prog. Bio. **97**(3), 241–256 (2010)
14. Kotas, M., Jezewski, J., Horoba, K., Matonia, A.: Application of spatio-temporal filtering to fetal electrocardiogram enhancement. Comput. Meth. Prog. Bio. **104**(1), 1–9 (2011)
15. Kupka, T., Jezewski, J., Matonia, A., Horoba, K., Wrobel, J.: Timing events in Doppler ultrasound signal of fetal heart activity. In: Proceedings of the 26th Annual International Conference of the IEEE Engineering in Medicine and Biology Society, pp. 337–340 (2004)
16. Leski, J.M., Henzel, N.: Time series of fuzzy sets in classification of electrocardiographic signals. In: Proceedings of the 8th International Conference on Computer Recognition Systems CORES 2013, Advances in Intelligent Systems and Computing, pp. 541–550 (2013)
17. Łęski, J.M., Henzel, N.: ECG baseline wander and powerline interference reduction using nonlinear filter bank. Signal Process. **85**(4), 781–793 (2005)
18. Matonia, A., Jezewski, J., Kupka, T., Horoba, K., Wrobel, J., Gacek, A.: The influence of coincidence of fetal and maternal QRS complexes on fetal heart rate reliability. Med. Biol. Eng. Comput. **44**, 393–403 (2006)
19. McManus, C.D., Neubert, D., Cramer, E.: Characterization and elimination of AC noise in the electrocardiogram: a comparison of digital filtering methods. Comput. Biomed. Res. **26**, 48–67 (1993)
20. Moody, G.B., Mark, R.G.: The impact of the MIT-BIH Arrhythmia Database. IEEE Eng. in Med. and Biol. **20**(3), 45–50 (2001)

21. Nimunkar, A.J., Tompkins, W.J.: EMD-based 60-Hz noise filtering of the ECG. In: Proceedings of the 29th Annual International Conference of the IEEE EMBS, pp. 1904–1907 (2007)
22. Nimunkar, A.J., Tompkins, W.J.: R-peak detection and signal averaging for simulated stress ECG using EMD. In: Proceedings of the 29th Annual International Conference of the IEEE EMBS, pp. 1261–1264 (2007)
23. Pal, S., Mitra, M.: Empirical mode decomposition based ECG enhancement and QRS detection. Comput. Biol. Med. **42**, 83–92 (2012)
24. Pahlm, O., Sornmo, L.: Software QRS detection in ambulatory monitoring – a review. Med. Biol. Eng. Comput. **22**, 298–297 (1984)
25. Suchetha, M., Kumaravel, N., Benisha, B.: Denoising and arrhythmia classification using EMD based features and neural network. In: 2013 International Conference on Communications and Signal Processing (ICCSP), pp. 883–887 (2013)
26. Thakor, N.V., Zhu, Y.S.: Application of adaptive filtering to ECG analysis: noise cancellation and arrhythmia detection. IEEE Trans. Biomed. Eng. **38**(8), 785–794 (1991)
27. Ungureanu, G.M., Bergmans, J.W., Oei, S.G., Ungureanu, A., Wolf, W.: Comparison and evaluation of existing methods for the extraction of low amplitude electrocardiographic signals: a possible approach to transabdominal fetal ECG. Biomed. Tech. **54**(2), 66–75 (2009)
28. van Alste, A., van Eck, W., Herrman, O.E.: ECG baseline wander reduction using linear phase filters. Comput. Biomed. Res. **19**, 417–427 (1986)
29. Velasco, M.B., Weng, B., Barner, K.E.: ECG signal denoising and baselinewander correction based on the empirical mode decomposition. Comput. Bio. Med. **38**, 1–13 (2008)
30. Vullings, R., Peters, C.H., Hermans, M.J., Wijn, P.F., Oei, S.G., Bergmans, J.W.: A robust physiology-based source separation method for QRS detection in low amplitude fetal ECG recordings. Physiol. Meas. **31**, 935–951 (2010)
31. Wrobel, J., Horoba, K., Pander, T., Jezewski, J., Czabanski, R.: Improving the fetal heart rate signal interpretation by application of myriad filtering. Biocybern. Biomed. Eng. **33**, 211–221 (2013)
32. Wrobel, J., Matonia, A., Horoba, K., Jezewski, J., Czabanski, R., Pawlak, A., et al.: Pregnancy telemonitoring with smart control of algorithms for signal analysis. J. Med. Imag. Health. In. **5**(6), 1302–1310 (2015)
33. Wu, Z., Huang, N.E.: Ensemble empirical mode decomposition: a noise-assisted data analysis method. Adv. Adapt. Data Anal. **1**(1), 1–41 (2009)
34. Zhao, Z., Chen, Y.: A new method for removal of baseline wander and power line interference in ECG signals. In: Proceedings of the Fifth International Conference on Machine Learning and Cybernetics, pp. 4342–4347 (2006)

Visual Mismatch Negativity as a Non-attentional Reaction to Change in Repetition Pattern

Karina Maciejewska[✉], Zofia Drzazga, and Agnieszka Trojankowska

Department of Medical Physics, Institute of Physics, University of Silesia,
Uniwersytecka Street 4, 40-007 Katowice, Poland
karina.maciejewska@us.edu.pl

Abstract. Mismatch negativity (MMN) is an event related potential generated by brain's electric activation as an automatic response to change in repetitive stimulation. Two scenarios of an oddball experiment were performed among 9 students of University of Silesia at the age of 20–25 years, with the use of standard, deviant and distractor events. Difference deviant-standard waveforms were obtained, which presented posterior negativity in the range 140–200 ms after stimulus onset. Subtraction of the standard from deviant ERP waveforms, irrelevance to participant's task, and independence from stimulus physical parameters imply that the posterior negativity evoked in this study seems to be a visual mismatch negativity as a result of pre-attentive central visual processing.

Keywords: Event related potentials · Visual mismatch negativity · EEG

1 Introduction

The sensory system of human organism has an ability to extract the regularities and form predictions of upcoming events, which is essential because it optimizes the accuracy and speed of perceptual and cognitive processes, and minimizes processing resources as well as computational demands for redundant predictable events in the brain [1–3]. One of the tools for consciousness, memory trace efficiency, lack of perceptual processing and processing accuracy measurements is mismatch negativity waveform - an ERP, which is a reaction of brain activity to violation of regular schema of presented stimuli [4]. Most often, this waveform is elicited by a discriminable change in auditory stimulation, when infrequent sound is presented in a homogeneous sequence of frequent sounds [5–8]. It seems that the temporo-prefrontal network compares the current incoming signal with a memory trace of previous stimuli [9–13]. The biological function represented by an aMMN (auditory mismatch negativity) is to monitor and detect any change in ongoing auditory stimulation, irrespective of where attention is directed, as it represents the brain's automatic process involved in encoding of the stimulus difference or change [14]. It has been revealed that this MMN waveform might

© Springer International Publishing AG 2017
M. Gzik et al. (eds.), *Innovations in Biomedical Engineering*, Advances in Intelligent
Systems and Computing 526, DOI 10.1007/978-3-319-47154-9_34

be associated with pre-attentive cognitive operations, what means it might be connected to 'primitive intelligence' in the auditory cortex [15].

Recently, there have been attempts to obtain a visual analog of auditory mismatch negativity–vMMN (visual mismatch negativity) waveform, distributed posteriorly, around 100–400 ms after stimulus onset. However, the existence of vMMN potentials has not been unambiguously confirmed yet, and an opinion about vMMN is divided in the scientific community [1,16–21,23–27]. The aim of our study was to evoke mismatch negativity with visual stimuli and to speak in a discussion about the existence of visual mismatch negativity.

2   Material and Method

2.1   Participants

The experiment was performed among 9 students of University of Silesia (5 males and 4 females) at the age of 20–25 years. They all were healthy, physically active, right-handed, non-smokers, with normal blood pressure and body temperature at the day of the study, with no neural disorders diagnosed. The subjects had normal or corrected to normal vision and normal hearing. The methodology was fully explained to the participants who gave their consent to perform the experiment. Information about their health condition and life style was gathered in a questionnaire.

2.2   Procedure

The study consisted of two experiments. The first scenario was based on [28], where the authors described visual mismatch negativity they managed to obtain. The second scenario was modified changing some physical parameters. The presented paradigm in both scenarios were two kinds of checkerboards: red-black and green-black, displayed alternately. The choice of used colors was determined by the high sensitivity of human eye on the contrast of red and green. The signal was gathered with the use of 32 Ag/AgCl electrode cap (using standard 10/20 EEG system) with AFz electrode as ground electrode and common reference, using Advanced Source Analysis system ASA-Lab (ANT) with ASA v.4.7.1 software. The impedances were kept below 5 kΩ.

The schema of red-black and green-black checkerboards in paradigm 1 is presented in Fig. 1. The checkerboards were displayed in pairs containing two red-black checkerboards and two green-black checkerboards (RRGGRRGG). After ten standard stimuli presented in such an order, the arrangement was disturbed by inserting from time to time, a deviant stimuli - the third checkerboard of the same color. Deviants were 10 percents of all stimuli.

In order to stimulate pre-attentive processes, which is the scope of evoking vMMN waveform, this block of stimuli contained a distractor, which was a red-black or green-black checkerboard with a white cross in the middle. The arms of that cross changed and the participants were instructed to pay attention to the

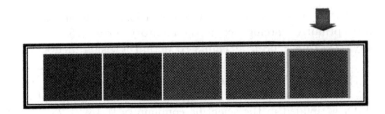

Fig. 1. Red-black and green-black checkerboards as standard stimuli with entered an additional checkerboard as a deviant stimuli used in an oddball paradigm in the first scenario (small checks and checkerboards presented in pairs) (Color figure online)

changes of length of arms of that cross. Time interval between stimuli (ISI) and presentation time were set to 400 ms and 20 ms, respectively, and the size of the checks was 0.4° with 1 m viewing distance.

In the second paradigm, the size of checks was increased to 1.5° and the checkerboards were presented one by one, not in pairs (RGRG). ISI and presentation time were kept as the same level as in the previous experiment. The aim of this change was to simplify the paradigm in order to check if it evokes any change in the signal.

2.3   Signal Processing

Recorded EEG signals were filtered using band-pass filter with frequencies 1–30 Hz and filter slope 24 dB/oct. Signals with amplitude over $\pm$ 75 μV were treated as artifacts (including electrooculography artifacts arised from eye movement) and removed from the analysis. After baseline correction and detrending using 100 ms prestimulus time window, the analyzed EEG epochs were averaged within 0.5 s time window. A difference waveform was created by subtracting standard signals from deviant ones and the data was grand averaged in order to establish mean values from the whole experimental group. The acquisition as well as processing of the signals were performed according to International Federation of Clinical Neurophysiology (IFCN) Guidelines for eliciting, recording, and quantifying mismatch negativity, P300, and N400 [14].

3   Results

3.1   Paradigm 1

Stimulation of the participants with red-black and green-black checkerboards resulted in evoking waveform with the highest amplitude in the posterior region. Figure 2 presents grand averaged ERPs at Cp1, Cp2, Pz, P3, P4 and POz elicited by standard and deviant stimuli.

The most evident is a positive peak in the 160–270 range with maximum at around 200 ms, dominating at POz, where the amplitude is 7.4 μv. The amplitudes at the other electrodes were between 1.06 and 5.86 μv. This waveform was

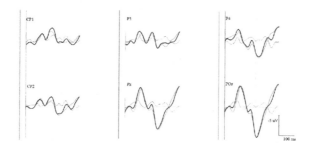

Fig. 2. Grand-averaged ERPs recorded from Cp1, Cp2, Pz, POz, P3 and P4 electrode site for standard (gray solid), deviant (black solid) and deviant-standard (black dot) stimuli evoked in the first scenario (small checks and checkerboards presented in pairs)

generated for both - standard and deviant stimuli, however the deviant stimuli generated smaller amplitudes. Second waveform generated in the experiment was a negativity in the 50–150 ms range with maximum at around 100 ms. It was also the highest at POz, where the amplitude was $-5.15\,\mu\text{V}$, while for the other electrodes the amplitudes were between -1 to $-4.51\,\mu\text{V}$. These peaks were not detected in the anterior regions. The waveforms were identified as P2 and N1 component, respectively. N1 is found to be a reaction to unexpected stimuli. There is also a second positivity seen between N1 and P2 around 130–150 ms - mostly seen at Pz, P4 and POz.

In order to obtain information about non-attentive reaction of the brain on the stimuli, a difference waveform was obtained by subtracting standard signals from deviant ones (black curve), which is presented in Fig. 3. This picture also presents a difference waveform obtained by subtracting standard signals from distractors (gray curve).

A negativity between 120 and 200 ms is well seen in the deviant-standard waveform, which is not present in the distractor-standard waveform. The amplitudes of this waveform are highest at 160–170 ms and amount to $0.94\,\mu\text{V}$ for P4 to $1.18\,\mu\text{V}$ for Cp1.

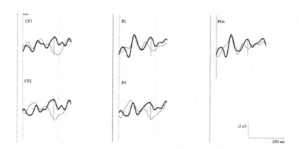

Fig. 3. Representative grand-averaged difference ERPs waveforms recorded from Cp1, Cp2, POz and P4 electrode site for deviant-standard (black) and distractor-standard (gray) stimuli evoked in the first scenario

3.2   Paradigm 2

The scenario used in the first experiment was modified to verify if these changes will affect the obtained waveforms. The size of checks was increased to 1.5° and the checkerboards were presented one by one, not in pairs. Figure 4 presents grand averaged ERPs at Cp1, Cp2, Pz, P3, P4 and POz elicited by standard and deviant stimuli using paradigm 2.

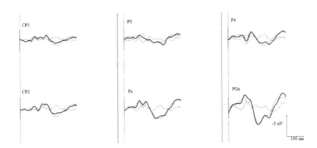

Fig. 4. Grand-averaged ERPs recorded from Cp1, Cp2, Pz, POz, P3 and P4 electrode site for standard (gray solid), deviant (black solid) and deviant-standard (black dot) stimuli evoked in the second scenario (big checks and checkerboards presented one by one)

In this experiment, we obtained a broad positivity around 200 ms with a 4.15 μV maximum at POz. The maxima from the other electrodes were in the range 1.3–2.53 μV. The negativity at around 100 ms was also seen, however it was not as well pronounced as in the first paradigm. The second negativity around 130–160 ms following N1 was also observed. These waveforms were evoked for both: standard and deviant stimuli, likewise in the first scenario. What is important, a standard-deviant difference waveforms was also obtained (negativity at around 140–200 ms), what is seen in the Fig. 4. The amplitudes were in the range 0.53–0.84 μV.

4   Discussion

The studies using MMN waveform give information about neurobiological substrate of central auditory or visual processing [29], which, according to Kahneman, are executed by two general systems. System 1 is automatic and fast, and works without effort of voluntary control, whereas System 2 uses attention to carry out effortful mental activities [30]. The main function of System 1 is to maintain and update our model of the world, which represents what is normal, i.e., what is predictable based on past events. The visual MMN can be described as the electrophysiological correlate of the automatic detection of unpredicted changes in our visual environment carried out by System 1 [31]. In previous studies it was shown that visual mismatch negativity has latency in the range 100–350 ms, however vMMN has been identified even in the range up to 400 ms

[7,18,20,21,23–27]. Such a wide latency range is connected to a wide range of different stimuli which may evoke a violation of regularity - colors, face and non-face objects, grating and many others, with emotions also included in some experiments. The MMN reflects central code of stimulus change and its amplitude and latency is related to the degree to which the deviant stimuli differ from the standard stimuli [4].

In order to properly interpret MMN waveform and what cognitive processes it represents, several conditions must be met. The sensory system must generate representations of the stimulus input, providing memory traces which represent the original sources and their regularities. It also has to up-date the representations to maintain integrity of the ongoing sources [29,32]. MMN waveform is correlated with non-attentional processes with substantial complex analysis outside the focus of perception. However, it might be argued that the posterior negativity observed in MMN studies is associated with attentional capture effect rather than memory-comparison-based change detection effect [22]. For that reason, it is important to eliminate impact of voluntary attention during stimulation. This is achieved by introducing to the scenario, a distractor, which dissuades attention of the subjects from the non-target stimuli. Furthermore, the MMN signal is presented as a difference waveform that arises from subtracting standard stimuli from deviant ones. In our experiment, we fulfilled both criteria using a white cross in the middle of the checkerboards as a target stimulus. Moreover, a difference deviant-standard stimulus waveform as a representation of MMN was calculated. What is noteworthy, we obtained a posterior negativity in the same latency range of the difference ERP waveform after changing checks to bigger ones and changing stimulation sequence to 'one-by-one', what confirms the irrelevance of the vMMN from physical character of the stimuli. Our results show a posterior negativity waveform appearing from 140 to 200 ms after the stimulus onset with maximum at 160–170 ms. Because of the fact that this is a difference waveform (deviant-standard) and it didn't involve participants' attention (the target stimuli were omitted from the analysis), it is likely that we managed to evoke visual mismatch negativity potentials - which are indications of automatic change detection system [22]. This seems to prove the independence of the pre-attentive processes from physical change of the upcoming signals. It may indicate that even with a slight modulation of signals coming from the surrounding world, brain still can maintain pre-attentive processes which administer receiving information.

5 Conclusions

Visual mismatch negativity, as an analogue to auditory mismatch negativity, is assumed to be connected with brain's automatic process involved in encoding difference or change of events upcoming from the surrounding world. In our study, irregular (deviant) repetition of red-black and green-black checkerboards elicited a posterior difference negativity waveform appearing from 140 to 200 ms after the stimulus onset. This is in agreement with results obtained by others [7,18,20–27].

Moreover, a change of physical parameters of the experiment (bigger checks and presentation of the stimuli one by one), still allowed to evoke a posterior negativity in the same latency range. The three aspects of the experiment: subtracting the standard from deviant ERP waveforms, irrelevance to participant's task, and independence from physical stimulus parameters make the posterior negativity evoked in this study seem to be a visual mismatch negativity as a result to pre-attentive central visual processing.

References

1. Kimura, M., Kondo, H., Ohira, H., Schroger, E.: Unintentional temporal context based prediction of emotional faces: an electrophysiological study. Cereb. Cortex **22**, 1774–1785 (2012)
2. Huettel, S.A., Mack, P.B., McCarthy, G.: Perceiving patterns in random series: dynamic processing of sequence in prefrontal cortex. Nat. Neurosci. **5**, 485–490 (2002)
3. Doherty, J.R., Rao, A., Mesulam, M.M., Nobre, A.C.: Synergistic effect of combined temporal and spatial expectations on visual attention. J. Neurosci. **25**, 8259–8266 (2005)
4. Sanju, H.K., Mohanan, A., Kumar, P.: Mismatch negativity. Indian J. Otol. **21**(2), 81–87 (2015)
5. Näätänen, R., Tiitinen, H.: Auditory information processing as indexed by the mismatch negativity. In: Sabourin, M., Craik, F.I.M., Robert, M. (eds.) Advances In Psychological Science. Biological and Cognitive Aspects, vol. 2, pp. 145–170. Psychology Press/Erlbaum Taylor and Francis, Hove (1998)
6. Winkler, I., Karmos, G., Näätänen, R.: Adaptive modeling of the unattended acoustic environment reflected in the mismatch negativity event-related potential. Brain Res. **742**, 239–252 (1996)
7. Czigler, I., Balazs, L., Winkler, I.: Memory-based detection of task-irrelevant visual changes. Psychophysiology **39**, 869–873 (2002)
8. Garrido, M.I., Kilner, J.M., Klaas, E.S., Friston, K.J.: The mismatch negativity: a review of underlying mechanisms. Clin. Neurophysiol. **120**(3), 453–463 (2009)
9. Näätänen, R.: Attention and Brain Function. Erlbaum, Hillsdale (1992)
10. Giard, M.H., Perrin, F., Pernier, J., Bouchet, P.: Brain generators implicated in the processing of auditory stimulus deviance: a topographic event-related potential study. Psychophysiology **27**, 627–640 (1990)
11. Rinne, T., Alho, K., Ilmoniemi, R.J., Virtanen, J., Näätänen, R.: Separate time behaviors of the temporal and frontal mismatch negativity sources. NeuroImage **12**, 14–19 (2000)
12. Opitz, B., Rinne, T., Mecklinger, A., von Cramon, D.Y., Schröger, E.: Differential contribution of frontal and temporal cortices to auditory change detection: fMRI and ERP results. NeuroImage **15**, 167–174 (2002)
13. Doeller, C.F., Opitz, B., Mecklinger, A., Krick, C., Reith, W., Schröger, E.: Prefrontal cortex involvement in preattentive auditory deviance detection: neuroimaging and electrophysiological evidence. NeuroImage **20**, 1270–1282 (2003)
14. Duncan, C.C., Barry, R.J., Connolly, J.F., Fischer, C., Michie, P.T., Näätänen, R., Polich, J., Reinvang, I., Van Petten, C.: Event-related potentials in clinical research: guidelines for eliciting, recording, and quantifying mismatch negativity, P300, and N400. Clin. Neurophysiol. **120**(11), 1883–1908 (2009)

15. Näätänen, R., Tervaniemi, M., Sussman, E., Paavilainen, P., Winkler, I.: "Primitive intelligence" in the auditory cortex. Trends Neurosci. **24**, 283–288 (2001)
16. Nyman, G., Alho, K., Laurinen, P., Paavilainen, P., Radil, T., Reinikainen, K.: Mismatch negativity (MMN) for sequences of auditory and visual stimuli: evidence for a mechanism specific to the auditory modality. EEG Clin. Neurophysiol. **77**, 436–444 (1990)
17. Astikainen, P., Ruusuvirta, T., Wikgren, J., Korhonen, T.: The human brain processes visual changes that are not cued by attended auditory stimulation. Neurosci. Lett. **368**, 231–234 (2004)
18. Czigler, I., Baläzs, L., Patö, L.G.: Visual change detection: event-related potentials are dependent on stimulus location in humans. Neurosci. Lett. **364**, 149–153 (2004)
19. Pazo-Alvarez, P., Cadaveira, F., Amenedo, E.: MMN in the visual modality: a review. Biol. Psychol. **63**, 199–236 (2003)
20. Zhao, L., Li, J.: Visual mismatch negativity elicited by facial expressions under non-attentional condition. Neurosci. Lett. **410**(2), 126–131 (2006)
21. Stagg, C., Hindley, P., Tales, A., Butler, S.: Visual mismatch negativity: the detection of stimulus change. Neuroreport **15**, 659–663 (2004)
22. Kimura, M., Katayama, J., Ohira, H., Schröger, E.: Visual mismatch negativity: new evidence from the equiprobable paradigm. Psychophysiology **46**, 402–409 (2009)
23. Wang, W., Miao, D., Zhao, L.: Automatic detection of orientation changes of faces versus non-face objects: a visual MMN study. Biol. Psychol. **100**, 71–78 (2014)
24. Berti, S.: The attentional blink demonstrates automatic deviance processing in vision. NeuroReport **14**, 664–667 (2011)
25. Kenemans, J.L., Grent's Jong, T., Verbaten, M.H.: Detection of visual change: mismatch or rareness? NeuroReport **14**, 1239–1242 (2003)
26. Maekawa, T., Goto, Y., Kimukawa, N., Taniwaki, T., Kanba, S., Tobimatsu, S.: Functional characterization of mismatch negativity to a visual stimulus. Clin. Neurophysiol. **116**, 2392–2402 (2005)
27. Wei, J.H., Chan, T.C., Luo, Y.J.: A modified oddball paradigm "cross-modal delayed response" and the research on mismatch negativity. Brain Res. Bull. **57**, 221–230 (2002)
28. Czigler, I., Weisz, J., Winkler, I.: ERPs and deviance detection: visual mismatch negativity to repeated visual stimuli. Neurosci. Lett. **401**, 178–182 (2006)
29. Naatanen, R., Sussman, E.S., Salisbury, D., Shafer, V.L.: Mismatch negativity (MMN) as an index of cognitive dysfunction. Brain Topogr. **27**(4), 451–466 (2014)
30. Kahneman, D.: Thinking, Fast and Slow. Macmillan, New York (2011)
31. Stefanics, G., Kremláček, J., Czigler, I.: Visual mismatch negativity: a predictive coding view. Front. Hum. Neurosci. **8**, 1–19 (2014)
32. Rahne, T., Bockmann, M., von Specht, H., Sussman, E.S.: Visual cues can modulate integration and segregation of objects in auditory scene analysis. Brain Res. **1144**, 127–135 (2007)

Device Based on EASI ECG Method as a Simple and Efficient Tool in Diagnostics of Patients Suffering from Noncommunicable Diseases (NCDs)

Wojciech Oleksy[✉], Ewaryst Tkacz, and Zbigniew Budzianowski

Faculty of Biomedical Engineering,
Department of Biosensors and Biomedical Signals Processing,
Silesian University of Technology, Gliwice, Poland
wojciech.oleksy@polsl.pl
http://www.polsl.pl

Abstract. Noncommunicable diseases (NCDs) kill 38 million people each year, 17.5 million among them die of cardiovascular diseases [1]. Although for over 100 years we know electrocardiography, technique which is essential tool in diagnosis of heart diseases, as well as other organs, still cardiovascular diseases are the deadliest from all NCDs. In XXI century we have all necessary tools, knowledge and technology to save more lives. Simple electronic device measuring and analysing ECG signal connected to smartphone could be a solution for this dramatic problem.

Electrocardiography is used to measure electrical activity of the heart as a function of time and presents it in digital or analogue form. The measurement is usually recorded from the body surface of the patient, which makes the standard electrocardiogram painless. Although the 12 lead ECG is the basic clinical procedure of heart diagnosis it has some drawbacks. Measuring all 12 leads is difficult and impractical, but most of all it restricts patient movement. In 1988, Gordon Dower developed a system of quasi-orthogonal lead called EASI, which uses only 5 electrodes in order to register standard 12 lead ECG signals [2]. The main goal of this work is to propose a simple electronic device based on EASI model, which transforms EASI electrocardiographic signals (ECG) into a standard 12-channel ECG. Such a device, which will have high correlation with standard 12 lead ECG would be easier and faster to use because of smaller number of electrodes and also would be a simple and efficient tool in diagnostics of patients suffering from noncommunicable diseases (NCDs).

Keywords: EASI · ECG · Artificial Neural Network · SVM · Linear regression · PACE regression · Least Median of Squares Regression · Gradient boosting

© Springer International Publishing AG 2017
M. Gzik et al. (eds.), *Innovations in Biomedical Engineering*, Advances in Intelligent Systems and Computing 526, DOI 10.1007/978-3-319-47154-9_35

1   Introduction

In Europe noncommunicable diseases (NCDs) are responsible for the largest share of mortality: about 80 % of deaths in 2009. Diseases of the circulatory system caused nearly 50 % of all of those deaths. This number is higher among men and it ranges in different countries from less than 30 % to more than 65 % of all deaths. In less wealthy countries those numbers are greater, because access to qualified medical personnel and the social awareness of the risks is limited. As a contrast, cancer is responsible for only 20 % of deaths, ranging from around 5 % to more than 30 % in some countries [3]. That is why it is so important to find ways to increase the availability of diagnostic methods which will assist in the detection of cardiovascular disease and to design such a device, which with help of appropriate algorithms and telemedicine, will allow more accurate or even automatic and remote diagnosis of the patient. All of those features we can find in a device measuring ECG using the EASI method. In 1988 Dower and his team introduced EASI ECG system, which derives standard 12 lead ECG using only 5 electrodes [4]. The E electrode is on the sternum while, the A and I electrodes are at the left and right mid-auxiliary lines, respectively. The S electrode is at the sternal manubrium. The fifth electrode G is a ground and is typically placed on one or the other clavicle, see Fig. 1. EASI was proven to have high correlation with standard 12 lead ECG, as well as with Mason-Likar 12-Lead ECG. Apart from that it is less susceptible to artefacts, it increases mobility of patients, it is also easier and faster to use because of smaller number of electrodes. What is more, smaller number of electrodes reduces cost of a device [5].

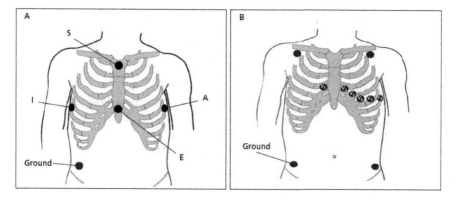

Fig. 1. Lead placement for the EASI system (A) and the Mason-Likar (B) 12-lead electrocardiogram.

2   Problem Description

In the classical approach introduced by Dower, using the EASI lead configuration, 3 modified vectorcardiographic signals are recorded from the following bipolar electrode pairs:

- A-I (primarily X, or horizontal vector component)
- E-S (primarily Y, or vertical vector component)
- A-S (containing X, Y, plus Z, the anteriorposterior component)

Each of the 12 ECG leads is derived as a weighted linear sum of these 3 base signals using the following formula:

$$\mathbf{L_{derive}} = a(A - I) + b(E - S) + c(A - S), \tag{1}$$

where $\mathbf{L}$ represents any surface ECG lead and a, b, and c represent empirical coefficients. These coefficients, developed by Dower, are positive or negative values, accurate to 3 decimal places, which result in leads very similar to standard leads. Our idea was to improve EASI ECG performance by finding a new model used for 12 ECG leads calculation. To do that we treated the system as a black box with 4 input variables: E, A, S, I and 12 output variables: I, II, III, aVR, aVL, aVF, $V1$, $V2$, $V3$, $V4$, $V5$, $V6$ and we used various machine learning and regression techniques to build a new model.

3   Proposed Device Solution

The system consists of a device that captures EASI signals and a smartphone connected via bluetooth, see Fig. 2.

Possible uses of the system include:

- diagnostic ECG;
- continuous supervision electrocardiographic patient, regardless of location as well as physical activity;
- ECG stress;
- ECG Holter independent of the location of the patient.

Advantages of this solution include:

- versatility of solution;
- possibility of sending data via Internet directly to medical center;
- unrestricted mobility;
- intuitive operation;
- high comfort;
- the low cost of the system.

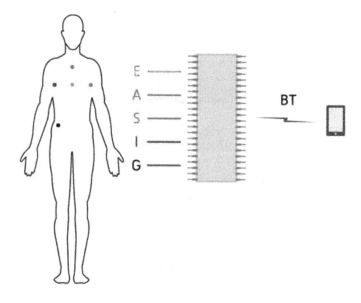

Fig. 2. Proposed device.

4   Methods Used

Our work was focused on improving Dower model by using some regression and machine learning techniques. Obtained model must have been easy to implement both in hardware and software. Several different methods were tested to find a best fitting model, namely LARS method, Lasso method, Forward Stagewise method [7], Linear Regression - Least Squares method [6], Least Median of Squares method [8], Regression Pace [9], Bagging Predictors method [10], Gradient Boosting method [11], Artificial Neural Networks - Multilayer Perceptron method [12–14] and Support Vector Machine method [15]. Some of them produced a linear model, other created a nonlinear one. Both models, linear and nonlinear, have different advantages and disadvantages. Linear models, so in other word models described by set of linear equations, usually are easier to understand and build, their total error could be easily estimated. However, they are less effective in most cases. Example of obtained model is given below:

5   Results

Improved model
Based on results obtained from all tested methods one linear model was generated:

$$\mathbf{aVF} = 0.21 \times E + 0.11 \times A - 1.09 \times S + 0.72 \times I - 3.06, \tag{2}$$

$$\mathbf{aVL} = -0.12 \times E + 0.59 \times S - 1.68 \times I + 2.30, \tag{3}$$

$$\mathbf{aVR} = -0.08 \times E - 0.11 \times A + 0.49 \times S + 0.94 \times I + 0.78, \tag{4}$$

$$\mathbf{I} = -0.03 \times E + 0.08 \times A + 0.07 \times S - 1.74 \times I + 1.00, \tag{5}$$

$$\mathbf{II} = 0.19 \times E + 0.15 \times A - 1.05 \times S - 0.14 \times I - 2.56, \tag{6}$$

$$\mathbf{III} = 0.22 \times E + 0.07 \times A - 1.12 \times S + 1.59 \times I - 3.57, \tag{7}$$

$$\mathbf{V1} = 0.63 \times E + 0.08 \times A + 0.50 \times S + 0.49 \times I + 4.04, \tag{8}$$

$$\mathbf{V2} = 1.08 \times E - 0.09 \times A + 0.52 \times S - 1.24 \times I + 13.66, \tag{9}$$

$$\mathbf{V3} = 0.80 \times E + 0.28 \times A + 0.09 \times S - 2.31 \times I + 5.06, \tag{10}$$

$$\mathbf{V4} = 0.37 \times E + 1.23 \times A + 0.09 \times S - 1.19 \times I - 2.24, \tag{11}$$

$$\mathbf{V5} = 0.14 \times E + 1.56 \times A + 0.09 \times S + 0.36 \times I + 0.02, \tag{12}$$

$$\mathbf{V6} = 0.04 \times E + 1.25 \times A - 0.15 \times S + 0.70 \times I - 1.23, \tag{13}$$

Results Comparison

Each calculated model was 10 fold cross validated. All results are based on data from PhysioNet database [16] and also on the data that were generated according to the following model (described in the paper "Investigation Of A Transfer Function Between Standard 12-Lead ECG And EASI ECG" [17]):

$$\begin{aligned}
\mathbf{E} = {} & -6.4073889 \times II - 4.58091464 \times aVR + 4.4236590 \times aVF \\
& + 1.4023342 \times V10.2316670 \times V2 + 0.63803224 \times V3 - 0.3104148 \\
& \times V4 - 0.5253245 \times V5 + 0.7453142 \times V6,
\end{aligned} \tag{14}$$

$$\begin{aligned}
\mathbf{A} = {} & 0.1205489 \times I + 0.1440902 \times aVL - 0.07460267 \times V1 \\
& - 0.005248586 \times V2 + 0.04413031 \times V3 - 0.001846735 \times V4 \\
& + 0.14529887 \times V5 + 0.5326776 \times V6,
\end{aligned} \tag{15}$$

$$\begin{aligned}
\mathbf{S} = {} & -0.9615144 \times II + 0.07950829 \times aVL + 0.21000511 \times aVF \\
& - 0.096557012 \times V1 + 0.3608502 \times V2 - 0.32692627 \times V3 + 0.252434208 \\
& \times V4 + 0.04650518 \times V5 - 0.1318653 \times V6,
\end{aligned} \tag{16}$$

Table 1. Correlation coefficient

	Obtained model	EASI dower approach	Improved EASI coefficients
aVF	0.939	0.984	0.776
aVL	0.966	0.955	0.922
aVR	0.984	0.985	0.966
I	0.985	0.971	0.973
II	0.964	0.994	0.894
III	0.941	0.963	0.786
V1	0.99	0.882	0.849
V2	0.984	0.968	0.872
V3	0.975	0.971	0.751
V4	0.971	0.981	0.851
V5	0.992	0.977	0.97
V6	0.997	0.888	0.985

Table 2. Root mean squared error [mV]

	Obtained model	EASI dower approach	Improved EASI coefficients
aVF	27.45	28.41	66.29
aVL	22.02	35.45	34.22
aVR	16.03	31.86	55.3
I	18.01	40.75	42.47
II	26.13	32.57	78.2
III	31.41	37.19	60.03
V1	21.01	99.24	86.42
V2	40.54	177.75	119.61
V3	46.62	120.25	141.69
V4	55.6	144.6	129.96
V5	24.66	119.93	49.9
V6	10.77	93.17	33.1

$$\mathbf{I} = -0.1494002 \times I - 0.24593780 \times aVL - 0.003465868$$
$$\times V1 - 0.1516211491 \times V2. \tag{17}$$

Calculated models were compared with results obtained using classical Dower approach and also with Improved EASI Coefficients described in the paper [18]. We have determined performance of all systems by calculating for each of them correlation coefficient (Table 1) and root mean squared error (Table 2). All obtained results are presented in tables below. Performance of the linear model is also shown on the plot (Fig. 3), where it is compared with original ECG

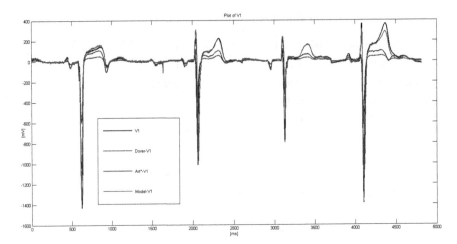

Fig. 3. Plot of measured and derived V1 signals.

signal as well as with two other EASI based signals, one generated using classical Dower method and other generated using Improved EASI Coefficients method.

6   Conclusion

Above results show that using various machine learning and regression techniques help to improve the basic EASI ECG model. The best performance was obtained for our linear model built using machine learning and regression techniques. It provides a significantly lower values of Root Mean Squared Error. Second best model was one created by Dower. Notably low performance was observed for model that was obtained using improved EASI coefficients method described in the paper [18]. Currently a prototype of a device is tested in a series of clinical trials on a group of volunteers, in which we want to compare a working EASI ECG system using our improved model with a standard ECG equipment.

References

1. WHO - Noncommunicable diseases. http://www.who.int/mediacentre/factsheets/fs355/en/
2. Dower, G.E., et al.: Deriving the 12-lead electrocardiogram from four (EASI) electrodes. J. Electrocardiol. **21**(Suppl), S182–S187 (1988)
3. WHO Europe - The European health report 2012: charting the way to well-being. http://www.euro.who.int/en/publications/abstracts/european-health-report-2012
4. Patent. http://www.google.com/patents/US4850370/
5. Redley, B.: EASI ECG Monitoring vs Traditional 12-Lead ECG. A Review of the Literature (2005)

6. Efron, B., Johnstone, I., Tibshirani, R.: Least angle regression. Ann. Stat. **32**, 407–499 (2004)
7. Hastie, T., Tibshirani, R., Jerome, F.: The Elements of Statistical Learning. Data Mining, Inference, and Prediction. Springer Series in Statistics. Springer, New York (2013)
8. Rousseeuw, P.J.: Least median of squares regression. J. Am. Stat. Assoc. **79**, 871–880 (1984)
9. Wang, Y., Witten, I.H.: Pace Regression. Working Paper Series (1999)
10. Braiman, L.: Bagging predictors. Mach. Learn. **24**, 123–140 (1996)
11. Friedman, J.H.: Stochastic gradient boosting. Comput. Stat. Data Anal. **38**, 367–378 (2002)
12. Simon, H.: Neural Networks: A Comprehensive Foundation. Prentice Hall, Englewood Cliffs (1999)
13. Bishop, C.M.: Neural Networks for Pattern Recognition. Oxford University Press, Oxford (1995)
14. Frank, E., Witten, I.H.: Data Mining. Practical Machine Learning Tools and Techniques. Morgan Kaufmann, San Fransisco (2005)
15. Smola, A.J., Schlkopf, B.: A tutorial on support vector regression. Stat. Comput. **14**, 199–222 (2004)
16. PhysioNet data. http://www.physionet.org/challenge/2007/data/
17. Oleksy, W., Tkacz, E.: Investigation of a transfer function between standard 12-Lead ECG and EASI ECG. In: BIOSIGNAL 2010, p. 35 (2010)
18. Feild, D.Q., Feldman, C.L., Horek, B.M.: Improved EASI coefficients: their derivation, values, and Performance. J. Electrocardiol. **35**, 23–33 (2002)

Detection of QRS Complex with the Use of Matched Filtering

Sandra Śmigiel[(✉)] and Tomasz Marciniak

Faculty of Telecommunications, Computer Sciences and Electrical Engineering,
University of Science and Technology, al. prof. S. Kaliskiego 7,
85-789 Bydgoszcz, Poland
{asandra.smigiel,btomasz.marciniak}@utp.edu.pl

Abstract. In recent years the ECG signal feature parameters play an important role in diagnosing, forecasting and analyzing heart diseases. In this paper, we present a new approach for using matched filtering method for the purpose of QRS complex detection. The method is based on the following steps: pre-processing, matched filtering and algorithm for QRS complex detection. To evaluate the proposed technique, the well known Physiobank Database: the PTB Diagnostic ECG database has been used. The proposed algorithm allows to achieve high detection of R-peak in ECG signal, as it will be shown in the last section. The application of the new method is a simple and efficient way to improve the accuracy of removal artefacts in ECG signal and QRS complex detection.

Keywords: ECG signal · QRS complex · Matched filtering

1 Introduction

Electrocardiography is an indirect method that relies on electrical registering of the heart muscle activity from patient's chest as potential (voltage) difference between two electrodes, which is then graphically represented as an electrocardiograph curve, i.e. electrocardiogram. Electrocardiogram (ECG) constitutes a graphic recording of potential shifts during depolarisation and repolarisation of patient's myocardial cells. It is one of the most basic tests in cardiology which provides data about patient's general health and functioning of the circulatory system [2].

The most frequently analysed electrocardiogram parameter is the R-peak (Fig. 1). During its evaluation certain difficulties occur resulting from the characteristics of the waveform: irregular intervals between waves, varied characteristics and heights, appearance of a constant component, low-frequency distortions and faults from electric power system.

Designing an effective way to detect diagnostic parameters in the ECG signal is undoubtedly problematic due to shifting morphology of particular waveform components. Even nowadays assessing the characteristics of the ECG signals

ⓒ Springer International Publishing AG 2017
M. Gzik et al. (eds.), *Innovations in Biomedical Engineering*, Advances in Intelligent Systems and Computing 526, DOI 10.1007/978-3-319-47154-9_36

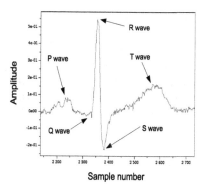

Fig. 1. ECG waveforms

proves to be a challenge to many researchers. Difficulties in processing and analysis stem from quality of the signal and its specificity [5,8]. Numerous techniques which introduce new approach to analysis of particular waveform components have appeared in recent years. One of them pertains to the use of Fourier [20] or wavelet transforms, employing various wavelets like Daubechies, Spline and Morlet in the pursuit of BPM [11,13] recognition and classification. Another method relies on the first order derivative of the Gaussian function as a converted wavelet transform to determine the form of the ECG curve [10,14]. Other algorithms used to describe the ECG signal at this stage were developed based on spectral transformations. These features were applied in the ECG classification via statistic methods [9], genetic algorithms or neural networks [1,22].

Aiming to resolve the aforementioned issues, this work distinguishes activities concerning the pre-processing of the ECG signal and devising new methods and algorithms for R-peak detection. This ought to improve the results and reduce the influence that interfering factors have on the analysis of the electrocardiograph curve.

2   Objective

This article reviews the use of matched filtering in the ECG signal analysis. The objective is to devise a new method of detecting heart rate based on the electrocardiogram assessment. This article does not, however, interpret the ECG signal through the prism of illnesses and other abnormalities. An attempt was made to represent R-peak locations in the ECG signal as accurately as possible without prior processing, and after pre-processing that removes occurring distortions.

The matched filter characteristic which corresponds to the R-peak has been artificially engineered based on Polish Cardiac Society's guidelines [3]. The undertaken research has aimed to answer whether employing matched filtering requires pre-processing which erases distortions from the ECG waveform.

3   Matched Filtering

Matched filtering [12] is a digital signal processing method, one of the tools that operate both within the time and frequency fields. Matched filtering algorithms retain the linear filter characteristics, which aim to achieve an optimal exclusion of the signal frequency components, interfering with the signal without altering its initial form. The basic matched filtering algorithm with regards to time is equivalent to a convolution which uses the following Eq. (1):

$$y_n = \Sigma_{m=0}^{N-1} x_{n-m} \cdot h_m \tag{1}$$

where:

$\{x_n\}_{n=0}^{N-1}$ – times series for signal witch matched filtering,
$\{h_n\}_{n=0}^{N-1}$ – weighting factors for filter's pulse characteristic,
$\{y_n\}$ – result of matched filtering,
T – number of readings for signal with matched filtering.

The concept of matched filter is rooted in recognising the resemblance between the signal in question and a pattern of reference, which is defined according to the convolution function. Filter pulse characteristic is created from the signal pattern samples recorded in reverse.

4   Description of the Implemented Method

4.1   Defining the Pattern

For the purpose of this article, a model containing parts of the ECG signal equivalent to the R-peak was designed. That model is being used for generating the matched filter pulse characteristic, delineated by a polynomial of a 3rd degree displayed below (2):

$$y = -6 \cdot 10^{-5} \cdot x^3 + 8 \cdot 10^{-4} \cdot x^2 + 4 \cdot 10^{-2} \cdot x + 9 \cdot 10^{-2} \tag{2}$$

Pattern generated by this interrelation is depicted in Fig. 2.

The pattern delineated by the polynomial can have its shape easily modified by alternation of its parameters. Tests with varied parameters have been conducted for the purpose of this article. These tests have used waveforms from the electrocardiographic database. Factors which have undergone modification include: R-peak width, its amplitude, its location in relation to other waveform components, the duration of the pattern, as well as R-peak appearance in the waveform or lack thereof.

R-peak distortions due to modifications to the primary pattern are shown in Figs. 3, 4, 5 and 6.

The testing was aimed at matching the pattern with the examined ECG samples as accurately as possible. During testing R-peak of the pattern was alternatively widened and narrowed, while the matched filter outlet was being evaluated. Figure 7 depicts the signal chosen from the examined waveforms with following markings: blue for the pattern which has been shortened 5 times, green for the unaltered amount of samples, and red for the pattern 5 times longer.

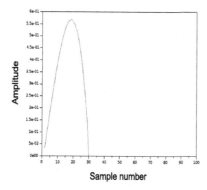

Fig. 2. Pattern for matched filtering

4.2   ECG Signal Pre-processing

Pre-processing has been conducted via a combination of low pass, high pass and FIR bandpass filters. They served in filtering out the frequencies interfering with the waveform which result from isoelectric line drift, cardiac artifacts and distortions produced by electrical power grids [4,17].

Pre-processing stage is portrayed in Figs. 8 and 9. Blue marks the original wave-forms and green is for the ones post matched filtering.

Literature on the subject presents a myriad of methods pertaining to heart rhythm detection. Their effectiveness is evaluated according to the number of accurately detected R-peaks. The literature analysis suggests the utmost complexity of the issue. It is the relatively high value of R-peak amplitude as compared to the other ECG components, and its appearance in regular, as well as irregular heart rate that makes R-peak the main point of reference for electrocardiograph signal analysis.

A QRS complex has so far been determined mainly by utilising algorithms that are based on artificial neural networks, genetic algorithms and wavelet transforms. Majority of testing has been conducted with the use of Matlab software. The distinct disadvantages of hitherto used methods, are their

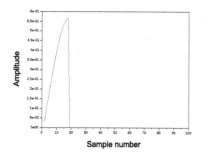

Fig. 3. Pattern shape

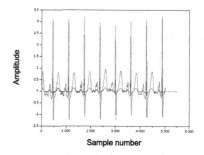

Fig. 4. Matched filtering results

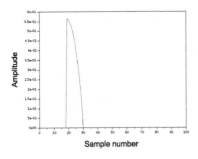

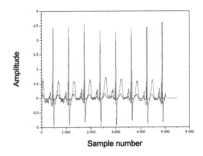

Fig. 5. Pattern shape

Fig. 6. Matched filtering results

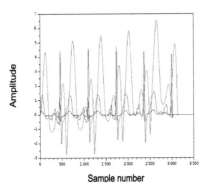

Fig. 7. R-peak distortions due to modifications to the primary pattern (Color figure online)

computational complexity, convoluted implementation, and their effectiveness being highly dependent on the ECG characteristic, which results from different disease entities [15,21].

This article portrays a new approach to locating the R-peak. The detection algorithm has been implemented by application of Scilab and Python. It exemplifies the optimal approach for detecting the R-peak which is derived from Slider Window solution [18]. It involves determination of a threshold for the entire examined waveform which, when exceeded, enables the researcher to locate the R-peak. Then each sample set, which values have exceeded the threshold and remained within the examined window width, is filtered for the samples with maximum value. They indicate where the R-peak is located.

A threshold of a sample has been calculated according to the interrelation (3):

$$t_i = T \cdot (max(s_{i-n}, s_{i+n}) - avg(s_{i-n}, s_{i+n})) + avg(s_{i-n}, s_{i+n}) \qquad (3)$$

where:
t_i - the threshold value for the sample i,
T - coefficient (value 0.65),
n - half the width of the window,

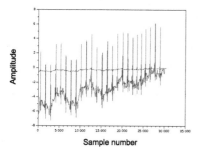

Fig. 8. ECG before the pre-processing (Color figure online)

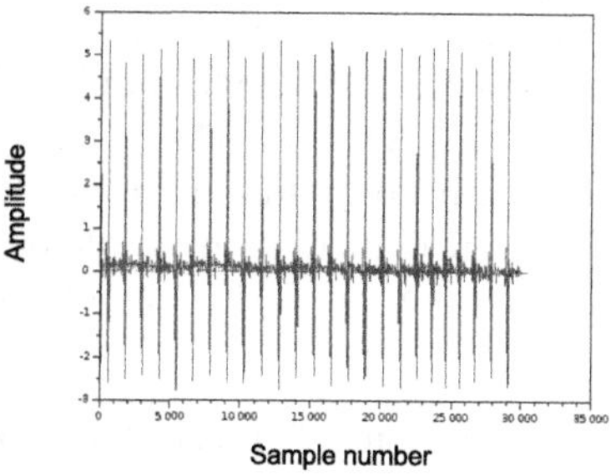

Fig. 9. ECG post the pre-processing (Color figure online)

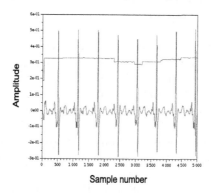

Fig. 10. An algorithm for R-peak detection

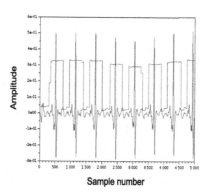

Fig. 11. Incorrectly calculated R-R interval for slider window

s_i - the sample value for the sample i,
$max(s_{i-n}, s_{i+n})$ - maximum value for samples,
$avg(s_{i-n}, s_{i+n})$ - average value for samples.

Figure 10 displays the R-peak detection algorithm results. A major factor necessary for the algorithm to work properly is the window width. It has been experimentally stated that the best results are achieved when the window width corresponds to 1500–2000 samples (for the examined signal sample of 1 kHz this equals 1.5 ms–2 ms). If the n value is too high, the algorithm will not react appropriately to rapid amplitude changes in the signal.

Figure 11 depicts an example of n value being lower than the R-R distance, for which some waveform components may be incorrectly recognised as R-peaks.

5   Experimental Results and Discussion

Electrocardiograph records from a cardiological database, consistent with global standards, have been used for the testing of the algorithm. Clinical data used for the purpose of this article originates from the Physiobank Database.

The testing of the method has been based on data acquired from the PTB Diagnostic ECG. The database stores records of the following cardiovascular diseases: myocardial infarction, heart block, cardiomyopathy, heart failure [16].

The analysis contained within this article has been conducted by examining 58 registered records of different patients. Each sample is represented in 1–5 channels, with the frequency of 1000 Hz. The duration of evaluated waveforms is 10 s.

After pre-processing, R-peak location is detected in the examined signal. R indexes are noted for two cases of analysis: before the pre-processing and afterwards. Each of them aims to assess the accuracy of R-peak location detected in the waveforms. The statistical analysis of R-R distances consists of the following parameters: the average R-R distance - an arithmetic mean of all detected R-peak locations in each case, standard deviation - set in relation to the average of all R-R distances within the examined period.

Table 1 compiles the R-peaks detected in an exemplary ECG waveform from the database. It includes the name of the ECG record which was evaluated on the grounds of: use or lack of pre-processing, and use of matched filtering. Analysed variants: variant I - real signal without pre-processing; variant II - signal after convolution without pre-processing; variant III - real signal with pre-processing, variant IV - signal after convolution with pre-processing. A graphic assessment of the set of R-peak locations (Table 1) that occur in a wave-form from the database is depicted in Figs. 12, 13, 14 and 15. An analysis of where the R-peaks are located enables to identify the variable characteristic of the ECG components in time, including the R-peak amplitude as detected by the algorithm.

The results for all waveforms are displayed in Table 2. An actual number of R-peak appearances have been determined for every waveform, which was evaluated on the grounds of: use or lack of pre-processing, and use of matched filtering. Additionally, each of the defined variants had values FP (false positive, i.e. the number of R-peak surpluses detected) and FN (false negative, i.e. the number of times the algorithm has failed to detect the R-peak) indicated.

Results from Table 2 have been verified by comparing them with the actual R-peak appearances in each ECG record. This allowed for a detailed evaluation of particular waveforms in the designated database. Thanks to the visual

Table 1. Number of QRS detections for the case s0134lre

Record no.	Analyzed variants	R-peak
s0134lre	I	293, 1126, 1944, 2764, 3585, 5197, 5964, 6715, 7457, 8204, 8952, 9705
	II	306, 1137, 1957, 2777, 3598, 5209, 5977, 6729, 7472, 8218, 8967, 9718
	III	356, 1187, 2007, 2827, 3648, 5259, 6027, 6779, 7521, 8268, 9017, 9768
	IV	371, 1202, 2022, 2842, 3663, 5274, 6042, 6794, 7536, 8283, 9032, 9783

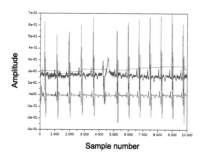

Fig. 12. Graphical marked R-peaks value in the ECG

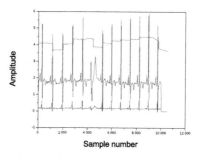

Fig. 13. Graphical marked R-peaks in the post-convolution waveform

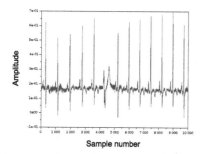

Fig. 14. Graphical marked R-peaks in the value with pre-processing

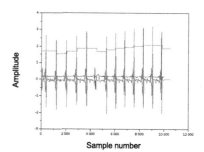

Fig. 15. Graphical marked R-peaks in the post-convolution waveform, with pre-processing

assessment, the most frequent occurrence of faulty R-peak detection in the pre-convolution waveform has been identified. It stems from a difference between samples ranged +30:−30 per R-peak. The issue is related to the distorted R-peak characteristic, which may contain more than a single maximum. In this waveform set a single R-peak may be detected as two separate ones with a similar amplitude (Figs. 16 and 17). A way to counteract this is to omit R-peaks that occur in close proximity (for the purpose of the experiment: up to 100 ms) to the

Table 2. Sample results of evaluation of QRS complex detection algorithm using matched filtering

No.	Real	R-peak real signal				R-peak real signal			
		Variant I		Variant III		Variant II		Variant IV	
		FP	FN	FP	FN	FP	FN	FP	FN
s0021bre	16	0	0	0	0	0	0	0	0
s0094lre	13	0	0	0	0	0	0	0	0
s0134lre	12	0	1	0	1	0	1	0	1
s0232lre	11	0	0	0	0	0	0	0	0

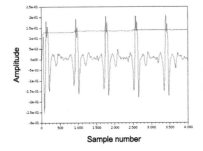

Fig. 16. Incorrectly marked R-peaks in the pre-convolution waveform, with pre-processing

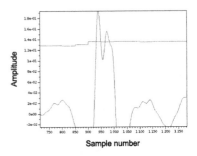

Fig. 17. Incorrectly calculated R-peak max value pre-convolution, without pre-processing

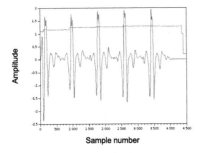

Fig. 18. Incorrectly marked R-peaks in the post-convolution waveform, with pre-processing

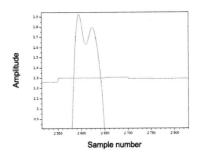

Fig. 19. Incorrectly calculated R-peak max value post-convolution, without pre-processing

detected R-peak. The proposed duration of 100 ms after the R-peak, in which the following ones ought to be ignored, is consistent with the norm describing the ECG components. The norm states that the R-peak should be no wider than 110 ms. An erroneous interpretation occurs in waveforms both with and without pre-processing. Waveforms that have undergone matched filtering are excluded, their the R-peak location is detected correctly in spite of many distortions (Figs. 18 and 19).

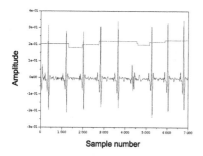

Fig. 20. R-peak variable amplitude in the pre-convolution waveform, with pre-processing

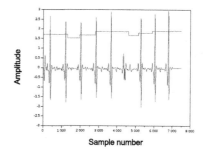

Fig. 21. R-peak variable amplitude in the pre-convolution waveform, without pre-processing

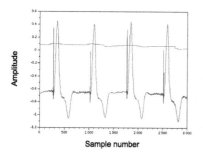

Fig. 22. Incorrectly marked R-peaks in the pre-convolution waveform, without pre-processing

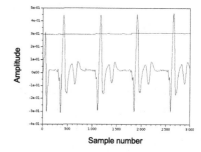

Fig. 23. Incorrectly calculated R-peak max value pre-convolution waveform, with pre-processing

   Issues of detecting R-peak locations in both: with and without pre-processing signals may stem from the R-peak variable amplitude. In some ECG records there may appear single R-peaks of a much lower amplitude compared to the adjacent ones, which may be omitted in the further analysis. Graphic evaluation of particular wave-forms reduces the possibility of faulty results (Figs. 20 and 21).

   Faulty results may also be obtained in waveforms in which neither the matched nor the pre-processing have been performed. The QRS complex may be omitted, if the amount of samples is drastically reduced and the amplitude in relation to the other ECG components is lowered, and the analysis will consider the succeeding T wave. This is of lesser importance when the heart rate is under consideration. However, when assessing particular R-peak locations, vital data regarding the waveform is lost and the achieved results are erroneous. Figures 22 and 23 displays a waveform in which R and T waves are identified as maximum in said waveform. In consequence, it is classified as two distinct R-peaks. The same waveform, after the pre-processing is per-formed, has a correct result. In the post-convolution waveforms the incorrect marking is avoided in both considered cases, i.e. with and without pre-processing (Figs. 24 and 25).

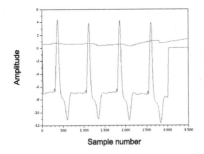

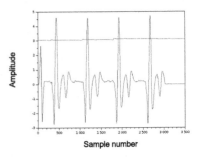

Fig. 24. Incorrectly marked R-peaks in the post-convolution waveform, without pre-processing

Fig. 25. Incorrectly calculated R-peak max value post-convolution, with pre-processing

6   Conclusions

This article presents the possible usage of matched filtering in locating the R-peak by examining distorted ECG signals. The analysis is first of its kind. Analysis of literature indicates that other researchers have focused exclusively on defining the QRS complex characteristic based on known methods such as wavelet analysis, Fourier transform, and application of genetic algorithms or neural networks.

As the performed tests indicate, it is possible to detect the R-peak by means of matched filtering, without performing the pre-processing that erases distortions.

Having reviewed the obtained results, this article validates the use of matched filtering in the ECG signal analysis. The tests have proven that it ensures the best accuracy, resistance to distortions and the correct electrocardiogram reading. This in turn allows for a proper diagnosis of heart rate.

The appropriate pattern needs to be applied for the analysis of cyclical shifts during the single R-R distance for the entirety of the recorded ECG waveform. This article proves by evaluation of the examined waveform set that artificially calculated pattern of reference, which does not lower the effectiveness of the R-peak detection, may be applied.

The main issues with the R-peak detection that have arisen during the testing stem from the influence of distortions exerted on the waveform recording. Most of the current algorithms are facing difficulties in detecting the QRS complex at as early as the pre-processing stage. Consequently, this may heighten the number of incorrect classifications of waveform components. The proposed method of R-peak detection allows for those mistakes to be omitted by employing the matched filtering, without the need for the pre-processing.

The lack of necessity to use the pre-processing and the simplicity of the execution of convolution function make this method very appealing, as it can be implemented on devices of low processing power like mobile phones [19].

Using the fact that proposed method is not computing power greedy this solution can also be implemented in the area of BSN (Body Sensor Network)

where thin nodes communicate with the powerful sink [7]. For the communication no infrastructure is required because we can use wireless or PLC technology or both of them simultaneously to ensure greater reliability [6].

References

1. Afsar, F., Arif, M.: Robust electrocardiogram beat classification using discrete wavelet transform. In: Bioinformatics and Biomedical Engineering. IEEE (2008)
2. Akker, T.J.: Computer Pre-processing of Some Electrophysiological Signals. Off-setdrukkerij Kanters B.V. (1984)
3. Baranowski, R., Wojciechowski, D., Maciejewska, M.: Zalecenia dotyczące stosowania rozpoznań elektrokardiograficznych. Kardiologia Polska **68**, 1–56 (2010)
4. Chan, M.: Filtering and signal averaging algorithms for raw ECG signals. In: 482 Digital Signal Processing, pp. 1–16 (2010)
5. Elgendi, M., Eskofier, B., Dokos, S., Abbott, D.: Revisiting QRS detection methodologies for portable, wearable, battery-operated, and wireless ECG systems. PloS One **9**(1), 5 (2014)
6. Kiedrowski, P.: Toward more efficient and more secure last mile smart metering and smart lighting communication systems with the use of PLC/RF hybrid technology. Int. J. Distrib. Sensor Netw. (2015)
7. Kiedrowski, P., Dubalski, B., Marciniak, T., Riaz, T., Gutierrez, J.: Energy greedy protocol suite for smart grid communication systems based on short range devices. In: Choraś, R.S. (ed.) Image Processing and Communications Challenges 3, vol. 102, pp. 493–502. Springer, Heidelberg (2011)
8. Kim, H., Yazicioglu, R.F., Merken, P., Van Hoof, C., Yoo, H.J.: ECG signal compression and classification algorithm with quad level vector for ECG holter system. IEEE Trans. Inf. Technol. Biomed. **14**(1), 93–100 (2010)
9. Kutlu, Y., Kuntalp, D.: Feature extraction for ECG heartbeats using higher order statistics of WPD coefficients. Comput. Meth. Prog. Biomed. **105**(3), 257–267 (2012)
10. Li, H., Wang, X., Chen, L., Li, E.: Denoising and R-Peak detection of electrocardiogram signal based on EMD and improved approximate envelope. Circ. Syst. Sig. Process. **33**(4), 1261–1276 (2014)
11. Mahmoodabadi, S.Z., Ahmadian, A., Abolhasani, M., Babyn, P., Alirezaie, J.: A fast expert system for electrocardiogram arrhythmia detection. Expert Syst. **27**(3), 180–200 (2010)
12. Marciniak, T.: Cyfrowa filtracja dopasowana sygnałów szerokopasmowych w dziedzinie czasu. Rozprawa doktorska (2006)
13. Narayana, K.V.L., Rao, A.B.: Wavelet based QRS detection in ECG using MAT-LAB. Innov. Syst. Des. Eng. **2**(7), 60–69 (2011)
14. Nouira, I., Abdallah, A.B., Bedoui, M.H., Dogui, M.: A robust R peak detection algorithm using wavelet transform for heart rate variability studies. Int. J. Electr. Eng. Inf. **5**(3), 270–283 (2013)
15. Pathoumvanh, S., Hamamoto, K., Indahak, P.: Arrhythmias detection and classification base on single beat ECG analysis. In: The 4th Joint International Conference and Communication Technology, Electronic and Electrical Engineering, pp. 1–4 (2014)
16. PTB Database. http://www.physionet.org/physiobank/database/ptbdb/

17. Singh, N., Ayub, S., Saini, J.P.: Design of digital IIR filter for noise reduction in ECG signal. In: 5 th International Conference on Computational Intelligence and Communication Networks, pp. 171–176 (2013)
18. Śmigiel, S., Ledziński, D.: ECG signal analysis for detection BPM. Zeszyty Naukowe Wydziału Telekomunikacja i Elektronika **263**(18), 23–31 (2014)
19. Śmigiel, S., Ledziński, D., Marciniak, T., Marchewka, A.: BPM detection algorithm implemented on a mobile device. Maintenance Probl. **96**(1), 101–109 (2015)
20. Uslu, E., Bilgin, G.: Exploiting locality based fourier transform for ECG signal diagnosis. In: International Conference on Applied Electronics, pp. 323–326 (2012)
21. Verma, S., Vashistha, R.: Efficient RR-interval time series formulation for heart rate detection. In: Multimedia, Signal Processing and Communication Technologies 2013 (IMPACT), pp. 84–87. IEEE (2013)
22. Zhu, H., Dong, J.: An R-peak detection method based on peaks of Shannon energy envelope. Biomed. Sig. Process. Control **8**(5), 466–474 (2013)

Survey of Wearable Multi-modal Vital Parameters Measurement Systems

Agnieszka Szczęsna[1](✉), Adrian Nowak[2], Piotr Grabiec[2], Marcin Paszkuta[1], Mateusz Tajstra[3], and Marzena Wojciechowska[2]

[1] Institute of Informatics, Silesian University of Technology, Gliwice, Poland
Agnieszka.Szczesna@polsl.pl
[2] Polish-Japanese Academy of Information Technology, Warsaw, Poland
[3] Silesian Center for Heart Disease, Zabrze, Poland

Abstract. Wearable systems with biomedical sensors have diagnostic, as well as monitoring applications. Parameters extracted from physiological measures in everyday situations can provide indicators of health status and can have diagnostic value, especially for cardiology telemedicine. The publication presents the review of reconfigurable, wearable or possible to adapt for wearing, multi-modal vital parameters measurement systems for use especially in cardiology telemedicine. From about 300 commercially available reviewed system, three selected systems have been studied in detail, the results of this comparison are also presented.

Keywords: Wearable system · Telemedicine · Biomedical sensors

1 Introduction

Main principle of medical wearable systems are built-in biomedical sensors, that after being applied on a biological material [1] enable conversion of the analog biosignals to pre-processed digital form, that can be later easily analysed and can provide many valuable information for patient diagnosis. Until recently, continuous on-line monitoring of physiological parameters was possible only in the hospital setting. But today, with many developments in the field of wearable technology, the possibility of accurate, continuous, real-time monitoring of physiological signals in patient home is not only more achievable, but also have a chance to become a part of rehabilitation process in near future. A key element is the need to use analytical methods that extract from raw data the digital value of the examined parameter relevant to diagnostic. Such a connection of microelectronics, system-on-chip, wireless communication and intelligent low-power sensors have allowed the realization of a Wireless Body Area Network [2].

The publication presents analysis of reconfigurable, wearable, multimodal vital parameters measurement systems for use especially in cardiology telemedicine. In Sect. 2, we define a set of features that will be a criterion for evaluation of systems.

M. Gzik et al. (eds.), *Innovations in Biomedical Engineering*, Advances in Intelligent Systems and Computing 526, DOI 10.1007/978-3-319-47154-9_37

2   Wearable System of Biomedical Sensors

The basic function of sensor layer is registering and transmitting chosen physiological life parameters of the patients for further analysis. This is the basis for identification of emergency situations, early diagnosis and monitoring of patient condition [3]. The following review of systems was conducted for easy application by the patient, thus wearable and non-invasive, systems that can be used in cardiac telemetry. An important feature was also the openness of the system and ability to create different configurations of sensors, adding other types of them, and possibility to gather data for different analysing procedures. Because of that, we excluded from the review all clinical and professional medical equipment, which is usually connected with high cost, need of qualified staff and have closed architecture, often difficult to develop. Next criterion was ability to measure possibly the most desired parameters [4]: velocity of pulse wave, frequency of cardiac rhythm, heart rhythm variability, physical activity, perspiration rate, arterial blood saturation, the temperature of the sternum skin surface, fluid retention in thorax, fluid retention in abdomen, percentage of fat tissue in thorax, percentage of fat tissue in abdomen.

In summary, required is comfortable, easy to use, wearable monitoring system, made in the form of clothing with built-in biomedical sensors, allowing acquiring of chosen parameters directly from the patient's body, without a problematic installation and calibration procedures. Very important parameter is the openness of the system.

3   Review of Commercially Available Wearable Systems

We analysed about 300 systems currently available for purchase. Our evaluation was based on technical documentation and web sites of products. We summarized them in terms of openness, the possibility to get measurement data and measurements of required parameters described in Sect. 2. We defined 11 parameters evaluated by 0–1. The Fig. 1 presents percentage of all analysed systems measured the given parameter. Most reviewed systems (about 80 %) measured frequency of cardiac rhythm. Only 3 systems measure 6 on 11 required parameters: BioRadio (Great Lakes Neurotechnologies), EQ02 LifeMonitor (Equivital) and BioHarness 3 (Zephyr Technology).

Based on research of biomedical sensors systems market, it can be concluded that at the moment, purchase of system, that meets all the assumed parameters is not possible. It was decided to adapt the existing system to requirement of integration, design and build universal wearable element with set of biomedical sensors. For this purpose more detailed analysis for 3 selected systems were prepared: Shimmer Set with Shimmer3 module (Shimmer)[1], Hexoskin Wearable Body Metrics (Hexoskin)[2] and EQ02 LifeMonitor (Equivital)[3]. That systems

---

[1] http://www.shimmersensing.com.

[2] http://www.hexoskin.com.

[3] http://www.equivital.co.uk/.

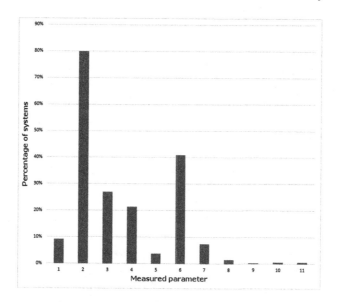

Fig. 1. Percentage of all analysed systems measured the given parameter. Parameters: pulse wave velocity (1), frequency of cardiac rhythm (2), heart rhythm variability (3), physical activity (4), perspiration rate (5), arterial blood saturation (6), the temperature of the breastbone skin surface (7), fluid retention in thorax - impedance spectroscopy (8), fluid retention in abdomen - impedance spectroscopy (9), percentage of fat tissue in thorax (10), percentage of fat tissue in abdomen (11)

are very different and do not measure all parameters but are representatives of the 3 groups of systems to monitoring vital parameters: modular and open, unprofessional with wearable element and more professional, close with medical certification. We evaluated the ease of installation and use, openness and made a rough analysis of captured ECG signal obtained in similar conditions. The main assessment of the signal quality in each system was subjective and based on characteristic elements of signal. The main aspects were: the stability of signal, maintainability, and possibility of measurement in motion. At the moment the tests are mainly descriptive.

4   Comparison of Selected Systems

Comparison of all mentioned systems is presented in Table 1.

The set called Shimmer3 is a set of Shimmer modules, that are connected by Bluetooth. System does not contain wearable element, sensors are attached by stripes (Fig. 2). Development kit used in tests consists of galvanic skin response sensor (GSR), ECG/EMG electrodes, inertial measurement unit (IMU), skin temperature sensor and optical pulse sensors (PPG) and gets 4 points in our evaluation.

Table 1. Comparison of five example analysed systems. Measured parameters: pulse wave velocity (1), frequency of cardiac rhythm (2), heart rhythm variability (3), physical activity (4), perspiration rate (5), arterial blood saturation (6), the temperature of the breastbone skin surface (7), fluid retention in thorax - impedance spectroscopy (8), fluid retention in abdomen - impedance spectroscopy (9), percentage of fat tissue in thorax (10), percentage of fat tissue in abdomen (11).

System	Points	1	2	3	4	5	6	7	8	9	10	11
Shimmer3	4	−	+	+	+	+	−	−	−	−	−	−
EQ02 LifeMonitor	6	−	+	+	+	+	+	+	−	−	−	−
Hexoskin wearable body metrics	3	−	+	+	+	−	−	−	−	−	−	−
BioRadio	6	−	+	+	+	+	+	+	−	−	−	−
BioHarness	6	−	+	+	+	+	+	+	−	−	−	−

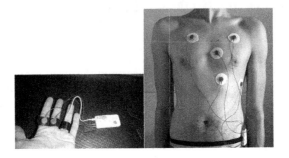

Fig. 2. Shimmer system - using electrodes and pulse sensor.

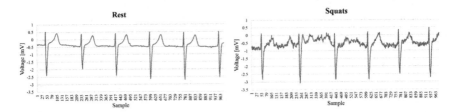

Fig. 3. Shimmer system - ECG signal captured during rest and performing squats (sampling frequency - 256 Hz).

The result ECG signal with 256 Hz frequency sampling, captured during static rest and performing squats are presented on Fig. 3. Observed signal comes from one of the chest leads (V2), it is clear and readable, but also very sensitive to any movement, which may be caused by the use of disposable electrodes. The system is modular and versatile, what usually is the basis for creating different measuring sets [5–7].

Second analysed system is EQ02 LifeMonitor (Equivital) which is more professional equipment with medical certificates (FDA Device Classification Class

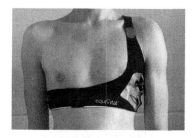

Fig. 4. EQ02 LifeMonitor elastic band with 3 textile electrodes.

II, EU Device Classification Class IIb, Device safety EN60601-1 Classification). System measures 6 parameters from our list and use a elastic belt with 3 textile ECG electrodes (Fig. 4). System has also skin temperature, breathe rate, inertial measurement unit (IMU) and galvanic skin response (GSR) sensors.

In Fig. 5 the ECG signals with 256 Hz captured during static rest and doing squats are presented. The signal is stable and clear, although sometimes there are little noise. Similar to previous system, signal captured during physical activity is noisy.

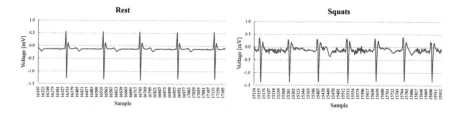

Fig. 5. Equivital system in ambulatory mode - ECG signal captured during static rest and performing squats (sampling frequency - 256 Hz).

Findings in [8] demonstrate the validity and reliability of the EQ02 for ambulatory monitoring of multiple physiological parameters and suggest that the system could be used to provide a complete human physiological monitoring platform for the study of occupational health.

Next tested system was Hexoskin Wearable Body Metrics (Hexoskin) which is low-cost and has wearable biometric shirt with 3 ECG textile electrodes (Fig. 6). The electrodes set does not have reference electrode. System has also breath rate and inertial measurement unit (IMU) sensors. The ECG signal during movement occurred drift of the baseline, even though it is possible to determine the proper heart rhythm. The signal is legible but has lower quality than signal obtained by previous presented systems (Fig. 7).

System was scientific validated for now only in [9] and provided reliable detection of an athlete's heart rate when lying, sitting, standing or walking slowly.

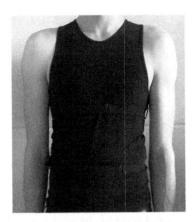

Fig. 6. Hexoskin wearable body metrics shirt.

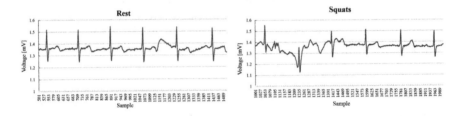

Fig. 7. Hexoskin system - ECG signal captured during static rest and performing squats (sampling frequency - 256 Hz).

The Shimmer set was the most flexible in terms of data acquisition as well as expansion (open architecture, full modularity). Its biggest drawbacks were a weak transmission of data between a large number of sensors and PC, and the absence of wearable element (T-shirt or vest). The system produced by Equivital showed the greatest stability measurements of the test systems. Its biggest drawbacks proved to be closed architecture which restricts the ability to obtain a direct measurement data and minimal possibility of expansion. The Hexoskin system obtained the lower quality results of the measurements.

5   Conclusion

We analysed about 300 commercially available systems and verified the functionality of 3 tested sets. It was confirmed that none of the systems meets 100 % of the defined objectives.

It was found that the market lacks universal wearable elements (vest, shirt, suit), equipped with a set of electrodes characterized by the following features: universality (the ability to connect different measuring devices, like ECG, ICG, GSR), comfortable for user (comfortable long-term wearing, washable, with good perspiration), relatively good quality of the obtained measurement signal. As part of the further work it was decided to design and build universal wearable element which can be connected with different systems and sensors sets.

Acknowledgements. This work was supported by project "The use of tele-transmission of medical data in patients with heart failure for improvement of quality of life and reduction of treatment costs (Monitel-HF)" (STRATEGMED 1/233221/3/NCBR/3/2014) funded by the National Centre for Research and Development under the program STRATEGMED.

References

1. Hogetveit, O.J.: Biomedical Sensors. Handbook of Research on Biomedical Engineering Education and Advanced Bioengineering Learning: Interdisciplinary Concepts: Interdisciplinary Concepts, vol. 2, p. 356 (2012)
2. Ullah, S., Higgins, H., Braem, B., Latre, B., Blondia, C., Moerman, I., Saleem, S., Rahman, Z., Kwak, K.S.: A comprehensive survey of wireless body area networks. J. Med. Syst. **36**(3), 1065–1094 (2012)
3. Baig, M.M., Gholamhosseini, H., Connolly, M.J.: A comprehensive survey of wearable and wireless ECG monitoring systems for older adults. Med. Biol. Eng. Comput. **51**(5), 485–495 (2013)
4. Daubert, J.C., Saxon, L., Adamson, P.B., Auricchio, A., Berger, R.D., Beshai, J.F., Breithard, O., Brignole, M., Cleland, J., DeLurgio, D.B., et al.: 2012 EHRA/HRS expert consensus statement on cardiac resynchronization therapy in heart failure: implant and follow-up recommendations and management. Europace **14**(9), 1236–1286 (2012)
5. Burns, A., Doheny, E.P., Greene, B.R., Foran, T., Leahy, D., O'Donovan, K., McGrath, M.J.: SHIMMER: an extensible platform for physiological signal capture. In: 2010 Annual International Conference of the IEEE Engineering in Medicine and Biology Society (EMBC), pp. 3759–3762 (2010)
6. Gradl, S., Kugler, P., Lohmuller, C., Eskofier, B.: Real-time ECG monitoring and arrhythmia detection using Android-based mobile devices. In: 2012 Annual International Conference of the IEEE Engineering in Medicine and Biology Society (EMBC), pp. 2452–2455 (2012)
7. Mamaghanian, H., Khaled, N., Atienza, D., Vandergheynst, P.: Compressed sensing for real-time energy-efficient ECG compression on wireless body sensor nodes. IEEE Trans. Biomed. Eng. **58**(9), 2456–2466 (2011)
8. Liu, Y., Zhu, S.H., Wang, G.H., Ye, F., Li, P.Z.: Validity and reliability of multiparameter physiological measurements recorded by the equivital LifeMonitor during activities of various intensities. J. Occup. Environ. Hyg. **10**(2), 78–85 (2013)
9. Villar, R., Beltrame, T., Hughson, R.L.: Validation of the Hexoskin wearable vest during lying, sitting, standing, and walking activities. Appl. Physiol. Nutr. Metab. **40**(9), 1019–1024 (2015)

Wearable Sensor Vest Design Study for Vital Parameters Measurement System

Agnieszka Szczęsna[1(✉)], Adrian Nowak[2], Piotr Grabiec[2], Piotr Rozentryt[3], and Marzena Wojciechowska[2]

[1] Institute of Informatics, Silesian University of Technology, Gliwice, Poland
Agnieszka.Szczesna@polsl.pl
[2] Polish-Japanese Academy of Information Technology, Warsaw, Poland
[3] Silesian Center for Heart Disease, Zabrze, Poland

Abstract. By using clothing with built-in biomedical sensors, the acquiring chosen parameters directly from the patient's body is available without a special and tiresome installation and calibration. The publication presents the stage of the design process of wearable element for vital parameters measurement system. The system is designed for use especially in cardiology telemedicine. The basic function of such a sensor layer is registering and transmitting chosen physiological life parameters of the patiences for further analysis. In the publication were defined the main issues to be addressed during the wearable element design and given propositions of solving them.

Keywords: Wearable system · Cardiology telemedicine · Textile electrode · Biomedical sensors

1 Introduction

Heart failure is emerging epidemic for 21st century. In Poland, the number of deaths from heart failure is higher than the most common cancers. Currently, heart failure is the leading cause of hospitalization in Poland, and the cost of hospital treatment of this group of patients account for 60–70% of the total cost of treatment failure reported by the National Health Fund. Therefore, urgent action is needed to reduce these costs through better use of the potential of ambulatory care. To achieve this goal, it is mandatory to develop a reliable monitoring system enabling remote continuous assessment of various parameters to predict cardiovascular events with the possibility of early intervention [1].

The introduction of home monitoring of patients will:

- Reduce of hospitalizations numbers;
- Reduce of visits to the clinic numbers;
- Improve quality of patients life;
- Lower treatment costs.

M. Gzik et al. (eds.), *Innovations in Biomedical Engineering*, Advances in Intelligent Systems and Computing 526, DOI 10.1007/978-3-319-47154-9_38

The publication presents the stage of the design process of wearable element for vital parameters measurement system. The system is designed for use especially in cardiology telemedicine. The basic function of sensor layer built-in wearing element is registering and transmitting chosen physiological life parameters of the patients for further analysis [2, 3].

Main idea is comfortable, easy to use, wearable monitoring system made in the form of clothing with built-in biomedical sensors, allowing acquiring chosen parameters directly from the patient's body, without a special and tiresome installation and calibration.

2 Design Study

The general concept is a system consisting of an integrator, which collect data from wearable units in different configurations and forwarded it to the server (by wireless network like WiFi or LTE), where data is analysed in order to recognize emergency situations. One wearable unit consist of control module (hub) and wearable element (shirt, suit or vest) with different biomedical sensors.

The integration of sensors with clothing, in a metrologically correct way, and making them, at the same time, patient friendly, is an important technological problem. The main difficulty is the realization and method of attachment of electrodes, including providing the required conductivity, its dependence on pressure (the degree of adhesion to the body) resistance to washing and cleaning. As a universal and wearable element of vital parameters measurement system, the designed vest should measure ECG and bioelectrical impedance signals, which it becomes increasingly important nowadays.

2.1 Textile Materials

The use of existing methods for electrical potential sensing (suction cup electrodes, adhesive or hand held electrodes) are not at a satisfactory level of comfort in applications of preventive ECG measurement and poorly applicable for long term ECG monitoring of patients [4].

For designed system we prepared project of textile electrodes (Fig. 6). The electrode material should be made of electrically conductive textile which guarantees high comfort for the user while ensuring good quality of ECG measurements. In [5] testing procedures and markers for suitable textile materials in terms of their performance as textile integrated electrodes for impedance measurements were presented. Using a test bench for objective evaluation and including subjective evaluations, 25 potential materials were analysed. Objected evaluation concerned static resistance, absolute value of the ac impedance at 100 kHz, electrode-skin contact impedance, influence of sweat on the electrode-skin contact impedance, pressure-dependence of the electrode-skin contact impedance, temperature-dependence of the electrode-skin contact impedance, static resistance change after 30 washing cycles, static abrasion resistance change after 10000 Martindale cycles. Because it can be assumed that during long-term application the electrodes will be moistened (to some extent) with sweat, the wet measurements are more important than dry electrolyte measurements. Subjective evaluation of the properties based on materials tactile properties and level of comfort.

From tests presented in [5] the best suited material is knitted fabric composition of polyamide, elastane and silver. Following on defined parameters we chose a material with similar properties. The selected material is stretch conductive fabric (Plug&Wear vendor), which is made from silver plated 92 % polyamide, 8 % elastane, fabric which offers the unique ability to stretch in both directions. Material has following properties: sheet resistance $<1\,\Omega/\mathrm{sq}$ (unstretched), conductivity increases when stretched, thickness 0.5 mm, weight $130\,\mathrm{g/m^2}$, temperature range -30 to $90\,^\circ\mathrm{C}$.

Suitable material for shirt should be breathable, comfortable, pleasant and stretchable textile. The electrode conductive material must be similar in structure and physical parameters to shirts material so that at comparable external factors behaved similarly. For example, different shrinkage of the electrode fabric, present after laundry/washing, can cause material distortion. Electrode material should be reasonably good water absorbent and slightly dry. By absorbing the sweat of the patient increases electrical parameters of contact with the skin. In our design the shirt textile material is composed of 80 % polyamide and 20 % elastan.

2.2 Placement of Electrodes

The ECG and bioimpedance electrodes placement should be adjusted to make it less prone to errors associated with a small displacement of the electrodes during the movement of the subject. We have chosen 5 electrodes pattern (Fig. 1). This is a scheme commonly used in the clinical observation of patients, uses 4 limb leads, and one of the precordial lead (V1–V6) [6].

The vest has also 6 pairs of bioimpedance electrodes for measurements of thoracic and abdomen electrical bioimpedance [7]. In addition to limit displacement, the electrodes are lined with sponge to form a soft bulge, better adhering to skin during movement (Fig. 6). A properly selected stretchable vest material also holds the electrodes in the right place.

2.3 Prototype Design Process

Based on the review of the products on the market we first tested the Shenzhen Yingda Strong Technology ECG T-Shirt (Fig. 2). In the shirt is integrated 10 textile electrodes in the Mason-Likar placement. The T-shirt has no bioimpedance electrodes and measurement of closely spaced 10 electrodes is difficult during movements. The electrodes connections are in the form of metal clips, that touch the body (the first textile electrode in Fig. 5). During long use, it can cause skin irritation. The electrodes are flat and poor adherent to the body, in order to obtain a signal had to be manually pressed to the body. The relatively

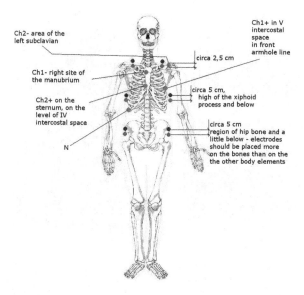

Fig. 1. Placement schema of ECG (green dots) and bioimpedance (blue and red dots) electrodes. (Color figure online)

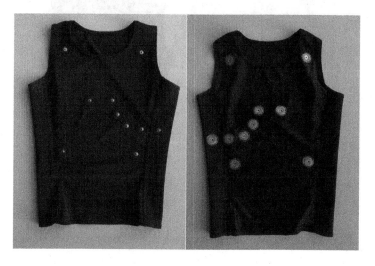

Fig. 2. The Shenzhen Yingda Strong Technology ECG T-Shirt - right and left side.

stiff material on the sides of the T-shirt caused a folding of material including electrodes, which reduced the adhesion during movement.

Next we prepared the first vest prototype version (Fig. 3). During carefully tests we were able to identify problems, which affect the measured signal and user comfort. In this version the bioimpedance electrodes have been added. The electrodes placement has been changed according to the design schema

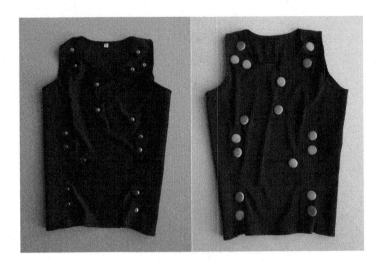

Fig. 3. The first vest prototype version - right and left side.

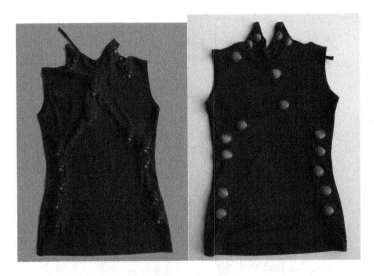

Fig. 4. The second vest prototype version - right and left side.

(Fig. 1, described in Sect. 2.2). The electrodes placed on the neck were put on the additional band. The textile electrodes were made in the form of special convex metal buttons, which were covered with a conductive material (the second electrode in Fig. 5). Unfortunately, metal button causes rapid drying of the electrodes. The rigid connection of the cable within the electrode still causes pulling away from the body. Fitted vest with stretchy material makes it difficult to put on and take off the shirt.

After extensive testing we have prepared the second vest prototype version (Fig. 4). This version introduces a number of changes. First set of changes improves wearing comfort. Rigid elements on the sides were removed and complete vest is flexible. The zip fastener was added on vest back to facilitate

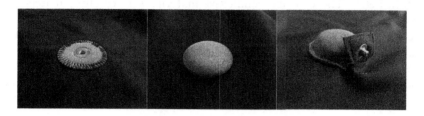

Fig. 5. The textile electrodes from: Shenzhen Yingda strong technology ECG T-Shirt, the first prototype vest version and the second prototype vest version.

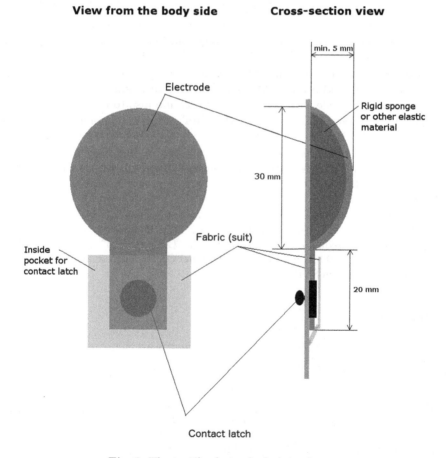

Fig. 6. The textile electrode design schema.

dressing/undressing. Instead of separate band on the neck a turtleneck collar was added. In order to improve the adhesion of the electrode to the body, connection is moved outside electrode area on a conductive material strip (the third textile electrode in Fig. 5). Metal part of electrode is replaced by electrode made from sponge which is springy and convex. Schema of the textile electrode is presented in Fig. 6. The vest and conductive material were carefully matched and selected as described in the Sect. 2.1.

As a result we have prototype version of wearable vest with ECG and bioimpedance textile electrodes. The vest is esthetic and comfortable for users and allows long-term measurement of biosignals during daily activities. With the introduction of a number of innovative improvements to vest and textile electrode design, measurements are legible even when performing movements.

3   Conclusion

A prototype measuring system wearable element is designed as a typical clothing with sewn in textile electrodes. This configuration will be evaluated for compliance with clinical requirements. Proposed solution resembles typical clothes and does not require attachment of electrodes to the body. Placement of ECG and bioimpedance electrodes in the clothing, provides adequate electrical contact with the skin and a possibility of skin irritation is minimized. The vest is designed as comfortable wear for prolonged use, and also to be easy to wash.

Such universal vest can be connected to vital parameters monitoring systems (for example like Shimmer[1]). In the future it is planned to replace the cable connections by conductive threads (like in our Inertial Motion Capture suit [8]) and add pockets for attaching additional sensors (like temperature, inertial measurement unit, etc.).

Acknowledgements. This work was supported by project "The use of teletransmission of medical data in patients with heart failure for improvement of quality of life and reduction of treatment costs (Monitel-HF)" (STRATEGMED 1/233221/3/NCBR/3/2014) funded by the National Centre for Research and Development under the program STRATEGMED.

References

1. Korewicki, J., Rywik, S., Rywik, T.: Management of heart failure patients in Poland. Euro. J. Heart Fail. **4**(2), 215–219 (2012)
2. Patel, S., Park, H., Bonato, P., Chan, L., Rodgers, M.: A review of wearable sensors and systems with application in rehabilitation. J. Neuroeng. Rehabil. **9**(1), 1 (2012)
3. Rodgers, M.M., Pai, V.M., Conroy, R.S.: Recent advances in wearable sensors for health monitoring. Sens. J. IEEE **15**(6), 3119–3126 (2015)
4. Vojtech, L., Bortel, R., Neruda, M., Kozak, M.: Wearable textile electrodes for ECG measurement. Adv. Electr. Electron. Eng. **11**(5), 410 (2013)

---

[1] http://www.shimmersensing.com.

5. Ulbrich, M., Mühlsteff, J., Sipilä, A., Kamppi, M., Koskela, A., Myry, M., Wan, T., Leonhardt, S., Walter, M.: The IMPACT shirt: textile integrated and portable impedance cardiography. Physiol. Meas. **35**(6), 1181 (2014)
6. Drew, B.J., Funk, M.: Practice standards for ECG monitoring in hospital settings: executive summary and guide for implementation. Crit. Care Nurs. Clin. North Am. **18**(2), 157–168 (2006)
7. Sherwood, A., Royal, S.A., Hutcheson, J., Turner, J.R.: Comparison of impedance cardiographic measurements using band and spot electrodes. Psychophysiology **29**(6), 734–741 (1992)
8. Kulbacki, M., Koteras, R., Szczęsna, A., Daniec, K., Bieda, R., Słupik, J., Segen, J., Nawrat, A., Polański, A., Wojciechowski, K.: Scalable, wearable, unobtrusive sensor network for multimodal human monitoring with distributed control. In: Lacković, I., Vasic, D. (eds.) 6th European Conference of the International Federation for Medical and Biological Engineering. IP, vol. 45, pp. 914–917. Springer, Heidelberg (2015). doi:10.1007/978-3-319-11128-5_227

Author Index

Printed in the United States
By Bookmasters